S0-BIF-894

Color Atlas and Text of

ADULT DEMENTIAS

Color Atlas and Text of

ADULT DEMENTIAS

David M. A. Mann
PhD MRCPath
Reader in Neuropathology
Department of Pathological Sciences
University of Manchester

David Neary
MD FRCP
Professor of Neurology
The Royal Infirmary
Manchester

Humberto Testa
MD PhD FRCP FRCR
Consultant Radiologist
The Royal Infirmary
Manchester

Mosby-Wolfe

London Baltimore Bogotá Boston Buenos Aires Caracas Carlsbad, CA Chicago Madrid Mexico City Milan Naples, FL New York Philadelphia St. Louis Sydney Tokyo Toronto Wiesbaden

Project Manager: Anton Lawrencepulle
Developmental Editor: Rachael Miller
Designer/Layout Artist: Lindy Van Den Berghe
Cover Design: Lara Last
Illustration: Lynda Payne
Production: Michael Heath
Index: Jill Halliday
Publisher: Harvey Shoolman

Published in 1994 by Mosby-Wolfe, an imprint of Times Mirror International Publishers Limited

Printed by Grafos, S. A. Arte sobre papel

ISBN 0 7234 1784 9

For full details of all Times Mirror International Publishers Limited titles, please write to Times Mirror International Publishers Limited, Lynton House, 7–12 Tavistock Square, London WC1H 9LB, England.

A CIP catalogue record for this book is available from the British Library.

Library of Congress Cataloging-in-Publication Data applied for.

Contents

Preface

I first 'discovered' Alzheimer's disease, or probably more accurately stumbled across Alzheimer's disease, in 1972 when, as a newly qualified postdoctoral researcher having completed a study concerning changes in the nucleic acids of nerve cells in human ageing, I was rummaging through the Departmental tissue archive in search of cases of neurodegenerative disease which could be compared with these 'normal' findings. At that time Alzheimer's disease languished in relative obscurity and, despite the pioneering work of the Newcastle group, still had the status of a clinical and pathological curiosity within the scientific community impinging little, if at all, on the awareness of society in general. All of this seems a distant cry from the present. Now, Alzheimer's disease, together with other causes of dementia, is globally recognised as one of the major disorders affecting mankind which tragically touches an ever increasing number of individuals and families.

On examining the histopathology of this particular case I was intrigued by the bizarre intracellular changes (tangles) and extracellular foci of degeneration (plaques) that are characteristic of the disorder and decided to investigate what effect these might have on nerve cell structure and function. Hence my journey into the world of dementia research was launched.

In 1977 I teamed up with David Neary, Julie Snowden, and Tito Testa at the Royal Infirmary. David had recently founded the Cerebral Function Unit. At this time at the Institute of Neurology, David Bowen, who had turned his attentions to the transmitter neurochemistry of the disease, also joined us. Our joint efforts led to descriptions of the clinical, pathological, and chemical correlative features of Alzheimer's disease. This 'three-way' association has prospered through the years, most recently taking on board aspects of these relationships in non-Alzheimer forms of dementia.

In 1978, the Manchester dementia 'brain bank' was set up in this Department. Since then well over 300 cases have been added to the collection, these coming mainly from those younger individuals who have received longitudinal clinical and neuropsychological assessment at the CFU during the last 15 years.

This text represents the fruits of our partnership and is based almost entirely upon the knowledge and experience we have gained, during this time, in the clinical and pathological investigation of dementia. The information and illustrations come, with only few exceptions, from our own case material. We have tried to not only record the clinical and neuropathological diagnostic features of the main disorders causing dementia but also to detail what is known of their natural history and evolutionary course. We have concentrated on the more common causes of dementia and have paid less attention to rarer ones; some of these have still to make an appearance within our study population.

Pathologists are often called upon by anxious family members or physicians to investigate the cause of dementia within patients. Yet many pathologists, although willing to co-operate with such wishes, may be somewhat reluctant to examine and diagnose the brains of patients affected in this way, possibly because there are relatively few central nervous system autopsies performed in their institutions or because they themselves have little experience of the histopathological staining methods or diagnostic criteria used to differentiate between the various causes of dementia. A practical protocol expressing and explaining the major features of such disorders can potentially be a great help. The purpose of this text is to provide just such an illustrative guide through the major neurodegenerative and other disorders that cause dementia in adult life. Rare or secondary conditions causing dementia will not be discussed or will be mentioned only briefly since these will infrequently, if at all, impinge upon the daily work of the intended reader. The text is not meant to be a formal review of the clinical and pathological features of every such condition; hence the reader will not find references or a recommended bibliography. This latter type of text is now beginning to flood the shelves of libraries and booksellers alike; it is not our intent to add further to this particular tide of knowledge.

Dementing disorders touch upon many groups of professionals and non-professionals alike. It is intended that this atlas will attract neurologists, psychiatrists, geriatricians and pathologists, as well as geneticists and biologists working on the molecular biology of these dementing diseases. It is anticipated that it will be of practical value, serving as a handy source of consultation to those studying at undergraduate or postgraduate level. Lastly, it is hoped that it will convey some of the enthusiasm and insight into this fascinating condition that we ourselves have been fortunate enough to gain during the past 20 years.

David M. A. Mann

Acknowledgements

In a publication of this kind the illustrations can be only as good as the material on which the authors' photographic record is based. Hence, it is only right and proper to thank first and foremost all those colleagues who over the years have spent many hours labouring over the microtome and staining bench to produce such excellent 'raw' material. In particular, in most recent times, I should like to thank Dr Paul Cooper, who kindly allowed me to use many of the immunostained specimens he had prepared for his research work. My special thanks are also due to Pauline Scullard and Gail Healey, my current 'right-hand women', for the preparation of the routine histological material that makes up the backbone of our post-mortem brain work-up. Also, the help of the many students and technicians, who over the years have lent technical and intellectual support to our work, is gratefully acknowledged. The hard work of the Department's and the Medical School's Photographic Unit is recognised, particularly the contribution to the photography of brain slices made by Jane Crosby. The help of Drs Paul Talbot and Alan Jackson in providing the CT and SPET brain imaging illustations is much appreciated. Last, but not least, I have to thank Margaret Barringer for her careful and patient preparation of the manuscript; her tolerance in the face of multiple revisions, mostly in my 'own fair hand', defies belief. At many points during the course of the work's preparation I am sure she must have felt that she would be chained to the microprocessor in this task for the rest of her natural life.

The clinical and research work carried out both in this Department and in the Cerebral Function Unit has for many years received generous support from the North Western Regional Health Authority, with significant contributions from The Medical Research Council, The Wellcome Trust, The Alzheimer's Disease Society, Research into Ageing, and the Motor Neurone Disease Association; without their assistance this work would not have been possible.

David M. A. Mann
David Neary
Humberto Testa

Introduction

Disorders leading to the syndrome of dementia usually affect older people, and dementia is now recognised as the fourth most common cause of morbidity and mortality among the elderly after cardiovascular disease, carcinoma, and cerebrovascular disease. Hence, about 10–15% of all persons over 65 years of age have dementia, and the very old are at greatest risk; as many as 25–45% may be affected. Before this age dementia is relatively uncommon, affecting less than 1 in 1000 people.

In the United Kingdom alone some 600,000 people have dementia and the proportion of the general population affected seems similar in most Westernized societies. The impact of so many, mostly old, people with dementia on relatives, carers, or society in general is incalculable, in both personal and social terms as well as in the narrow perspective of economic support. The terms 'epidemic' and 'disease of the century' are by no means overstatements of the implications and repercussions of the condition.

In most instances the disorders causing dementia appear to arise spontaneously, or at least there may not appear to be any clear family history. In others, particularly those occurring during middle age, there is a well-defined family history and the disorder is usually inherited as an autosomally dominant disorder.

Women seem to be affected more frequently than men, even when allowances are made for different patterns of mortality between the sexes leading to a larger proportion of females in the elderly population. However, this pattern of gender distribution varies according to the pathological cause of the dementia and in some situations males outnumber females.

Clinically, dementia is a syndrome comprising a constellation of symptoms that can encompass memory disturbances, personality changes, mood alterations, disorientation, and lack of concentration and motivation. These aspects are, however, neither represented equally nor are all necessarily present in the clinical profile associated with any one of the many underlying pathological causes. Hence the 'popular' view of dementia as a global and irretrievable breakdown in brain function, that is broadly similar irrespective of the underlying pathological cause, is erroneous; distinct neuropsychological profiles are associated with particular patterns of pathology. This means that each disease entity will have its own clinical characteristics, which are dictated more by the anatomical distribution of the brain damage than by the kind of change induced, and which set it apart from other pathological forms. In this way it becomes possible to diagnose the cause of dementia with confidence according to the clinical and pathological profiles described and discussed in this book.

1. Clinical features

Dementia is not a disease, it is the neuropsychological deficit resulting from chronic brain disease (encephalopathy). Chronic encephalopathies may be progressive or non-progressive. Incomplete recovery from brain trauma or cerebral hypoxia, for example, results in a chronic but non-progressive dementia. The subject of this book is progressive encephalopathy and its manifestations in a variety of dementia syndromes.

Chronic progressive encephalopathies can be classified into three subtypes.

- Extrinsic.
- Metabolic.
- Intrinsic.

Extrinsic brain disorders

Extrinsic brain disorders are the neurological conditions that lead to compression of the brain and require neurosurgical treatment. There are two major clinical syndromes associated with extrinsic cerebral disease.

- A focal neuropsychological syndrome associated with the symptoms and signs of raised intracranial pressure.
- The syndrome of hydrocephalus.

The diagnosis of these disorders forms part of the service requirement of a neuroscientific centre with appropriate brain imaging techniques. These neurosurgical disorders will not be discussed further.

Metabolic encephalopathy

In metabolic encephalopathy the efficient function of a primarily intact nervous system is compromised by the imposed effects of systemic disease. The degree of cerebral impairment fluctuates according to the relative severity of the general medical disorder and constitutes a distinct syndrome, often referred to as a 'confusional state', intermediate between full arousal and unresponsive coma (**Table 1.1**).

Table 1.1 Features of metabolic encephalopathy

Features
Fluctuating arousal
Incoherent thought and anomia
Illusions and hallucinations
Constructional apraxia
Disorientation in time and place
Social and personal misconduct

The reduced level of arousal leads to a quantitative rather than a qualitative reduction in the efficiency of the processes of language, perceptuo-spatial function, praxis, memory, and the regulation of behaviour. Disturbed arousal is manifest as mental and physical slowness, impaired concentration, and vigilance, drowsiness, and sleepiness. Fluctuations of alertness occur from moment to moment. Before coma supervenes behaviour may be overactive and purposeless (delirium). Language does not break down into aphasia, but there is an inability to maintain a coherent train of thought and there are verbal misunderstandings. Written expressions are more incoherent than speech. Nonspecific naming errors are made. Perceptual errors lead to illusions and hallucinations, which are often fearful. Complex spatial functions are impeded so that constructional tasks such as copying and maze-trailing are failed. Memory suffers and there is disorientation, first for time, then later for place, but never for personal identity. The purposeful regulation of behaviour becomes impossible, leading to erratic responses and motiveless wandering.

Neurological signs that often accompany metabolic encephalopathy are postural tremor, asterixis, and myoclonus. The electroencephalogram (EEG) typically shows diffuse slow large amplitude wave forms. The systemic diseases producing a metabolic encephalopathy are summarised in **Table 1.2** and the main features of the syndrome in **Table 1.3**. In addition to the characteristic neuropsychological syndrome there will be evidence of systemic disease on clinical, haematological, biochemical and endocrine investigation.

Table 1.2 Causes of metabolic encephalopathy

Cause	Example
Toxic state	Systemic infection Alcohol Drug overdose
Deficiency state	Vitamin B12 deficiency
Hepatic encephalopathy	
Renal encephalopathy	
Cardio-respiratory encephalopathy	
Endocrine disorder	Diabetic ketoacidosis Hypoglycaemia Hypothyroidism
Electrolyte imbalance	Hyper- and hyponatraemia Hyper- and hypocalcaemia

Table 1.3 Features of metabolic encephalopathy

Psychological syndrome	Neurological signs	EEG
Fluctuating disorder of arousal	Tremor Asterixis Myoclonus	Diffuse high amplitude slow wave forms

The disorders giving rise to metabolic encephalopathy are not the main subject of this book, but it is essential that the major features of the syndrome are understood so that they can be clearly distinguished from those of dementia due to progressive intrinsic brain disease. This distinction is therapeutically important since the metabolic encephalopathies are essentially treatable. Diagnosis and treatment of systemic disease, especially in the early stages, can lead to a complete resolution of metabolic encephalopathy. This reversible state of affairs stands in contrast to the lack of any specific and effective treatments for the dementia due to intrinsic brain damage. It must however be borne in mind that patients with progressive dementia due to intrinsic brain disease, are not immune, but are indeed more susceptible, to the development of metabolic encephalopathy since they have less cerebral reserve and are more likely to be old and frail. The development of fluctuations in arousal and especially nocturnal confusion should instigate a search for systemic complications such as drug intoxication and infection.

Dementia due to chronic progressive intrinsic encephalopathy

Dementia has traditionally been defined as a global deterioration of intellectual function, but two considerations indicate that this definition is erroneous:

- Cerebral diseases do not affect the brain uniformly, but preferentially affect certain brain regions and spare others.
- Psychological processes are regionally organised and depend on the functioning of specific brain regions. Different cerebral diseases or encephalopathies are therefore associated with distinctive characteristic neuropsychological syndromes.

Dementia must be seen as a generic term embracing a variety of distinct neuropsychological syndromes characteristic of particular diseases. A useful empirical classification of chronic encephalopathies and their associated neuropsychological syndromes can be based on the major distribution of pathology within the brain (**Table 1.4**).

Table 1.4 Classification of chronic encephalopathies

Cortical
Subcortical
Cortical-subcortical
Multifocal

Some disorders affect chiefly cerebral cortex, others predominantly subcortical structures, or cortex and subcortex together. Only a minority have a multifocal distribution with no respect for functional anatomical systems. Within this classificatory framework, prototypical syndromes will be described in terms of the following features:

- The neurological symptoms and signs.
- The nature of the psychological breakdown.
- The distribution of cerebral pathology as demonstrated by functional single-photon emission tomographic imaging (SPET).
- The results of the associated electroencephalographic recordings.

This process of syndrome analysis permits a differential diagnosis of the different forms of dementia and provides clinical information that can be correlated with the pathological descriptions of individual diseases.

Cortical encephalopathies

Functional topography of the cortex

Psychological functions are regionally organised in the cerebral cortex and specific diseases have affinities for certain regions. Knowledge of this organisation allows an appreciation of the way neuropsychological syndromes reflect clinico-pathological relationships (**Fig. 1.1**).

- The posterior hemispheres are critical for perceptual and spatial functions; that is, recognition of the nature of objects in the environment and their spatial relationships to each other and to the individual. Breakdown in visual perception leads to a failure to recognise objects (agnosia) and individual faces (prosopagnosia), whereas spatial impairment leads to an inability to navigate external surroundings (spatial disorientation).
- Language is dependent on the areas around the sylvian fissure, extending from the frontal into the parietal and temporal lobes in the left hemisphere. Breakdown of language leads to an inability to communicate and comprehend speech and writing (aphasia), to calculate (acalculia), and to communicate by gesture (gestural apraxia).
- The superior parietal areas are important for the organisation of skilled movements. Failure of executive functions leads to difficulties in the purposeful use of limbs, face and mouth (apraxia).
- The medial portion of both hemispheres, designated the limbic system, which includes the hippocampus and amygdala, is essential for the acquisition and storage of information in the act of memorising. In amnesia there is an inability to learn new information (anterograde amnesia) and to recall past experience (retrograde amnesia).
- The anterior, or prefrontal, cortex is essential for regulation of mental life, including strategic planning and evaluation of actions taking place over periods of time. Breakdown in regulation leads to aberrant personal and social behaviour, change in personality, and inability to conceive and achieve successfully appropriate behavioural goals.

Neuropsychological syndromes associated with cortical encephalopathies

Three main psychological syndromes are associated with cortical encephalopathy (**Table 1.5**).

The distribution of three major diseases producing a cortical encephalopathy are shown in **Fig. 1.2**.

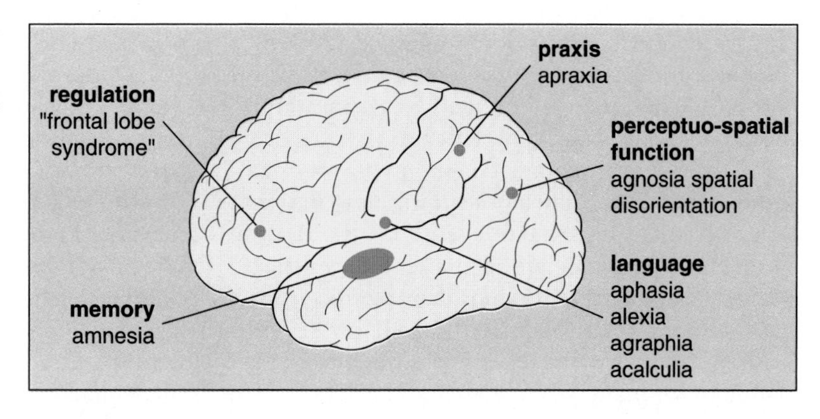

Fig. 1.1 Functional topography of the cerebral cortex and the psychological syndromes arising from breakdown of function of particular cortical areas.

Table 1.5 Profile of neuropsychological disorders associated with cortical encephalopathies. Primary (primary abnormality); secondary (secondary consequence of patient's primary deficits).

Areas of cortex involved	Language	Perceptuo-spatial function	Praxis	Memory	Regulation
Anterior	Primary			Secondary	Primary
Posterior	Primary	Primary	Primary	Primary	Secondary
Medial				Primary	

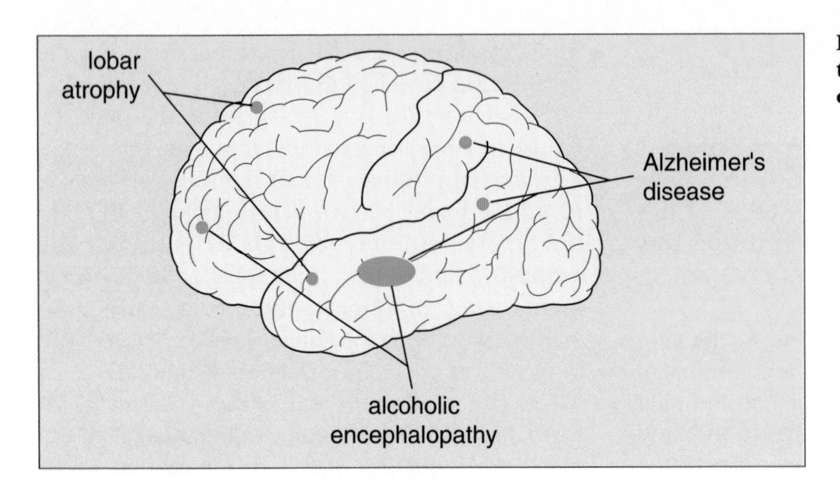

Fig. 1.2 Topographical distribution of impaired function in the cortical encephalopathies.

- Predominantly posterior and medial syndromes are seen in Alzheimer's disease.
- The anterior syndrome is associated with frontotemporal lobar atrophy of non-Alzheimer's disease type.
- A medial and anterior syndrome characterise alcoholic encephalopathy.

Alzheimer's disease

Alzheimer's disease is a predominantly cortical disease characterised by impaired function, particularly of the medial and posterior cortices. Evidence for this comes from studies of regional cerebral blood flow and pathological and biochemical findings at necropsy.

The earliest symptom is commonly memory failure: patients have difficulty learning new information and forget day-to-day events. As the disease progresses memories are also affected, but information from the distant rather than the recent past may appear to be relatively well preserved. Amnesia may be the exclusive psychological symptom for many years, with additional cognitive deficits emerging at late stages.

Memory disorder is not invariably the earliest symptom. Perceptuo-spatial problems are characteristic in Alzheimer's disease and difficulties with aligning cutlery when laying a table or folding clothes correctly may be the earliest apparent abnormality. Because they fail to negotiate and appreciate the spatial layout of the environment, patients may become lost in unfamiliar, and later in familiar, surroundings. People with Alzheimer's disease are unable to dress themselves because they do not orientate clothing correctly. Perceptual abnormalities result in failure to recognise faces of others and eventually his/her own face in the mirror.

When language areas around the peri-sylvian fissure are involved, language skills are affected. Utterances are halting, reflecting difficulty in finding words and failure to maintain a line of thought. Repetition and comprehension, reading, writing and calculation are impaired. Alexia, agraphia and acalculia are compounded by spatial difficulties, because the written word and numerals are poorly organised in space. Breakdown of skilled movements of the arms and legs may be secondary to spatial disorientation, which results in difficulty copying drawings and designs (constructional apraxia) and dressing (dressing apraxia). Sometimes there may be severe executive difficulties, disproportionate to perceptuo-spatial impairment, that are sufficient to prevent manual use of objects and the adoption of postures and appropriate movements on attempted walking.

In contrast to the specific psychological deficits, social graces are often well preserved into the advanced stages of the disease and profound cognitive problems are often masked by the patient's normal social facade. Patients rarely complain of symptoms, but may be aware of and admit to difficulties when confronted by test failures. The extent of insight is variable and seems to be inversely related to the severity of the patient's amnesia.

The neurological signs of Alzheimer's disease consist of akinesia, rigidity and myoclonus, which emerge with progressive involvement of subcortical structures. Physical problems, however, are dwarfed by the momentous psychological disturbance and may be absent until the relatively late stages of disease.

The EEG shows progressive slowing of wave forms. Computed tomography (CT) reveals non-specific cerebral atrophy (**Figs 3.1** and **3.2**), but functional imaging techniques, such as positron emission tomography (PET) and single-photon emission tomography (SPET), reveal characteristic abnormalities of the parietal regions (**Fig. 3.3**) (see pages 20, 24).

Lobar atrophy of non-Alzheimer's disease type

Fronto-temporal lobar atrophy is associated with a number of syndromes determined by the distribution of pathology within the anterior hemispheres (**Fig. 1.3**).

- Bilateral and chiefly frontal lobe involvement is characterised by fronto-temporal dementia.
- Asymmetrical involvement of predominantly the left dominant fronto-temporal lobes leads to the syndrome of progressive non-fluent type aphasia.
- Predominant involvement of both temporal lobes leads to a syndrome of fluent aphasia with associative visual agnosia (semantic dementia). All of these syndromes can be complicated by the amyotrophic form of motor neurone disease.

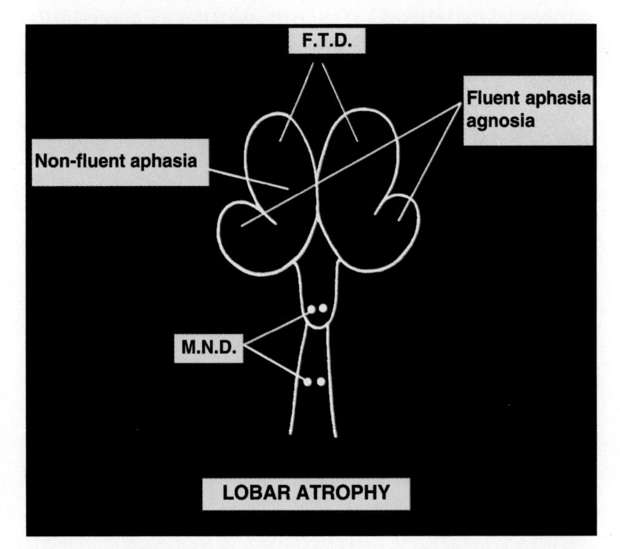

Fig. 1.3 The clinical syndromes of lobar atrophy. F.T.D. refers to fronto-temporal dementia; M.N.D. to motor neurone disease.

Fronto-temporal dementia

Fronto-temporal dementia is more common than generally recognised and may account for about 20% of younger patients with primary cerebral atrophy. Patients show altered personality and social and personal behaviour, becoming incapable of managing their own affairs, losing their jobs through irresponsibility and impaired judgement. They may appear apathetic and lacking motivation, or overactive and disinhibited. Insight is lost. Stereotyped behaviour is not uncommon, ranging from simple repetitive hand movements, repetitive utterances, and singing, to complex rituals involving cleaning, dressing, and eating. Over-eating and food fads are characteristic. Language becomes more economical and concrete, with verbatim copying of what is said by others (echolalia) and repetition of their own responses (perseveration), leading finally to mutism. Patients exhibit gross abnormalities, on psychological testing, of frontal lobe dysfunction, but despite their disturbed behaviour and mutism, they remain orientated in their environment and show no spatial abnormalities even into the terminal stages of the disorder.

Neurological signs are minimal and consist of primitive reflexes in the early stages. Akinesia and rigidity occur very late. The EEG is normal throughout the early stages, while CT confirms cerebral atrophy, which may be more evident in frontal regions (**Fig. 3.191**). SPET confirms selective abnormalities in the frontal and temporal lobes (**Fig. 3.192**) (see pages 20, 71).

Progressive aphasia

Lobar atrophy leads to two prototypical language syndromes depending on the distribution of pathology in the fronto-temporal lobes.

Non-fluent aphasia

A progressive decline in language occurs in the relative absence of other psychological deficits until many years have elapsed. Speech becomes non-fluent with effortful utterances and loss of prosody. Repetition is poor, consisting mainly of phonological word errors known as literal paraphasias (e.g. 'tig' for 'big'). Naming difficulties arise and writing is impaired in form and content. Oral and reading comprehension are relatively preserved. The form of speech disturbance most closely resembles that of Broca's aphasia in relationship to focal brain lesions.

CT reveals progressive atrophy of the left cerebral hemisphere (**Fig. 3.264**) while SPET shows asymmetrical abnormalities in the left dominant hemisphere (**Fig. 3.265**) (see pages 20, 88).

Later, behavioural irregularities develop akin to fronto-temporal dementia, when SPET imaging exposes the spread of pathology to both fronto-temporal lobes. The EEG reveals asymmetrical slow waves over the dominant cerebral hemisphere.

Fluent aphasia and associative agnosia

Patients develop profound problems in understanding verbal and, later, visual material (semantic dementia). Spontaneous speech is fluent, but contaminated by semantic word errors known as verbal paraphasias (e.g. 'green' for 'big'). Utterances are rapid and exhibit normal prosody, but are difficult to comprehend. There is anomia and a profound lack of comprehension of speech and reading. However, repetition is strikingly preserved, as is reading aloud and writing to dictation. Such a pattern of speech disturbances closely resembles the transcortical sensory aphasia of focal lesions.

Later, patients develop an inability to recognise objects and faces despite a preserved ability to copy accurately and match objects and faces (associative agnosia). The lack of understanding of the meaning of verbal and non-verbal material has been termed 'semantic dementia'.

CT reveals (**Fig. 3.287**) either nonspecific cerebral atrophy or more selective widening of the inter-hemispheric and sylvian fissures, suggesting fronto-temporal atrophy – especially involving the temporal lobes. SPET shows a bilateral reduction in metabolism in the anterior hemisphere (**Fig. 3.288**). The EEG is usually normal.

Lobar atrophy and motor neurone disease

The syndromes of fronto-temporal dementia and progressive aphasia can be complicated by the development of the amyotrophic form of motor neurone disease. This is most often associated with fronto-temporal dementia. Usually the neurological symptoms and signs commence after the development of the dementia and within two years the patients die of respiratory complications. In patients who survive longer, the extrapyramidal signs, seen in the late stages of fronto-temporal dementia, can make an appearance.

Motor neurone disease is amyotrophic with bulbar palsy, weakness, wasting and fasciculations of the limbs, in the absence of significant muscle spasticity. The bulbar palsy leads to the fatal complications.

Electrophysiological studies demonstrate widespread denervation of muscles.

Alcoholic encephalopathy

Both the frontal lobes and the limbic system are damaged by alcohol abuse and therefore alcoholics may exhibit a medial or anterior cortical syndrome, or both.

The medial cortical or amnesic syndrome usually arises as an aftermath of an acute neurological crisis (Wernicke's encephalopathy). The patient sinks into a stupor or coma, develops ocular palsies, irregular pupils, and ataxia. A proportion of individuals who survive are left with profound amnesia in the absence of the posterior cortical symptoms of aphasia, spatial disorientation, or apraxia. They may perform normally on tests sensitive to frontal lobe dysfunction. This syndrome is termed Korsakoff's amnesia or the Wernicke–Korsakoff syndrome.

A proportion of chronic alcohol abusers who neglect their diet, present with a progressive dementing syndrome in which there are features of both frontal lobe disturbance and amnesia.

Korsakoff's amnesic syndrome is associated with gradual improvement, although this may not be complete in all cases, whereas the more insidious presentation is associated with a chronic decline in mental function.

CT evidence of cerebral atrophy is seen in the majority of individuals who suffer from both the acute and chronic alcoholic syndromes.

Subcortical encephalopathies

Several diseases affect predominantly subcortical structures with relative sparing of the cerebral cortex. These include degenerative disorders such as Parkinson's disease, Huntington's disease, and progressive supranuclear palsy. A similar syndrome also occurs when the subcortical white matter is destroyed by multiple infarcts or is stretched and damaged secondary to chronic repeated head trauma and hydrocephalus.

Subcortical structures and their projections to the cerebral cortex seem to exert a quantitative and regulatory effect on the pace and organisation of its functions. Psychological events need to happen at an appropriate rate, in orderly sequence with flexible responses; that is, they require an organised strategy. Patients with subcortical disorders exhibit slowness and rigidity of thinking (bradyphrenia) with inflexibility and difficulty in switching responses (perseveration). Although forgetful they do not exhibit severe amnesia. They have difficulties in planning and sequencing mental events and may fail on tests sensitive to frontal lobe dysfunction. They do not show the specific abnormalities of language, visual perception and spatial functioning seen in cortical disorders. Social conduct and personality are generally preserved. The exception to this is Huntington's disease in which severe change of personality and behaviour occur. The bizarre behaviour of such patients may pre-date any cognitive changes, which are insufficient to account fully for the disturbed conduct.

The neuropsychological profile of subcortical disorders (**Table 1.6**) shows that there is some similarity to the anterior cortical encephalopathy in terms of the disorder of regulation and mild memory impairment, but without the progressive personality and linguistic impairment of anterior cortical disorder.

In subcortical disorders the neuropsychological deficits are overshadowed by profound and characteristic neurological symptoms and signs.

- Akinesia, rigidity, and tremor in Parkinson's disease.
- Involuntary and purposeless jerking movements in Huntington's disease.
- Paralysis of eye movements in progressive supranuclear palsy.

The EEG may be normal or show slight slowing of wave forms, but is of no diagnostic significance. CT may also exhibit normal or nonspecific cerebral atrophy (**Figs 4.1** and **4.25**). In progressive supranuclear palsy, PET and SPET reveal abnormalities in the frontal cortex similar to those of frontotemporal dementia (**Fig. 4.2**) (see pages 20, 97).

Cortical-subcortical encephalopathy

Two disorders display features of both cortical and subcortical syndromes determined by the spread of pathology to both structures. In Lewy Body disease the distribution of pathology is symmetrical, whereas in cortico-basal degeneration it is highly asymmetrical.

Table 1.6 Profile of neuropsychological disorders associated with subcortical and cortical-subcortical encephalopathies. Primary (primary abnormality); secondary (abnormality secondary to the patient's primary deficits).

Areas of cortex involved	Language	Perceptuo-spatial function	Praxis	Memory	Regulation
Subcortex				Secondary	Primary

Lewy Body disease

Lewy Body disease is a disorder of old age with no reported familial incidence. Mental changes develop before or after Parkinsonian symptoms and signs of akinesia, rigidity and tremor, which are responsive to the administration of L-dopa. Changes in the cerebral cortex may account for cortical symptoms of aphasia, agnosia and apraxia, but the dominant feature of the illness is a fluctuating confusional state with visual illusions and hallucinations leading to secondary delusions. Such fluctuations, presumably due to a simultaneous disorder of cortex and subcortex, are not characteristic of the cortical or subcortical encephalopathies. When confusion does occur in these latter disorders it usually relates to systemic complications, drug toxicity, anaesthesia, or the relative sensory deprivation of night time or unfamiliar surroundings.

The EEG characteristically reveals a severe slowing of wave forms and sometimes periodic wave complexes. CT shows cerebral atrophy. SPET (**Fig. 5.1**) (pages 20, 115) reveals reduced uptake in the cerebral cortex, especially in the posterior hemispheres.

Cortico-basal degeneration

The asymmetrical distribution of pathology in subcortical and cortical sites is mirrored by the development of neurological signs of a basal ganglia disorder together with cortical symptoms reflecting fronto-parietal lobe dysfunction, against a background of a subcortical neuropsychological syndrome.

Asymmetrical akinesia and rigidity predominantly affect the upper limbs, which are also the site of tremor, dystonic movements, and myoclonus. Psychologically, there is slowing, inflexibility, and perseveration concordant with a subcortical syndrome. Moreover, an asymmetrical cortical syndrome emerges, particularly a profound apraxia of the most affected side. The limbs progressively lose all executive functions and may develop autonomous movements (alien limb).

CT shows cerebral atrophy. Functional imaging (PET and SPET) (pages 20, 121) reveals asymmetrical abnormalities of the basal ganglia and associated fronto-parietal cortex (**Fig. 5.23**). EEG changes are of nonspecific asymmetrical slow waves.

Vascular encephalopathy

Recurrent completed strokes lead to an accumulated neurological and psychological deficit. The ictal nature of the evolution of the disorder, together with evidence of multiple infarctions or haemorrhages on brain imaging, is not likely to lead to diagnostic confusion.

When vascular lesions predominantly affect the subcortical white matter, a characteristic subcortical syndrome (subcortical arteriosclerotic dementia) emerges, which is often progressive and lacking ictal events. This syndrome requires differentiation from subcortical neurodegenerative diseases and from communicating hydrocephalus.

In a proportion of patients vascular events occur in both the cortex and the subcortex, but again without apparent historical stroke-like events. The clinical picture of multiple (cortical and subcortical) infarct dementia may superficially resemble Alzheimer's disease.

CT, MRI and functional brain imaging reveal asymmetrically distributed focal lesions in the cerebral hemispheres (**Figs 5.77, 5.78** and **5.79**) (page 133).

Multifocal encephalopathy

Subacute spongiform encephalopathies (prion disease), such as Creutzfeldt–Jakob disease, are rapidly progressive disorders, with low familial incidence, which are often terminal within approximately six months. Longer survival may occur in familial disease forms like Gerstmann– Sträussler–Sheinker syndrome.

The aggressive disease process does not seem to respect anatomical boundaries or functional systems, so a wide variety of psychological and neurological deficits rapidly emerges (**Fig. 1.4**). Some patients present with neurological symptoms such as a cerebellar syndrome, cortical blindness, sensory motor deficits, myoclonus, and epileptic seizures. Focal psychological syndromes including aphasia and ataxia may herald the onset of the disease. When thalamic structures are preferentially involved the predominant picture may be of progressive somnolence (fatal insomnia).

Despite the apparent heterogeneity of symptoms, in the early stages there is a characteristic disorder, rarely seen in other encephalopathies.

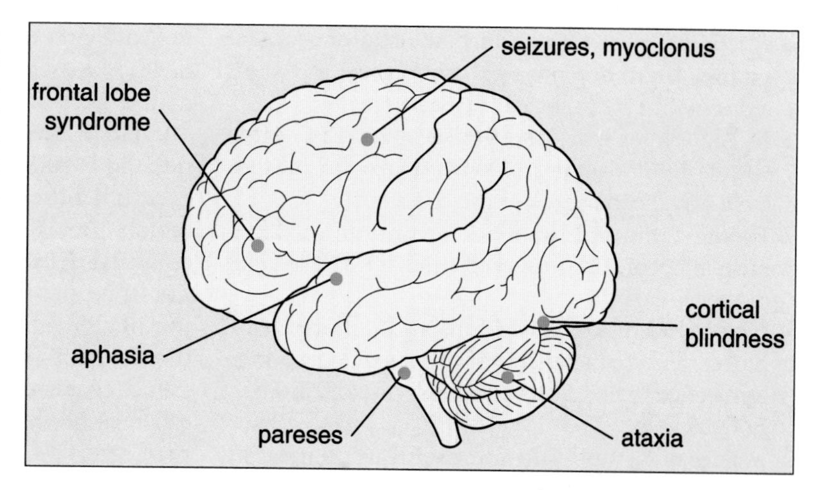

Fig. 1.4 Neurological and psychological disorders associated with multifocal encephalopathy. There is widespread cerebral involvement, which is not restricted to cortical and subcortical areas, but involves the cerebellum and brain stem as well, leading to ataxia (unsteadiness) and paresis (paralysis).

Responsiveness fluctuates dramatically. For long periods patients may be immobile with open staring eyes and catatonic posturing of the limbs. They then begin to move and speak, stop posturing, and comment on events that have occurred during their non-responsive state, indicating that they are conscious. As the disease progresses the islands of responsiveness become progressively attenuated until akinetic mutism supervenes.

The severe neurological and psychological disorder is reflected in the grossly disturbed EEG: there is a profound slowing of wave forms and characteristic periodic triphasic wave complexes emerge. CT is either normal (**Fig. 6.1**) or reveals nonspecific cerebral atrophy. SPET imaging shows a patchy reduction of tracer uptake in the cerebral cortex (**Fig. 6.2**) (page 144).

Diagnostic considerations

The relative prominence of associated mental and physical changes in the evolution of the disease differs for the four encephalopathic syndromes (**Table 1.7**). This distinction forms a basis for the differential diagnosis of these disorders, especially when the results of electroencephalography are taken into account.

- Cortical encephalopathies are characterised by profound mental changes and the relative absence of neurological signs, particularly in the early stages of the disease.
- Subcortical encephalopathies are associated with striking physical signs, while mental changes may be of relatively less significance and tend to occur later in the disease.

Table 1.7 Nature and relative severity of the psychological, neurological and EEG disorders associated

Encephalopathy	Psychological syndrome	Neurological signs	EEG
Anterior cortical	Severe, specific	Mild, late	Normal
Posterior medial cortical	Severe, specific	Mild, late	Progressive, slowing
Subcortical	Mild, specific	Moderate, early	Moderate, slowing
Cortical-subcortical	Fluctuating, asymmetrical	Moderate, early	Moderate, slowing
Multifocal	Severe, diffuse	Severe, diffuse	Severe, slowing. Periodic complexes

- In cortical-subcortical and multifocal encephalopathies there are physical symptoms and signs along with psychological disturbance.
- In Alzheimer's disease the standard EEG often shows mild slowing of wave forms in moderately advanced stages of the disease.
- Fronto-temporal dementia is unique in that a normal record is preserved until the later stages of the disease.
- Gross slowing of wave forms and periodic complexes are characteristic of the subacute spongiform encephalopathies and also of cortical Lewy Body disease.

Whereas CT and MRI are useful in delineating structural changes such as the presence of vascular diseases or hydrocephalus, they are less useful in the differential diagnosis of neurodegenerative disorders when they may be normal or reveal non-specific cerebral atrophy.

SPET imaging demonstrates functional change in the brain, which is of high diagnostic value in the neurodegenerative disorders because the abnormalities closely reflect the topographical distribution of pathology within the cerebrum (**Table 1.8**). The radioactive tracer crosses the blood–brain barrier and is taken up by cerebral tissue reflecting the cerebral blood flow and perfusion, and hence regional metabolic function (page 176). In fronto-temporal dementia the characteristic abnormality in the fronto-temporal lobes contrasts strikingly with the bilateral parietal defects seen in Alzheimer's disease. An asymmetrical dominant hemispheric defect characterises progressive non-fluent aphasia, whereas predominantly bitemporal defects underly progressive non-fluent aphasia and associative agnosia. Subcortical disorders such as progressive supranuclear palsy display an anterior cerebral defect, which is less severe than in lobar atrophy. An asymmetrical fronto-parietal defect is seen in cortico-basal degeneration, whereas multifocal lesions are demonstrated in subacute spongiform encephalopathy.

Table 1.8 SPET abnormalities

Syndrome	Disease	Abnormality
Anterior	Fronto-temporal dementia	Anterior
Posterior	Alzheimer's disease	Posterior
Subcortical	Progressive supranuclear palsy	Anterior subcortical
Cortical-subcortical	Cortico-basal degeneration	Asymmetrical fronto-parietal
Multifocal	Subacute spongiform encephalopathy	Diffuse and focal

2. Pathological causes of dementia

A cortical dementia will emerge as a dominant syndrome when fundamental regions of the temporal lobe (hippocampus, amygdala, entorhinal cortex), frontal lobe (orbitofrontal and convex cortex), or posterior parietal lobe are damaged or their functions disrupted (see **Fig. 1.1**). Additional or secondary damage to the temporal neocortex and anterior parietal and insular cortices, in association with certain ascending subcortical projection systems based on regions such as the nucleus basalis of Meynert, locus caeruleus, dorsal raphe and ventral tegmentum will exacerbate the clinical picture and provide subcortical signs and symptoms.

The number and range of disorders that can cause destruction of one or more of these key brain regions is diverse. Indeed, as if to emphasise this point, about 50 conditions have been identified, to date, in which a definable dementia has been considered to make up a part, or to constitute the whole, of the clinical symptomatology. The great majority of conditions are associated with clear pathological changes within the brain, though in other instances where the dementia relates to a toxic or metabolic cause, pathological changes may not be obvious, or at least definable, by conventional neurohistological procedures.

The terminology describing several of these disorders has changed in recent years. For example, the terms presenile and senile dementia were used for many years and applied rather indiscriminately to dementias of varying pathological origins. Presenile dementia was commonly equated with Alzheimer's disease; senile dementia was vaguely used to describe the presence of dementia in the elderly and could be applied with equal inconsistency to those cases due to Alzheimer's disease and those due to cerebrovascular disease. The term 'senile dementia of Alzheimer-type' was coined in an attempt to obviate some of this confusion. Now the terms senile and presenile dementia are in less common use, partly because of the need for consistency in terminology and partly because of the fact that, in some instances – for example, Alzheimer's disease – the disorder can occur at any time of life with apparently similar changes being produced in the brain regardless of age of onset. Moreover, it is now clear that not all 'presenile' disease is due to Alzheimer's disease, and that not all 'senile' disease is due to either Alzheimer's disease or cerebrovascular disease, or some combination of the two.

The entities of fronto-temporal dementia, a condition encompassing what has often been loosely equated with Pick's disease, and the dementias with extrapyramidal features such as Huntington's disease, Parkinson's disease, progressive supranuclear palsy and cortico-basal degeneration are all significant contributors to dementia in younger people. Likewise, the appearance of cortical Lewy Body disease as a major cause of dementia in the elderly has widened the possible diagnoses in this age group.

The common identification of a particular abnormal protein within the brain has collectivised certain rare disorders, such as Creutzfeldt–Jakob disease, kuru, and Gerstmann–Sträussler–Sheinker syndrome, (formerly known as the human spongiform encephalopathies), into what is now termed 'prion disease'. Increasing knowledge concerning their aetiology and pathogenesis has led to the virtual elimination of an 'infective' cause for these disorders, and with that a redundancy of the terms 'latent viral' or 'slow viral' as a disease descriptor.

The causes of dementia can be broadly categorized on pathological grounds as follows:

- Neurodegenerative.
- Vascular.
- Infective.
- Traumatic.
- Neoplastic.
- Toxic.
- Metabolic.

The more common disorders in these categories are listed in **Table 2.1**.

Table 2.1 Major pathological causes of dementia

Category	Example
Neuro-degenerative	Alzheimer's disease Down's syndrome Fronto-temporal dementia Pick's disease Fronto-temporal dementia with motor neurone disease Progressive aphasia Creutzfeldt–Jakob disease Gerstmann–Sträussler– Sheinker syndrome Familial fatal insomnia Kuru Huntington's disease Parkinson's disease Cortical Lewy Body disease Cortico-basal degeneration Progressive supranuclear palsy
Vascular	Multiple (cortical and subcortical infarction) Chronic hypertensive encephalopathy Binswanger's disease Congophilic angiopathy Subarachnoid haemorrhage
Infective	Acquired immune deficiency syndrome Subacute sclerosing panencephalitis Herpes simplex encephalitis Neurosyphilis Postencephalitic
Traumatic	Acute diffuse/focal brain injury Dementia pugilistica Subdural haematoma
Toxic and metabolic	Wernicke–Korsakoff syndrome Chronic hepatic encephalopathy Vitamin B_{12} deficiency Hypothyroidism Hypoglycaemia
Neoplastic	Primary intracranial tumour Metastatic carcinoma Hydrocephalus Limbic paraneoplastic change

This text is a guide to the clinical and pathological features of those conditions that are likely to be investigated because of their primary psychological or behavioural manifestations. Not all conditions listed in **Table 2.1** will therefore be discussed. For example, conditions in which mental changes are secondary to, or late aspects of, systemic disease or acute neurological illness will not be covered because the underlying cause of the cerebral changes will already have been investigated, diagnosed, and possibly treated. Such conditions do not provide difficulties in the differential diagnosis of primary dementia. Viral infections that cause an acute encephalopathy, which may resolve with appropriate treatment or may produce a form of chronic brain damage following recovery, are also excluded. Among these the most notable are subacute sclerosing panencephalitis associated with measles reactivation, and AIDS encephalopathy due to HIV infection. Likewise, the effects of carcinoma or carcinoma-like conditions are not discussed.

The principal demographic, radiological and neuropathological aspects of most of the major conditions causing a primary dementia (see **Table 2.1**) are presented in the following chapters. Molecular genetic and molecular biological features are described if known; and also if pertinent, nosology and clinico-pathological relationships. Interpretations of change in terms of disease cause (aetiology) and progression (pathogenesis) are presented and an overview of treatment (or at least patient management) is provided.

The results of virtually all epidemiological surveys into the prevalence of dementia point to Alzheimer's disease as the single major cause of dementia, accounting for about 55% of all cases by itself, and contributing along with other cerebral pathologies to a further 20%. It is therefore discussed first. Descriptions of other neurodegenerative conditions causing cerebral cortical pathology and a cortical encephalopathy will follow, and lead on to those producing subcortical, cortico-subcortical, and multifocal encephalopathies.

3. Cortical encephalopathies

ALZHEIMER'S DISEASE

Aetiology and demography

Alzheimer's disease is the most common dementing illness and can occur at any age over 30. It tends to affect women more than men, even when survival differences among the elderly are taken into account. It is relatively uncommon before 65 years of age, affecting about 0.1% of the population, but its incidence and prevalence rise rapidly thereafter. About 5% of all old people have severe and 10% mild-to-moderate Alzheimer's disease; and as many as 25–45% of over-80-year-olds are affected.

Familial cases are seemingly uncommon, being best defined when the onset is before 60 years of age, but a genetic involvement in older people could be more common than appears due to early death before the age of onset or before diagnosis, masking individuals at risk of disease and leading to only modest familial clustering. Point mutations producing amino acid substitutions in the amyloid precursor protein (APP) encoded by a gene located on the long arm of chromosome 21 have been clearly linked to the disorder in certain families with early onset of disease. Linkage to loci on chromosomes 14 and 22 has been demonstrated in other early onset families, although in families where onset usually occurs after 60 years of age, linkage to chromosome 19 has been reported.

Clearly, Alzheimer's disease is aetiologically heterogeneous with distinct genetic and apparently non-genetic (environmental) causes, though even in these latter instances a genetic trait may facilitate development of disease. Nonetheless, irrespective of aetiology, all types of Alzheimer's disease seem to share a common pathology, implying that a single pathogenetic mechanism operates despite these diverse aetiologies (see page 63).

The clinical picture is a cortical encephalopathy, and the duration of the disease is variable and depends on age of onset, premorbid health, and susceptibility to intercurrent disease. Consequently, it can vary from a year or two up to 15–20 years, longer courses of illness occurring mainly in younger individuals with better premorbid health.

Pathological features

Gross changes in the brain

The extent of changes seen on brain imaging are often age-dependent. CT scanning, especially in younger individuals, can show atrophy of the cerebral cortex that is particularly pronounced in perisylvian regions (**Fig. 3.1**); there is usually enlargement of the lateral ventricles (**Fig. 3.2**). However, many patients, more often the elderly, show an indistinct pattern of atrophy or may have a scan that is normal for their age.

Psychological symptoms (early)
Amnesia
Perceptuo-spatial disorder
Aphasia

Neurological signs (late)
Akinesia and rigidity
Myoclonus

Investigations
EEG: abnormal
SPET: parietal lobe abnormality

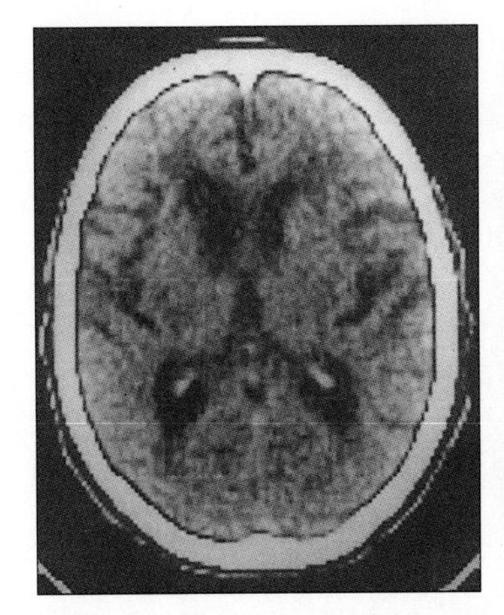

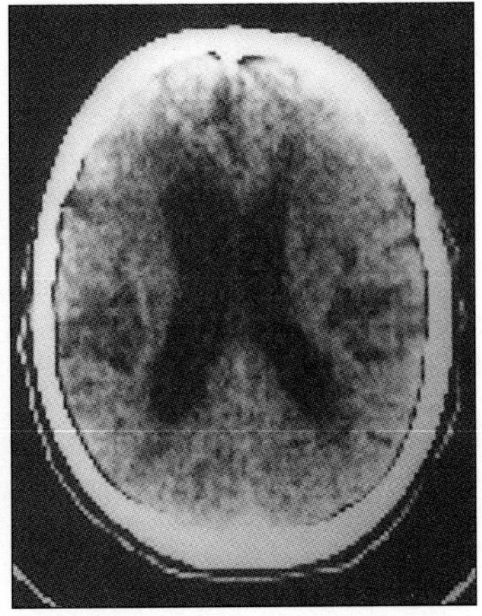

Figs 3.1 and 3.2 Perisylvian atrophy and dilatation of the lateral ventricles. CT scans of a 58-year-old man.

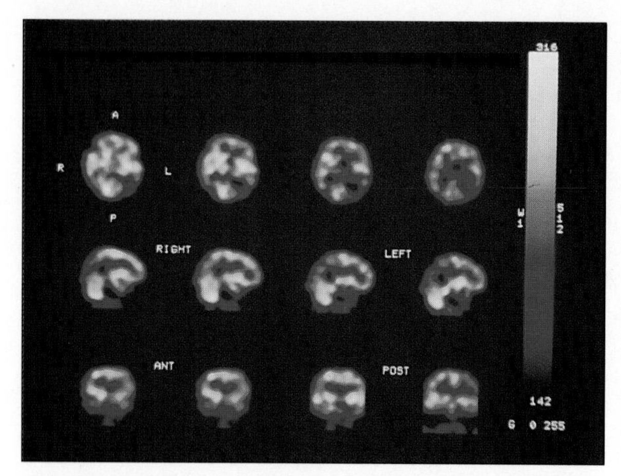

Fig. 3.3 Bilateral posterior hemisphere hypometabolism in a 62-year-old woman as seen with SPET imaging.

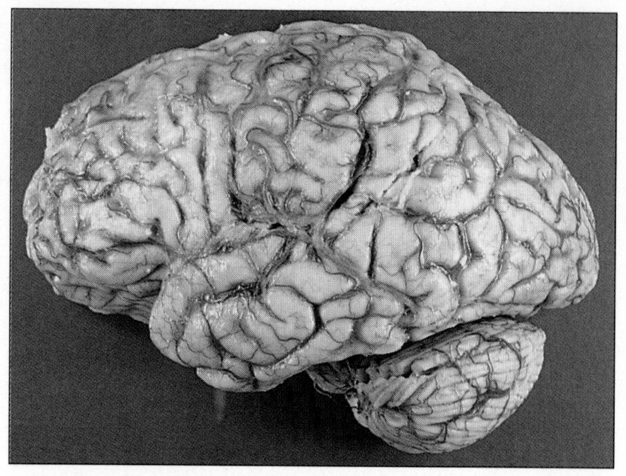

Fig. 3.4 Lateral view of the brain of a 65-year-old woman. This shows atrophy within the frontal and temporal lobes and perisylvian regions.

However, many patients, more often the elderly, show an indistinct pattern of atrophy or may have a scan that is normal for their age.

On SPET imaging there is a consistent pattern of hypometabolism bilaterally affecting the temporal lobe and the posterior parietal cortex (**Fig. 3.3**). These changes on functional imaging are usually apparent even when the CT scan reveals no unusual or localised structural features.

In terms of brain weight the degree of atrophy is extremely variable and is again usually age-dependent, with younger individuals showing a greater degree of atrophy, the brain often being reduced in weight to around 1000 g. In older individuals a reduction in brain weight is less apparent; indeed, in many surveys of mostly older people only a slight, and usually non-significant, reduction in brain weight has been recorded, though there is much individual variation.

Likewise, the distribution of the atrophy is variable. Typically, in younger persons, atrophy affects the frontal, fronto-parietal and temporal lobes, especially within perisylvian regions (**Fig. 3.4**). When sliced, a gross enlargement of the lateral ventricles is seen, particularly within the posterior hemisphere and temporal horns (**Figs 3.5** and **3.6**). The hippocampus (see **Fig. 3.6**), parahippocampal gyrus and the amygdala (see **Fig. 3.5**) are consistently and severely atrophic. The basal ganglia are frequently reduced in overall size (see **Fig. 3.5**), but do not usually show any discernible abnormality on gross inspection. The brain stem and cerebellum are normal, though in severely atrophic disease some reduction in size of both regions is apparent, while the third and fourth ventricles and the aqueduct are enlarged. In many older patients little atrophy beyond that of their age is noted (**Fig. 3.7**), though in others atrophy, when present, is limited to temporal lobe structures.

Morphometric measurements confirm this pattern of atrophy, with most involvement in the temporal lobe and fewer changes in frontal and parietal regions (**Figs 3.8** and **3.9**). In contrast to that seen on SPET imaging, the posterior parietal cortex shows relatively little gross atrophy; this latter region is probably, in the main, functionally deafferented without there being major intrinsic pathology. The basal ganglia are involved (**Fig. 3.9**), with the thalamus and caudate nucleus being affected more than the putamen and globus pallidus. Cerebral cortical grey and white matter are affected equally and there are no changes in the ratio between grey and white matter.

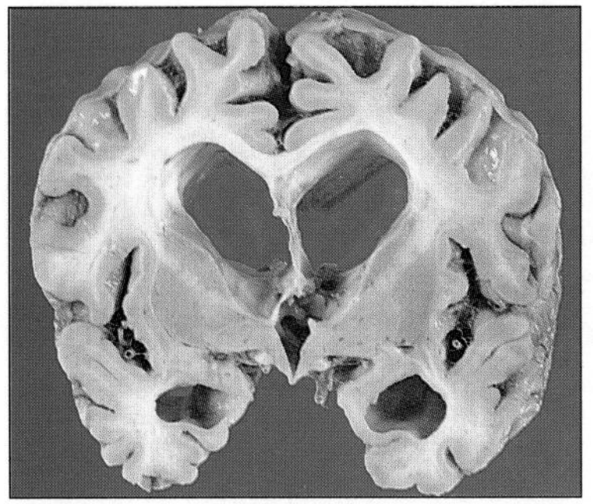

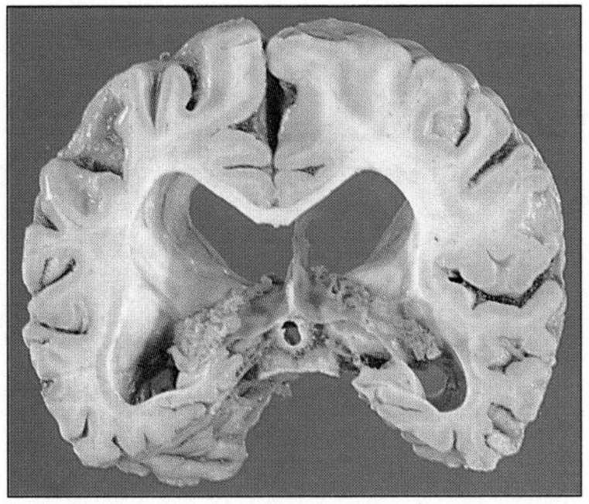

Figs 3.5 and 3.6 Coronal slices of the brain of a 62-year-old man showing cortical atrophy and ventricular dilatation. Note the severe atrophy of the amygdala and hippocampus.

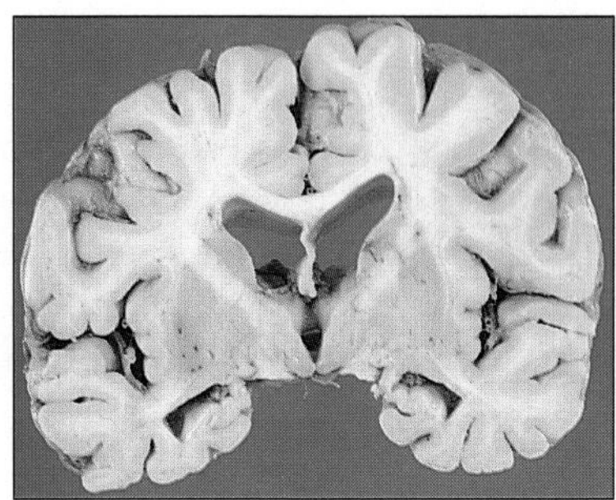

Fig. 3.7 Coronal slice of the brain of an 83-year-old woman shows less severe atrophy mostly within the temporal lobes.

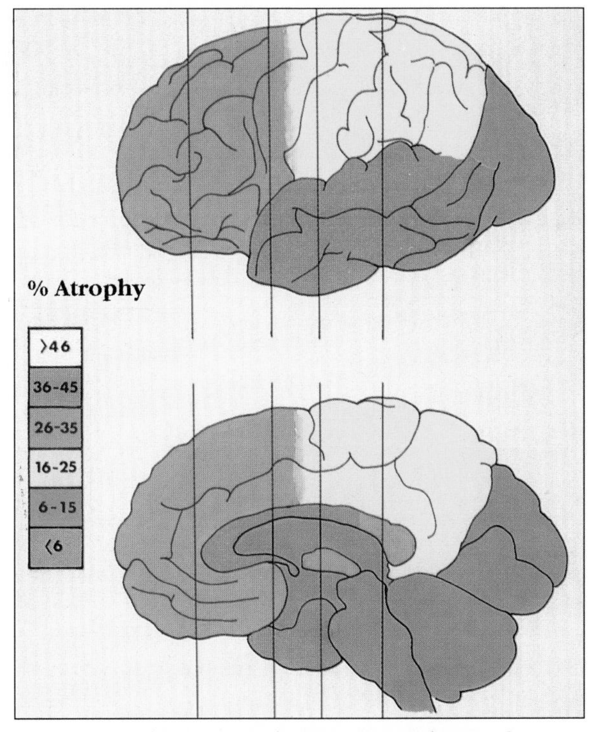

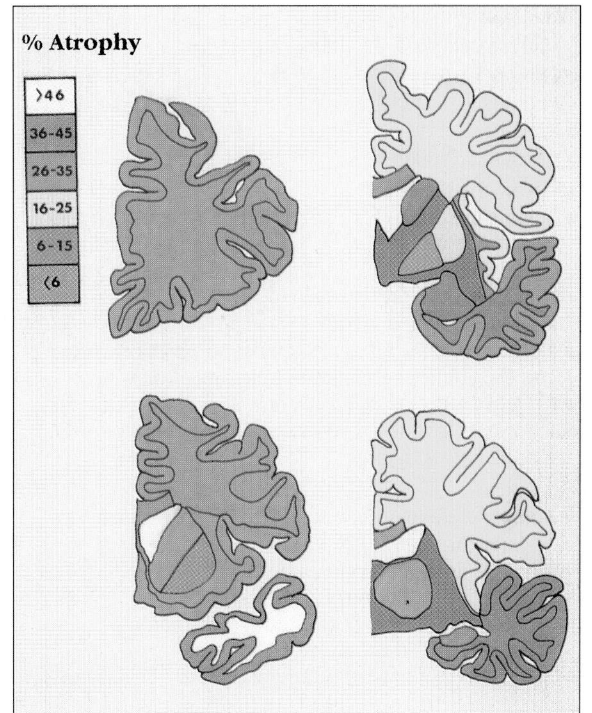

Figs 3.8 and 3.9 Morphometric analysis of regional brain atrophy. Note the preference for temporal lobe structures.

Although Alzheimer's disease may be suspected from clinical assessment, there are no particular changes on brain imaging, or in brain weight or in the distribution of atrophy, that might be regarded as unequivocally diagnostic for the disease; diagnosis can be made with certainty only from histopathological inspection of the tissues.

Histopathological features

Alzheimer's disease is associated histologically with the presence of 'numerous' so-called 'senile plaques' and 'neurofibrillary tangles' within the cerebral cortex, hippocampus and amygdala. These are intracellular and extracellular degenerative changes that damage nerve cells causing their dysfunction and lead eventually to their death and disappearance from the tissue.

Age of onset
Any age from 30 years onwards
Most common after 65 years of age.

Sex incidence
Affects females more than males.

Duration
Variable, usually 2–10 years.

Gross features
Generalized cortical atrophy with temporal lobe preference
Ventricular dilatation.

Histopathology
- Numerous deposits of amyloid β/A4 protein in the cerebral cortex, many with dystrophic neurites (neuritic plaques)
- Amyloid β/A4 protein deposits in cerebellar cortex and basal ganglia
- Numerous neurofibrillary tangles in cerebral cortex and hippocampus containing tau and ubiquitin
- Amyloid angiopathy; β/A4 protein in vessel walls
- Hirano bodies and granulovacuolar degeneration in hippocampus

Genetics
- Point mutations in codons 670/671 and codon 717 of gene for amyloid precursor protein, located on the long arm of chromosome 21
- Other genetic loci on chromosome 14 (unidentified), 19 (apolipoprotein E), and 22 segregate with the disease
- Autosomal dominant inheritance

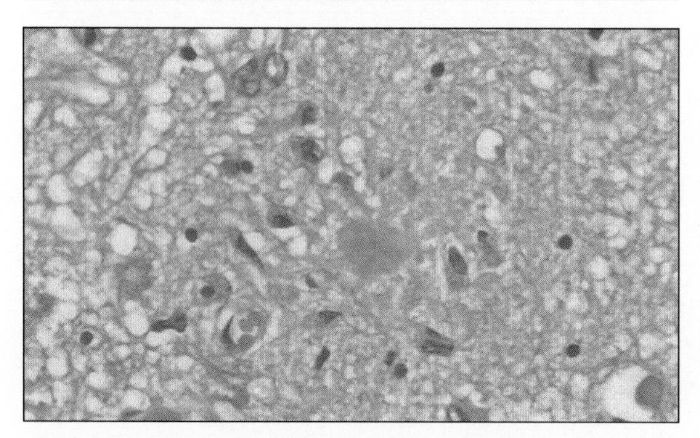

Fig. 3.12 A 'cored' type of senile plaque in the temporal cortex. (*Haematoxylin–eosin × 400.*)

Senile plaques

Appearance
Senile plaques are complicated foci of tissue degeneration containing a variety of molecular and cellular elements (**Fig. 3.10**). Consequently, they present a spectrum of morphological appearances and a wide-ranging numerical density, depending on which component is sought histochemically.

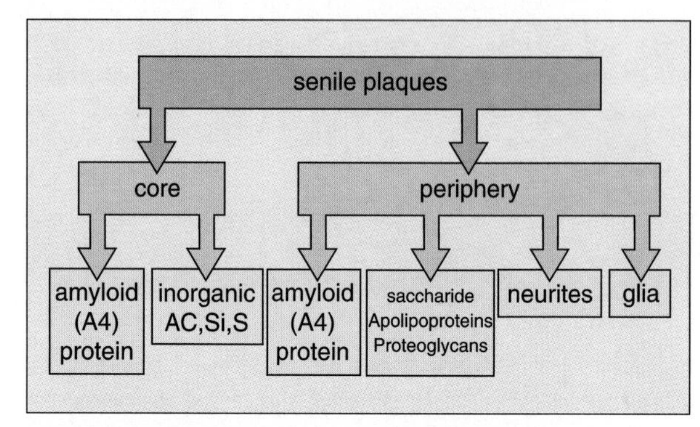

Fig. 3.10 Molecular and cellular components of senile plaques.

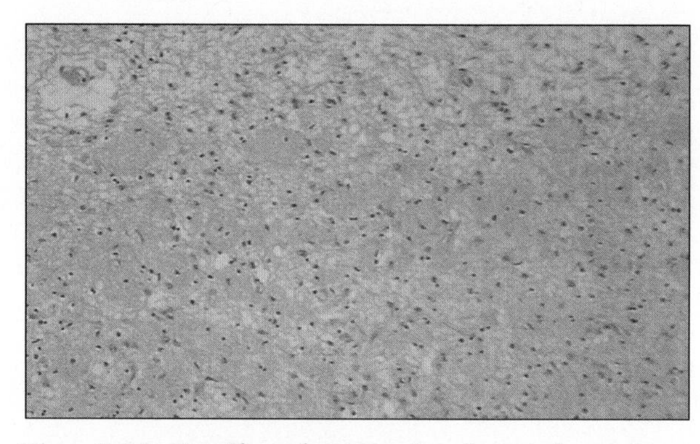

Fig. 3.11 Senile plaques in frontal cortex. (*Haematoxylin–eosin × 100.*)

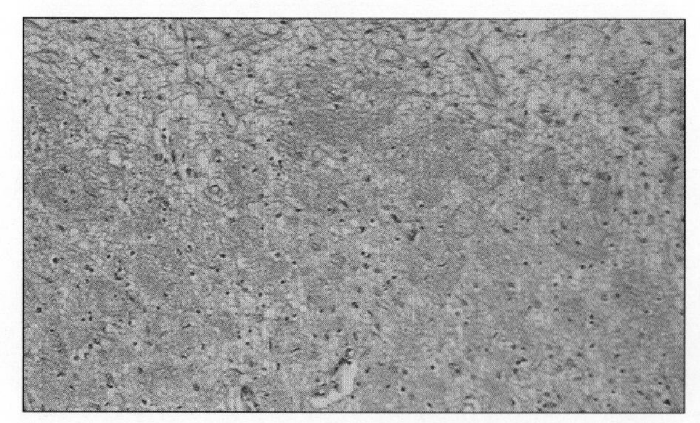

Fig. 3.13 Senile plaques in the frontal cortex. (*Phosphotungstic acid–haematoxylin × 100.*)

Routine staining (e.g. haematoxylin–eosin, phosphotungstic acid–haematoxylin) usually fails to reveal senile plaques, but occasionally they can be picked out using these methods (**Figs 3.11–3.13**). They can be demonstrated more often by the periodic acid–Schiff reaction (**Fig. 3.14**), though the efficacy of this varies from case to case.

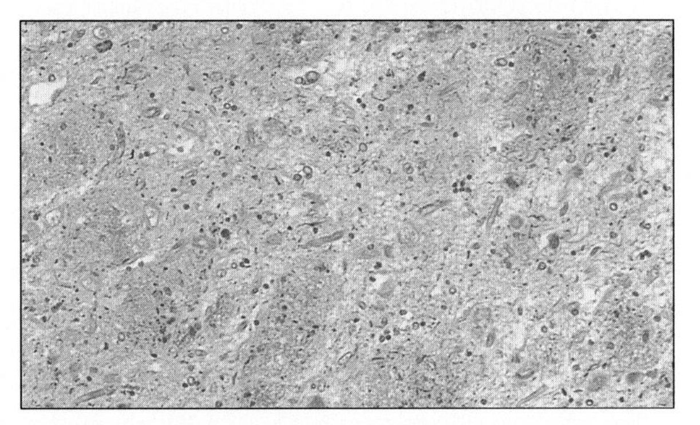

Fig. 3.14 Senile plaques in the frontal cortex. *(Anti-tau with periodic acid Schiff counterstain × 100.)*

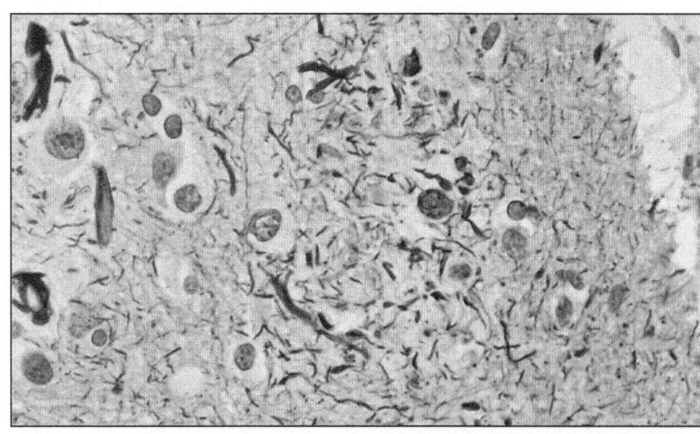

Fig. 3.15 'Neuritic' type of plaque in the temporal cortex. *(Palmgren silver method × 200.)* Note the blackened fibrillary structures (neurites), which give this type of plaque its name. Neurofibrillary tangles within the cells are also stained.

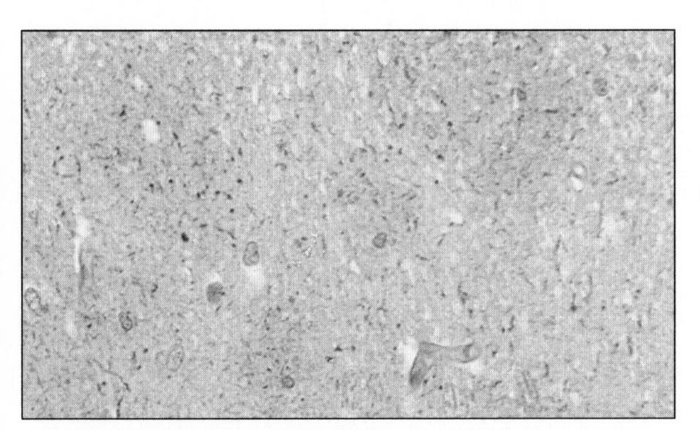

Fig. 3.16 Presence of tau protein within the brain. This exists as a widespread network of fibres (neurites) throughout the neuropil, with more focal aggregation within plaque regions. *(Anti-tau with periodic acid–Schiff counterstain × 100.)*

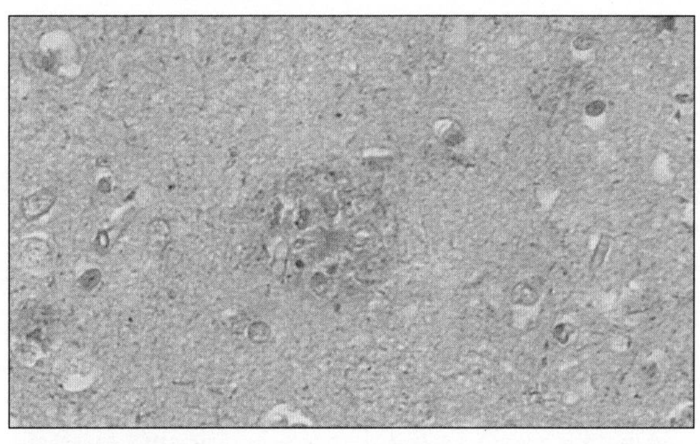

Fig.3.17 Tau-immunoreactive neurites around a cored plaque. *(Anti-tau with periodic acid–Schiff counterstain × 100.)*

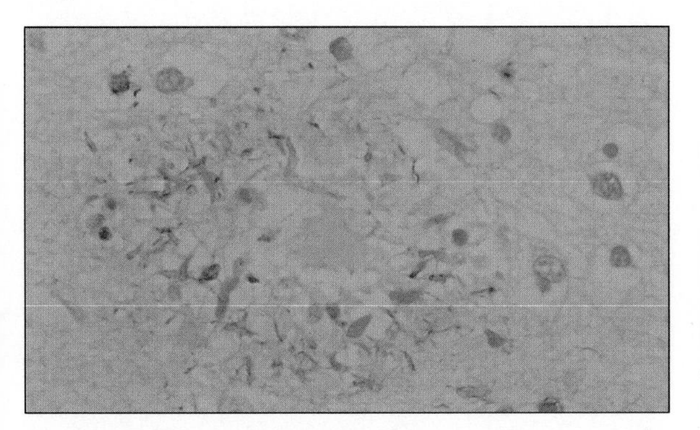

Fig. 3.18 Tau-immunoreactive neurites around a cored plaque. Note the unstained core. *(Anti-tau with haematoxylin counterstain × 400.)*

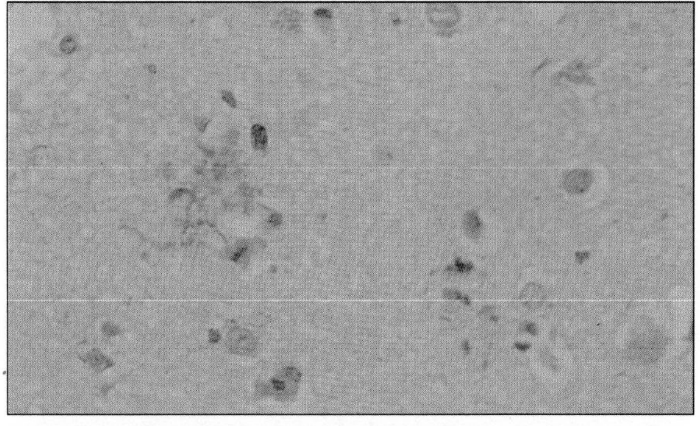

Fig. 3.19 Ubiquitin-immunoreactive neurites within plaques. *(Anti-ubiquitin × 200.)*

'Classic' silver impregnation methods such as Bielschowsky, Bodian and Palmgren have been most widely used to detect plaques and reveal the 'classical' or 'neuritic' type (**Fig. 3.15**), so-called because of the presence of filamentous structures corresponding to altered nerve terminals or 'neurites', which are 'blackened' by these techniques. Such neurites contain 'paired helical filaments' (PHF), which are also found in nerve cell bodies (as neurofibrillary tangles) and nerve cell processes (as neuropil threads) (see **Fig. 3.15** and page 39). PHF are composed mainly of the microtubule-associated protein, tau, and the

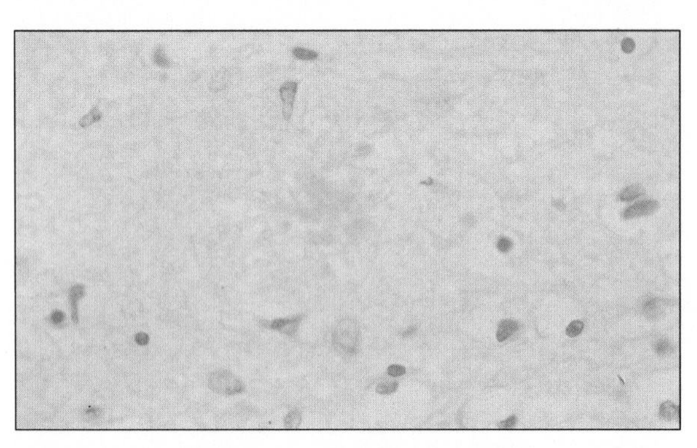

Fig. 3.20 Amyloid core of plaque. *(Congo red × 400.)*

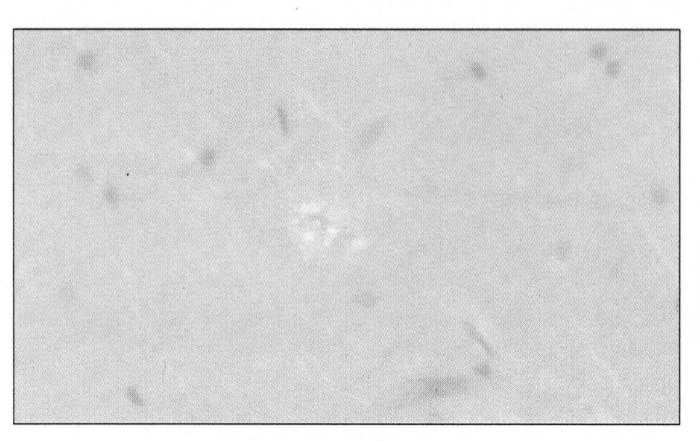

Fig. 3.21 Amyloid core of the same plaque stained with Congo red and viewed under cross-polarised light. Note the characteristic green-gold birefringence in the form of a Maltese cross. *(× 400.)*

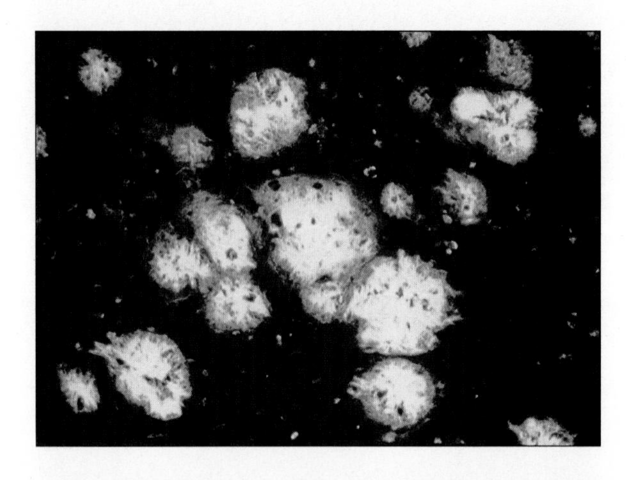

Fig. 3.22 Amyloid plaques stained with thioflavin S and viewed under fluorescent light. *(× 200.)*

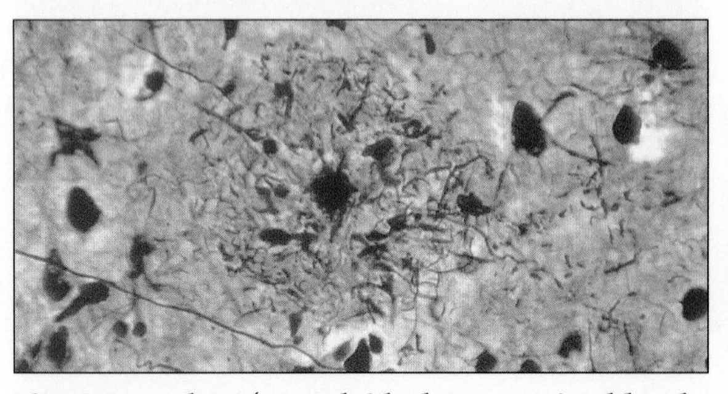

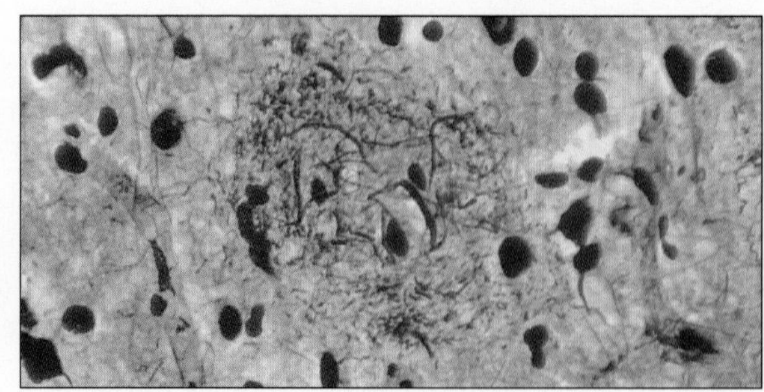

Figs 3.23 and 3.24 Amyloid plaques stained by the Von Braunmuhl method. *(× 400.)*

'stress' protein, ubiquitin. Antibodies directed against these particular molecules therefore reveal these same neuritic plaque structures (**Figs 3.16–3.19**) in immunohistochemical staining procedures.

The major non-cellular element of the senile plaque is a polypeptide variously known as A4-amyloid, β-amyloid or β/A4 amyloid according to its molecular weight (39–42 amino acids, molecular weight 4.2 KDa) and its capacity to aggregate spontaneously into a β-pleated configuration recognisable with Congo red (**Figs 3.20** and **3.21**) or thioflavin S (**Fig. 3.22**). When aggregated it forms twisted fibrils of 4–8 nm thickness with a periodicity of 30–40 nm. Other silver-type stains such as the Von Braunmuhl method on frozen sections (**Figs 3.23** and **3.24**) or the modified Bielschowsky and methenamine silver techniques on paraffin sections (**Figs 3.25** and **3.26**) also detect these 'amyloid plaques'. The latter three staining methods, as well as immunohistochemical procedures using antibodies raised against the β/A4 protein, show that cerebral cortical amyloid plaques have a wide variety of morphological appearances. Some have a well-defined compacted core with a peripheral 'halo' of staining (**Figs 3.23**, **3.25** and **3.27**)whereas in others the β/A4 protein is distributed in a more even granular manner throughout the plaque (**Figs 3.24**, **3.26** and **3.28**); the latter have been termed 'diffuse' plaques.

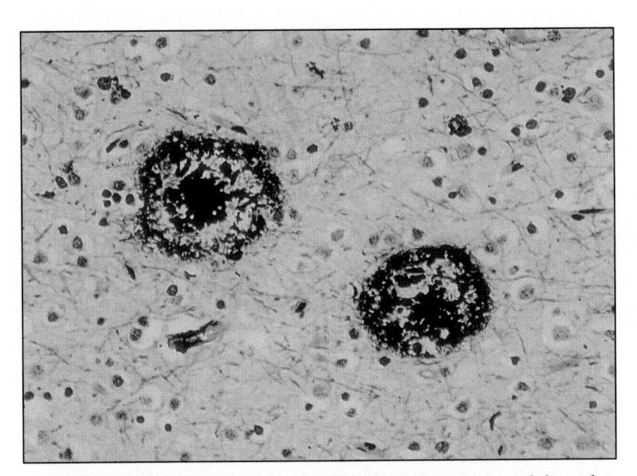

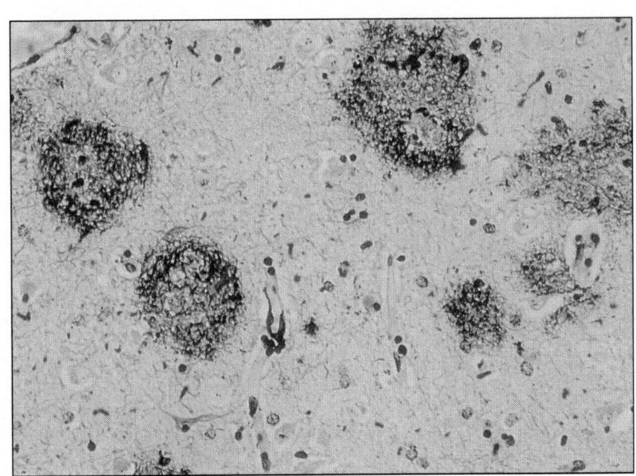

Figs 3.25 and 3.26 Amyloid plaques stained by the methenamine silver method. *(× 200.)*

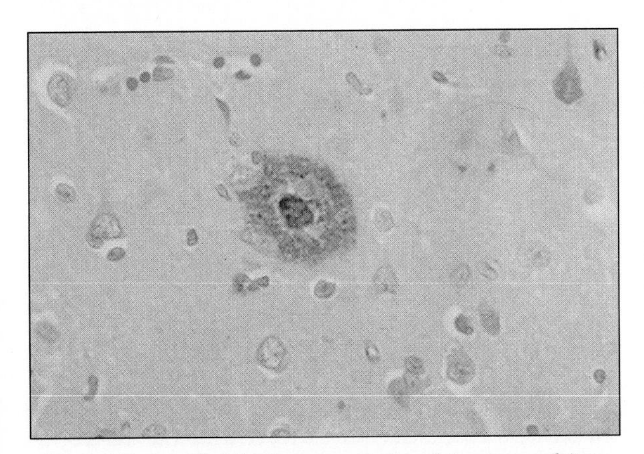

Fig. 3.27 Amyloid plaques stained immunohistochemically using an antibody to β/A4 protein showing a well-defined core with a halo. *(Anti-β/A4 × 400.)*

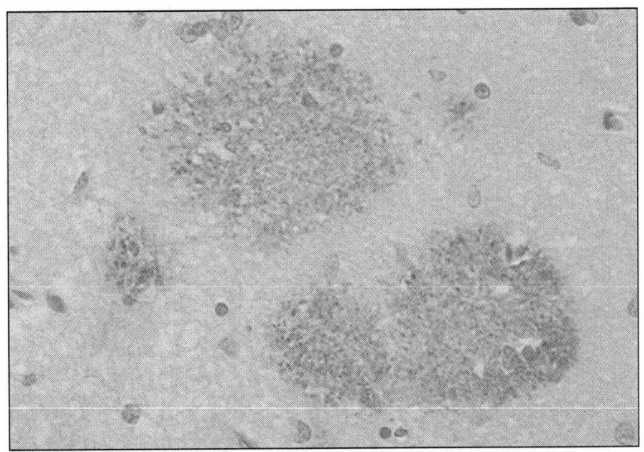

Fig. 3.28 Amyloid plaques stained immunohistochemically using an antibody to β/A4 protein showing the amyloid protein deposited more diffusely. *(Anti-β/A4 × 400.)*

Other plaques produce intermediate forms (**Fig. 3.29**). Often the plaques merge into large conglomerates enveloping neurones and other tissue elements (**Fig. 3.30**). Subpial deposits of amyloid protein are also present (**Fig. 3.31**). These diffuse kinds of plaques are not demonstrated, or at least only poorly demonstrated, using thioflavin S or Congo red, presumably because the β/A4 peptide in such plaques, although filamentous, is either not, or is only minimally, stacked into the β-pleated fibrillar form necessary for dye-binding. Moreover, such plaques do not stain with the usual silver methods for neuritic changes and neurofibrillary tangles (i.e. Palmgren, Bodian and unmodified Bielschowsky) due to the absence of PHF within nerve processes in the plaque region, although they can contain many tau-positive structures (see **Figs 3.19** and **3.21**).

The presence of large quantities of aluminium and silicon in plaque cores has been emphasised by some studies (**Fig. 3.32**). However, not all workers have been able to confirm this statement.

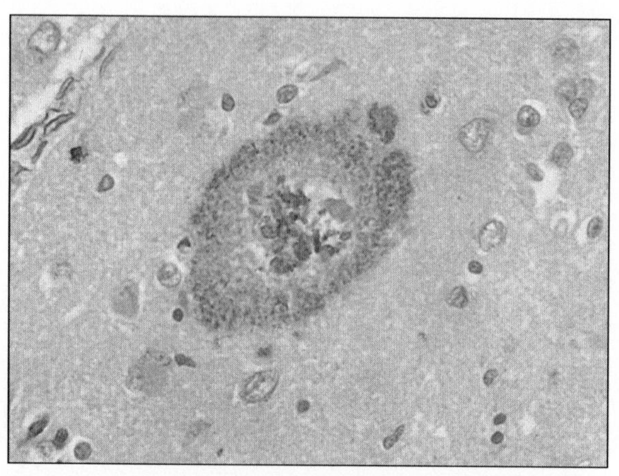

Fig. 3.29 Amyloid plaques stained immunohistochemically using an antibody to β/A4 protein showing an intermediate form. *(Anti-β/A4 ×400.)*

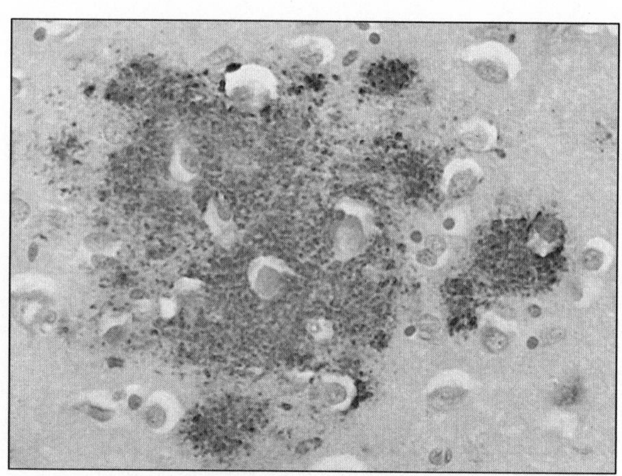

Fig. 3.30 Amyloid plaques stained immunohistochemically using an antibody to β/A4 protein showing a conglomerate form. *(Anti-β/A4 ×400.)*

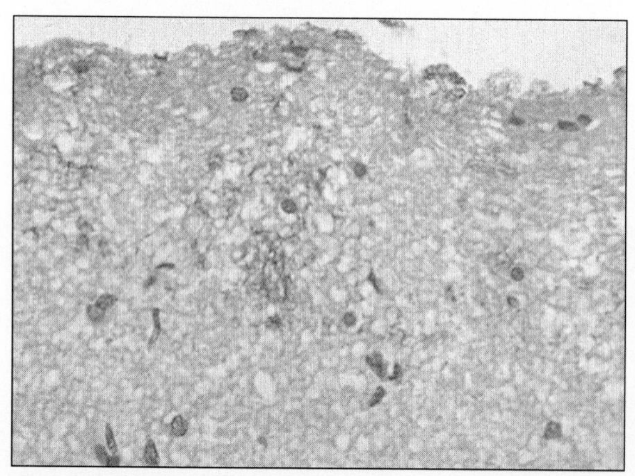

Fig. 3.31 Subpial deposits of β/A4 protein. *(Anti-β/A4 ×400.)*

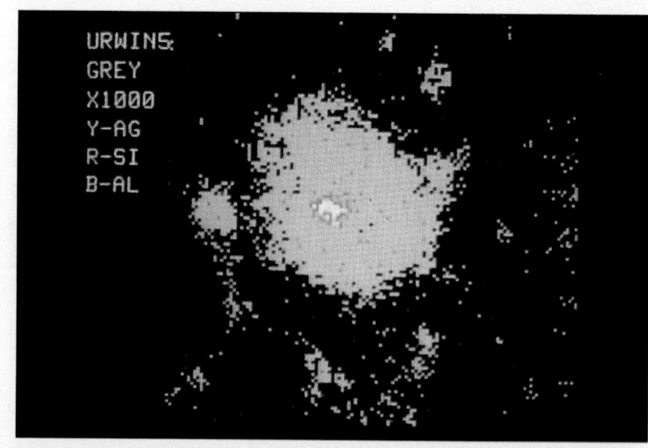

Fig. 3.32 'Digimap' showing localisation of silicon (red) and aluminium (blue) in a silver-stained (yellow) plaque of the cerebral cortex. Co-localisation of silicon and aluminium appears as white. (Courtesy of Prof. J. Edwardson.)

Lectin histochemistry reveals a large amount of carbohydrate in the form of oligosaccharides in plaques (**Figs 3.33** and **3.34**), especially in the cored type. This is both intracellular and extracellular and in part may represent accumulated amyloid precursor protein (see **Fig. 3.159**). Heparan sulphate proteoglycan is also strongly associated with the amyloid deposits (**Figs 3.35** and **3.36**), as are other molecules such as amyloid P component and Apolipoprotein E (**Figs 3.37** and **3.38**).

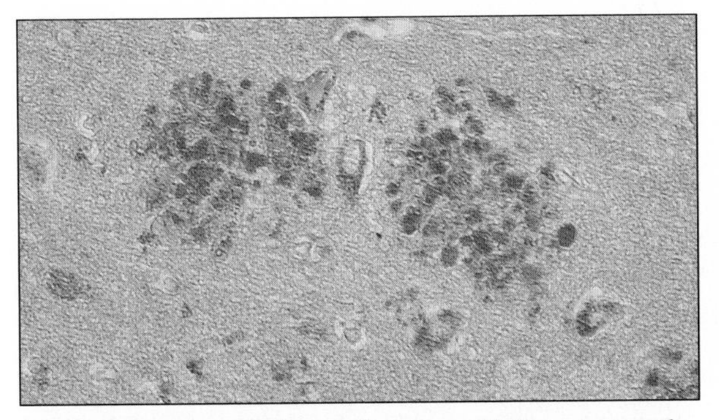

Fig. 3.33 Intracellular and extracellular accumulations of glycoconjugates in diffuse amyloid plaques of the temporal cortex. Demonstrated using lectin histochemistry with the marker lectin concanavalin A. *(× 400.)*

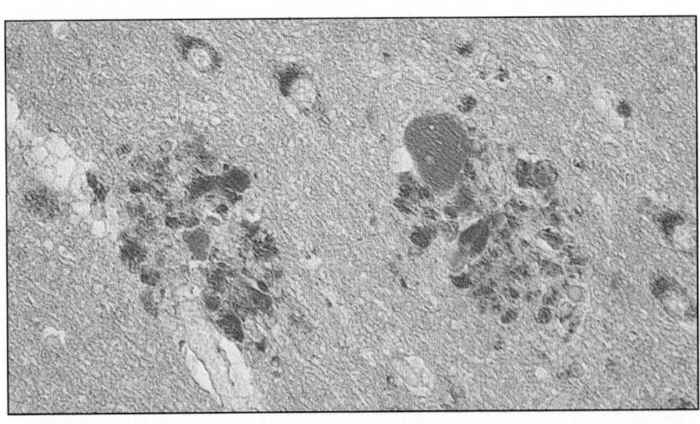

Fig. 3.34 As for 3.33, but within cored, neuritic plaques in the CA1 region of the hippocampus. *(× 400.)*

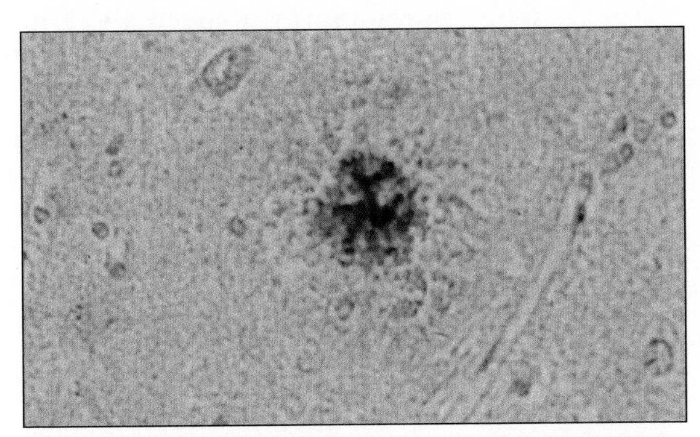

Fig. 3.35 Heparan sulphate proteoglycan within a cored amyloid plaque. *(Sulphated Alcian blue × 400.) (Courtesy of Dr A. Snow)*

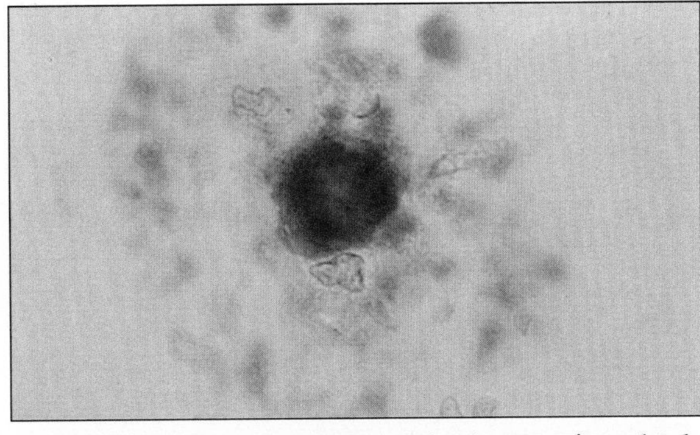

Fig. 3.36 As for 3.35 using antibody HK-249, which recognises heparan sulphate proteoglycan. *(Anti-heparan sulphate proteoglycan.) (Courtesy of Dr A. Snow.)*

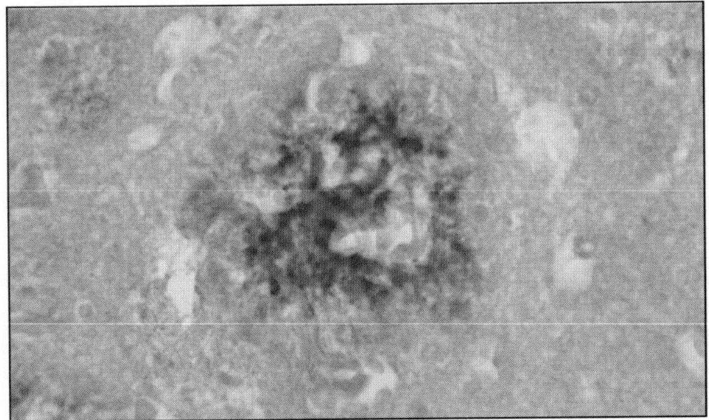

Fig. 3.37 Apolipoprotein E immunoreactivity within a cored plaque. *(Anti-apolipoprotein E × 400.)*

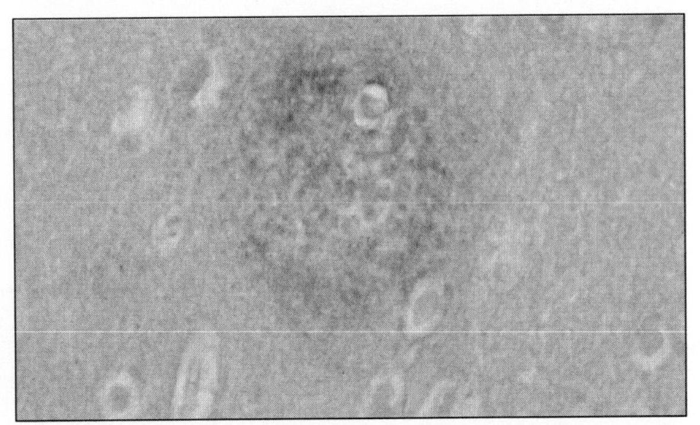

Fig. 3.38 Apolipoprotein E immunoreactivity within a diffuse plaque. *(Anti-apolipoprotein E × 400.)*

Non-neuronal cellular elements relating to microglial cells (**Figs 3.39** and **3.40**) and astrocytes (**Figs 3.41** and **3.42**) are also well represented in cored plaques, though both these cell types are less common or even absent in diffuse plaques (see page 62). Sometimes, the amyloid deposits adopt a 'stellate' appearance, reminiscent of the kuru-type of plaque seen in Creutzfeldt–Jakob disease (see page 152), particularly in the end-folium region of the hippocampus (**Figs 3.41–3.44**), in the cortical nuclei of the amygdala, or in the cerebellum (see **Figs 3.65–3.73**).

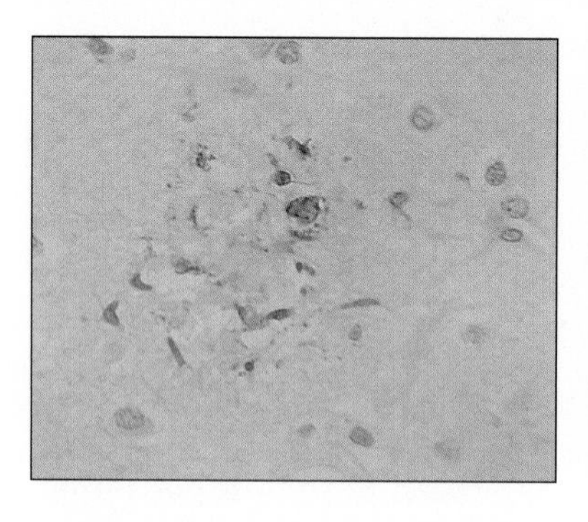

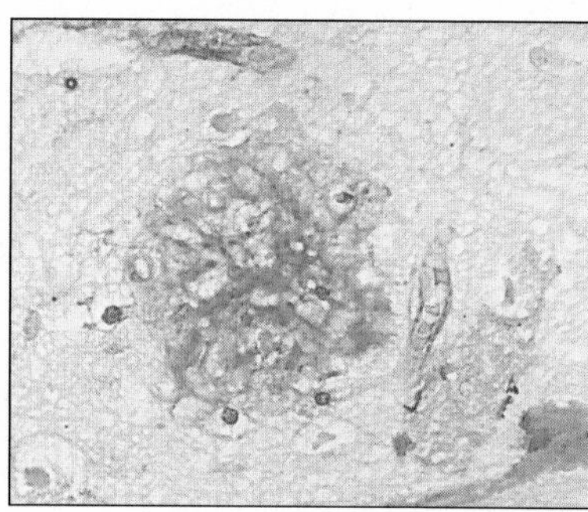

Fig. 3.39 (left) Microglial cells within an amyloid plaque, using anti-ferritin as a marker. *(× 400.)*

Fig. 3.40 (right) Double-stained section showing microglial cells (brown) within a cored amyloid plaque (red). Microglial cells are stained by lectin histochemistry using the marker lectin *Sambucus nigra*. The β/A4 is stained histochemically. *(× 400.)*

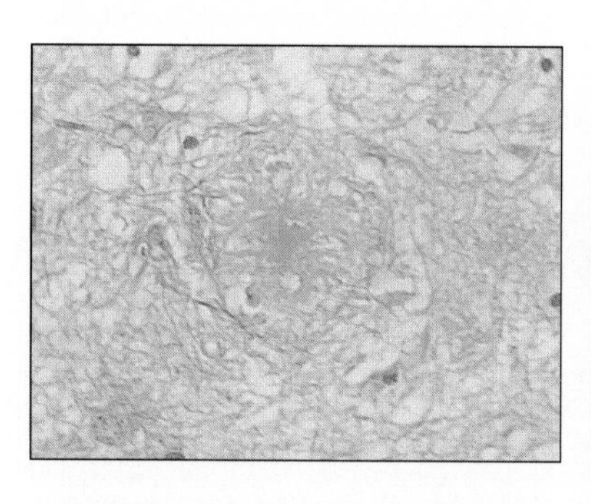

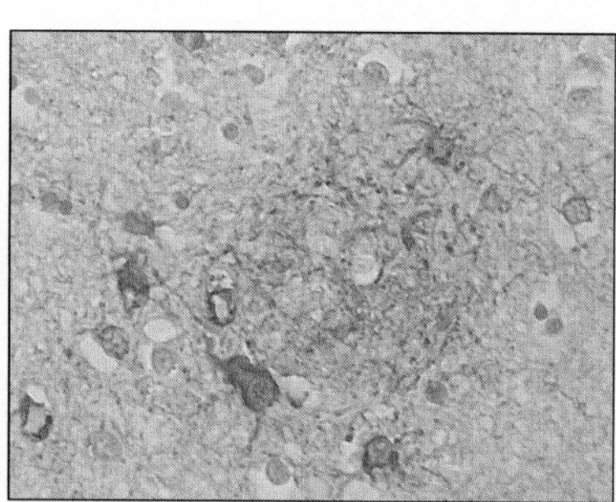

Fig. 3.41 (left) Astrocytic fibres surrounding a cored amyloid-plaque. *(Phosphotungstic acid–haematoxylin × 400.)*

Fig. 3.42 (right) Astrocyte cell bodies and processes surrounding and penetrating an amyloid plaque. *(Anti-GFAP × 400.)*

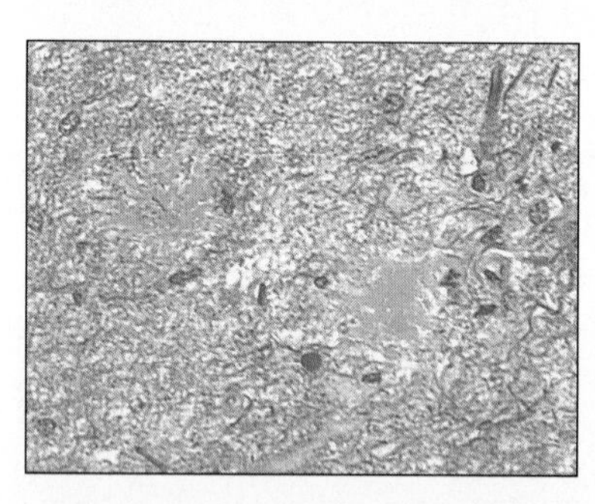

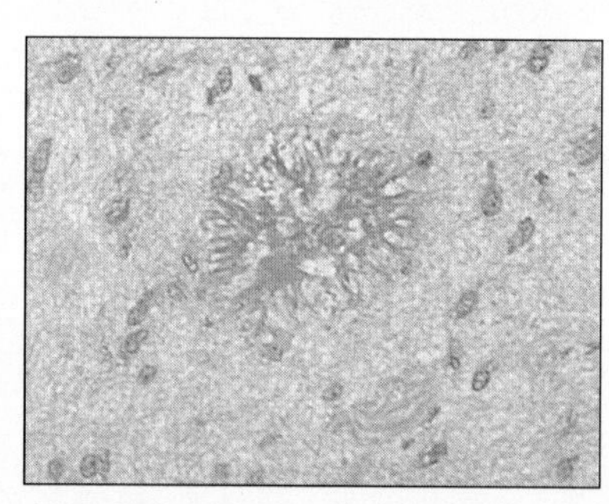

Fig. 3.43 (left) 'Stellate' type of amyloid plaque in the end-folium of the Ammon's horn region of the hippocampus in a 45-year-old man. Note the intense reactive astrocytosis. *(Phosphotungstic acid–haematoxylin × 400.)*

Fig. 3.44 (right) As in Fig. 3.43, but anti-GFAP, counterstained with periodic acid–Schiff. *(× 400.)*

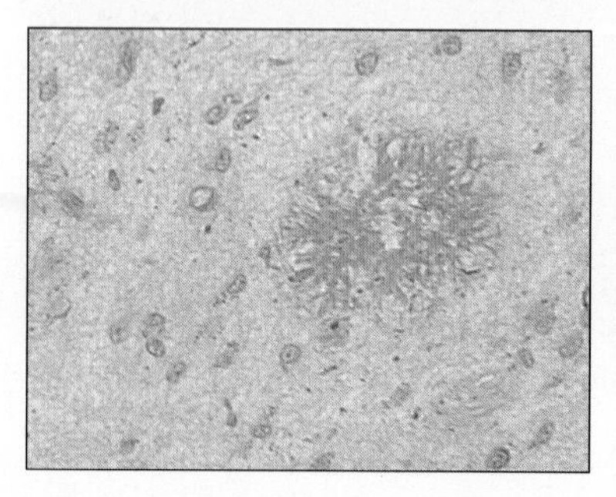

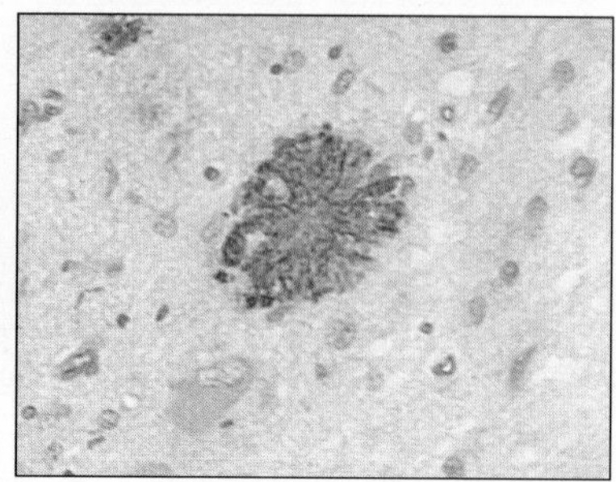

Fig. 3.45 (left) As in Fig. 3.43, but anti-tau, counterstained with periodic acid–Schiff. *(× 400.)*

Fig. 3.46 (right) As in Fig. 3.43, but anti-β/A4 staining. *(× 400.)*

To avoid confusion it is recommended that the term senile plaque is not used because it does not describe the morphology of the lesion, nor is is the lesion confined to the elderly. Plaque is used here as a generic term, and is qualified according to whether it refers mainly to extracellular (amyloid) or intracellular (neuritic) components of the lesion.

Ultrastructurally, cored or stellate amyloid plaques comprise a central mass of amyloid fibrils radiating peripherally (**Fig. 3.47**). Around this are many swollen (dystrophic) nerve processes containing PHF and dense bodies (**Fig. 3.48**). Glial processes, some containing filaments and relating to astrocytes, others with dense cytoplasm rich in organelles, and relating to microglia, are seen. In other plaques, particularly diffuse amyloid ones where there is no apparent central core (**Figs 3.49** and **3.50**), the amyloid fibres are loosely woven between the neuritic and glial elements (**Figs 3.50** and **3.51**).

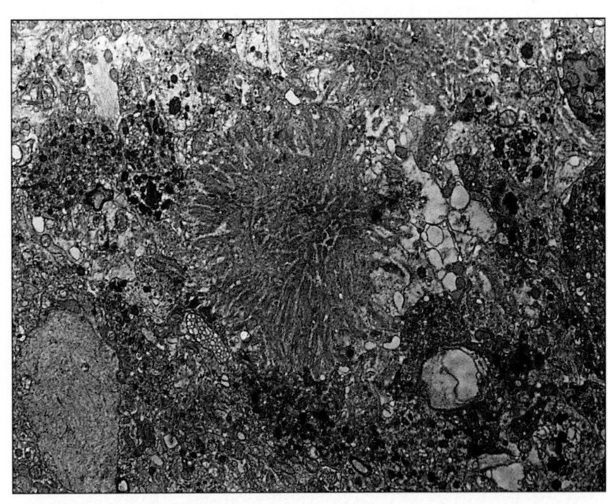

Fig. 3.47 Ultrastructure of cored plaques. This shows amyloid fibrils radiating peripherally. The amyloid is surrounded by swollen dystrophic neurites, containing electron-dense lamellar bodies derived from degenerating mitochondria, and glial cell processes. *(Circa 1000.)*

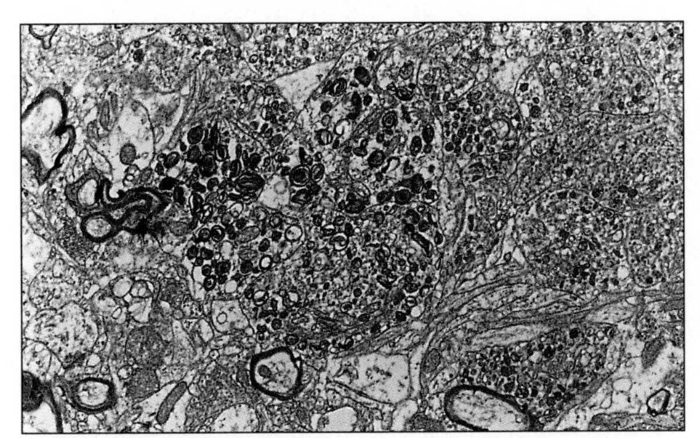

Fig. 3.48 Dystrophic neurites containing many dense bodies. *(Circa 5000.)*

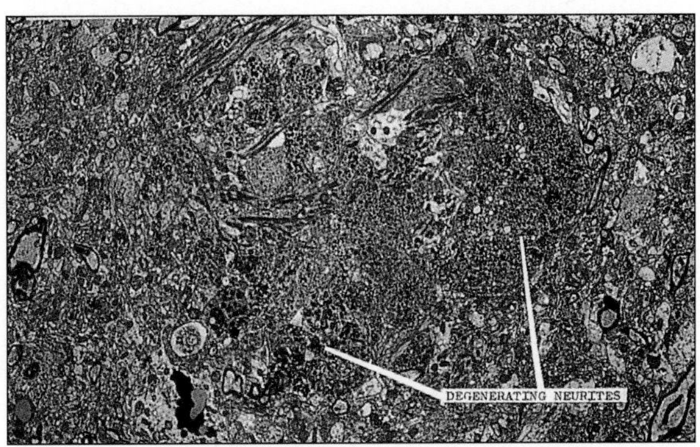

Fig. 3.49 A diffuse plaque. The amyloid fibrils are freely dispersed between the neuritic and glial structures. *(Circa 1000.)*

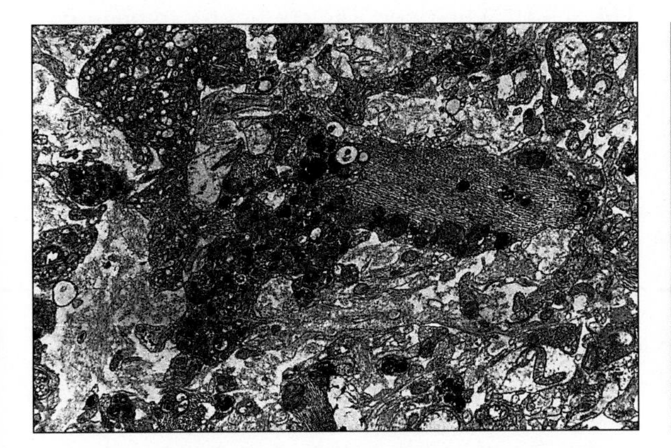

Fig. 3.50 Amyloid fibres within diffuse plaques. These are always single or bundles of filaments not arranged in the β-pleated conformation of cored plaques. *(×4500.)*

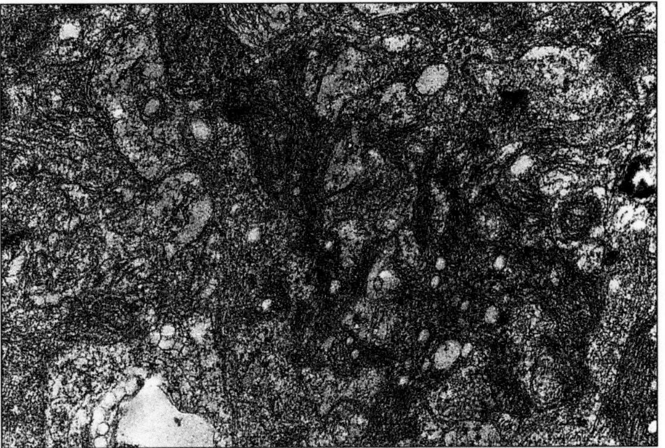

Fig. 3.51 A diffuse plaque. Amyloid fibrils are immunogold-labelled using antibody to β/A4 protein. *(×19,000.)*

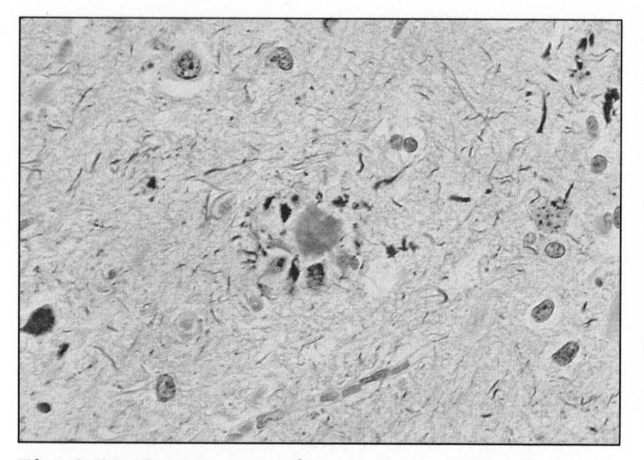
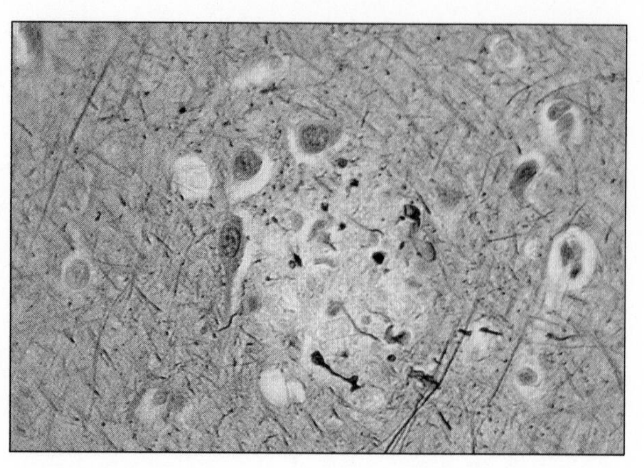

Fig. 3.52 'Burnt-out' plaques in temporal cortex (left and right). *(Palmgren silver stain × 400.)*

Evolution of plaques

It is clear, even when a single staining method is used, that plaques display a diversity of structure. It has been proposed that they undergo a series of evolutionary changes during their natural history and it has been widely suggested that diffuse plaques are the morphological 'forerunners' of neuritic plaques (page 60). It is still not clear whether each form can arise *de novo* and independently, with the former never actually progressing into the latter. The true neuritic plaque probably undergoes some evolutionary changes during which the amyloid 'coalesces' and the neuritic element diminishes, leaving a 'compact' or 'burnt-out' plaque (**Figs 3.52** and **3.53**). This comprises an amyloid mass with glial processes, but with little if any residual neuronal elements.

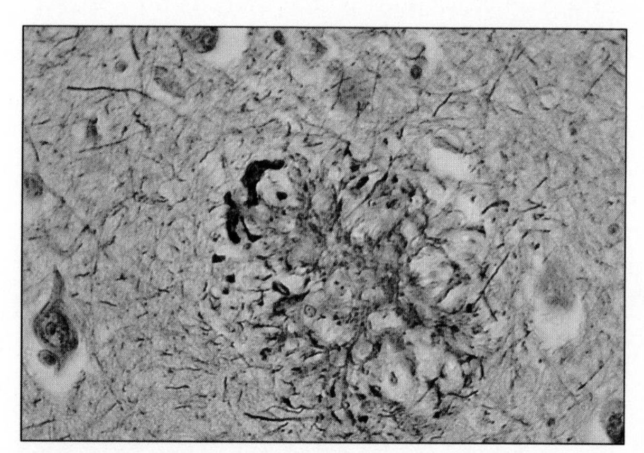

Fig. 3.53 A 'burnt-out' plaque in the amygdaloid nucleus. *(Palmgren silver stain × 400.)*

Distribution of plaques

Plaques are present throughout the cerebral cortex, and particularly in the association areas of the frontal, temporal and parietal cortex (**Figs 3.54–3.56**) and within the hippocampus (**Figs 3.59–3.61**) and amygdala. They are less common in primary sensory and motor regions of the cortex.

The plaques are not randomly distributed, but exist in laminar fashion with layers I–III often containing more than the deeper cortical layers (see **Fig. 3.54**). When deposits are not too numerous a columnar arrangement can sometimes be seen (see **Figs 3.55** and **3.56**). Higher concentrations of plaques are present in the sulcal depths rather than at the crests of the gyri. In the occipital cortex there is an apparent predilection for layer IV (see **Fig. 3.57**), and in the entorhinal cortex (see **Fig. 3.58**) deeper cortical layers (III and IV) are preferentially affected.

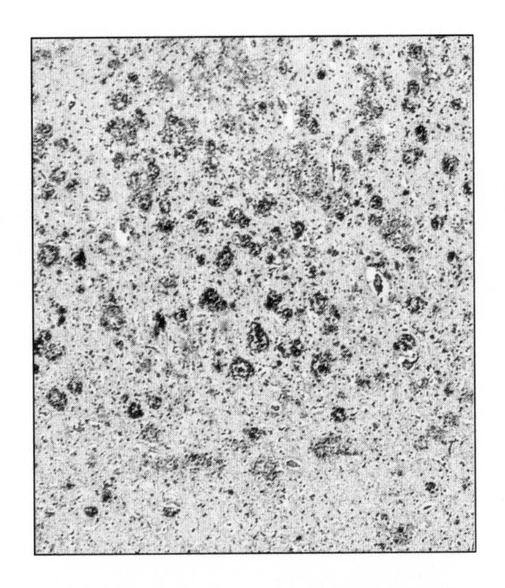

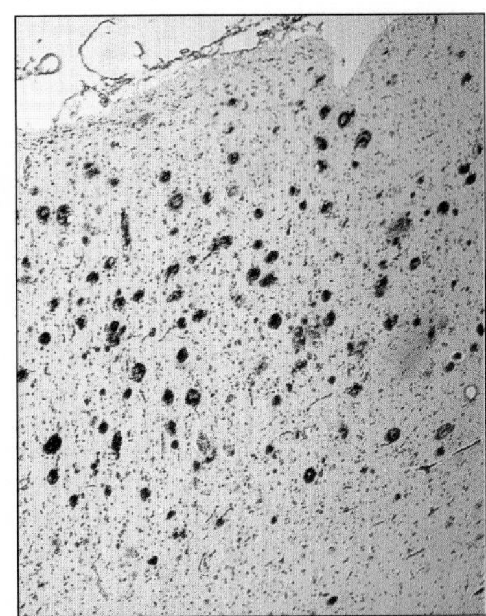

Fig. 3.54 (left) Topographic distribution of amyloid deposits in the frontal cortex. Note that more deposits are present in the outer cortical laminae than in the deeper laminae, though those in the latter are larger and contain more compacted amyloid. *(Methenamine silver stain × 40.)*

Fig. 3.55 (right) Amyloid deposits in the temporal cortex. These also exist in a columnar, as well as in a laminar, distribution, this being clearer when the overall deposition is less severe. *(Methenamine silver stain × 40.)*

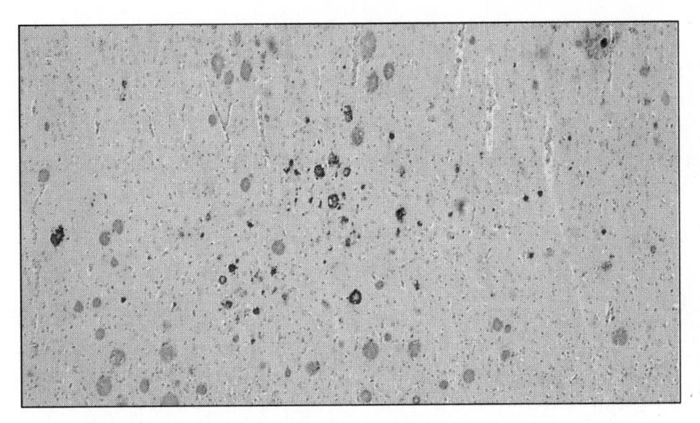

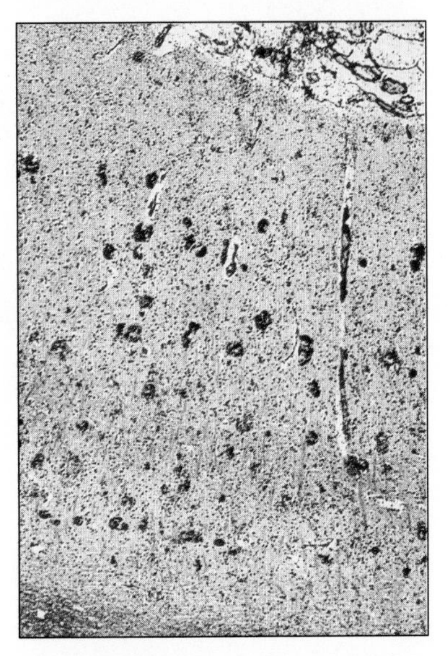

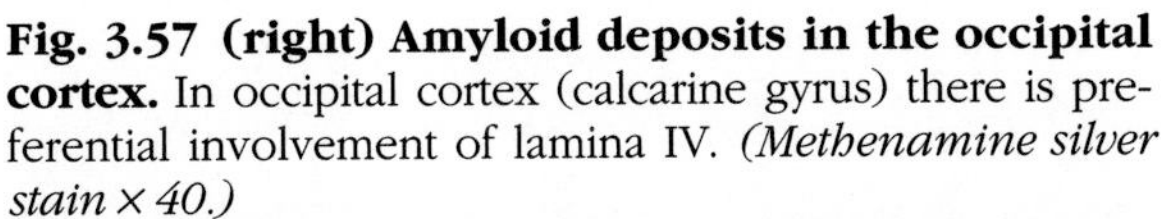

Fig. 3.56 Amyloid deposits in the temporal cortex. As **Fig. 3.55**, but anti-βA4 immunostaining. *(× 40.)*

Fig. 3.57 (right) Amyloid deposits in the occipital cortex. In occipital cortex (calcarine gyrus) there is preferential involvement of lamina IV. *(Methenamine silver stain × 40.)*

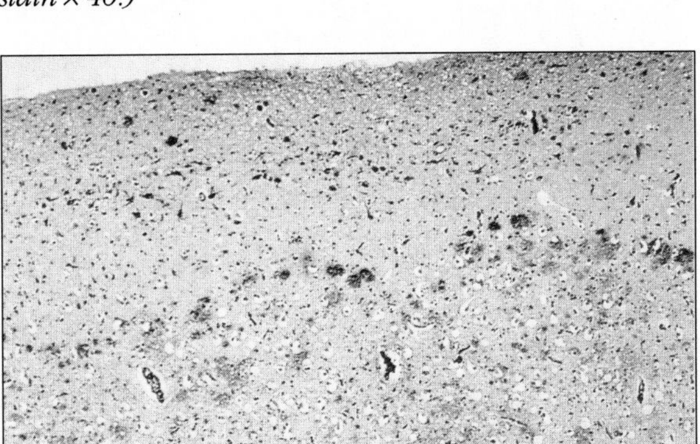

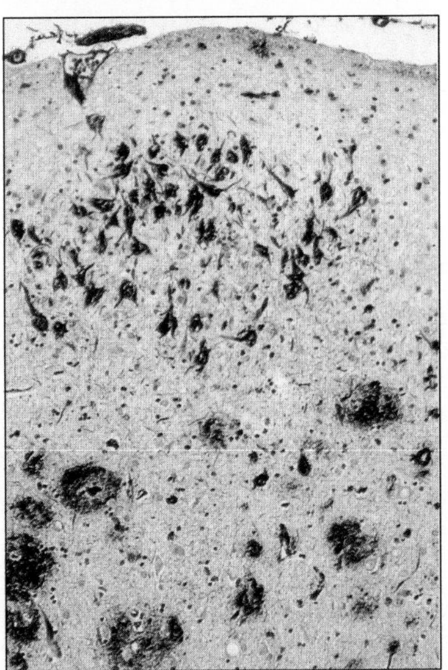

Fig. 3.58 Entorhinal cortex (above). In the entorhinal cortex amyloid deposits are present mostly in layer III. *(Methenamine silver stain × 20.):* **(right)** Note the intense neurofibrillary degeneration involving the stellate neurones of layer II. *(Methenamine silver stain × 40.)*

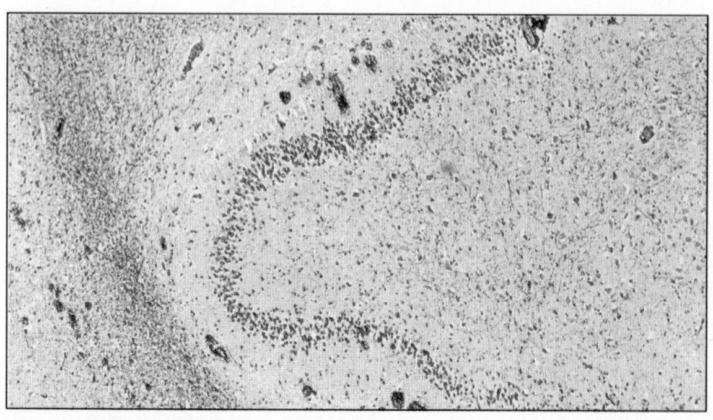

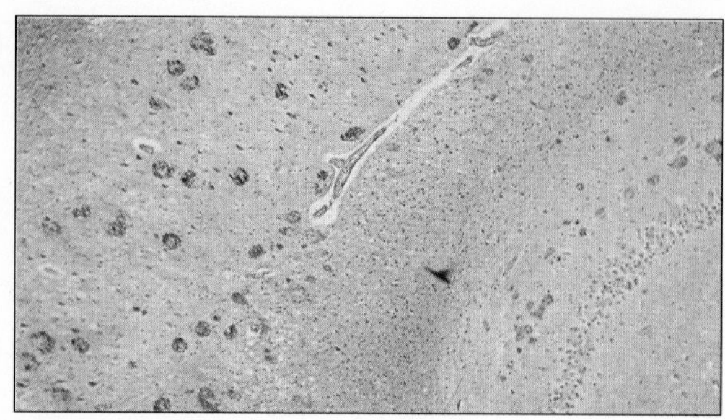

Figs 3.59 and 3.60 Amyloid deposits in the hippocampus. Amyloid deposits are seen preferentially around the dentate gyrus (**Fig. 3.59**) and in areas CA1 and the subiculum (**Fig. 3.60**). *(Methenamine silver stain × 40.)*

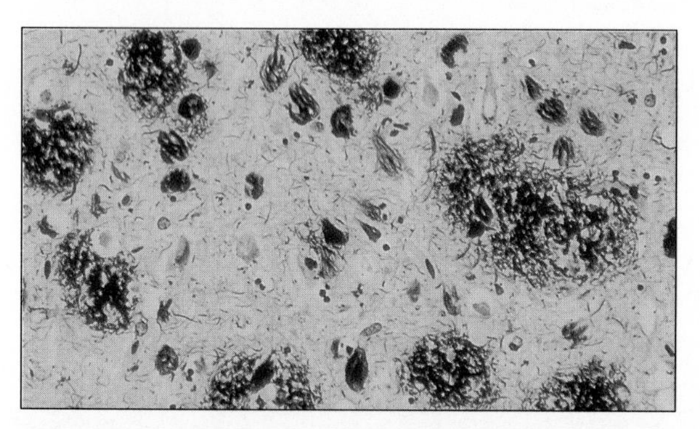

Fig. 3.61 Amyloid deposits in the hippocampus. Many amyloid plaques and neurofibrillary tangles in the subiculum of the hippocampus. *(Methenamine silver stain × 100.)*

In the hippocampus, the molecular layer of the dentate gyrus (see **Fig. 3.59**) and areas CA1 and subiculum (**Figs 3.60** and **3.61**) are favoured, while in the amygdala cortical and medial nuclei are affected more than basal and lateral regions.

The cerebellum does not contain neuritic plaques, but a diffuse form of amyloid deposit is widely present in the molecular layer of the cerebellar cortex (**Figs 3.62–3.64**) of many patients. Here, the amyloid occurs usually as finely dispersed, radially arranged, masses that closely parallel the dendritic tree of a Purkinje cell (see **Figs 3.62** and **3.63**), though on other occasions 'flat sheets' of deposit are aligned along the folium

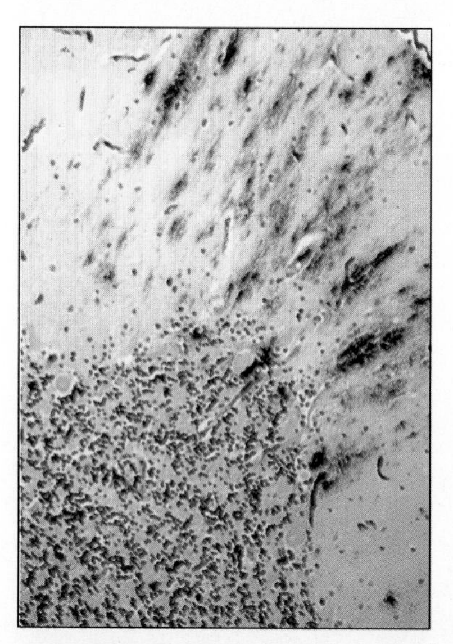

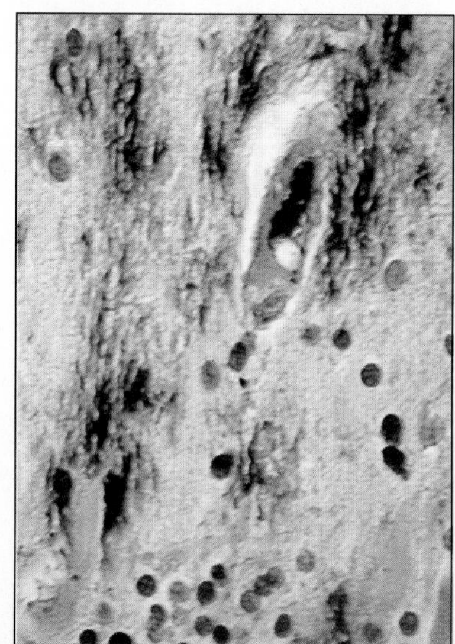

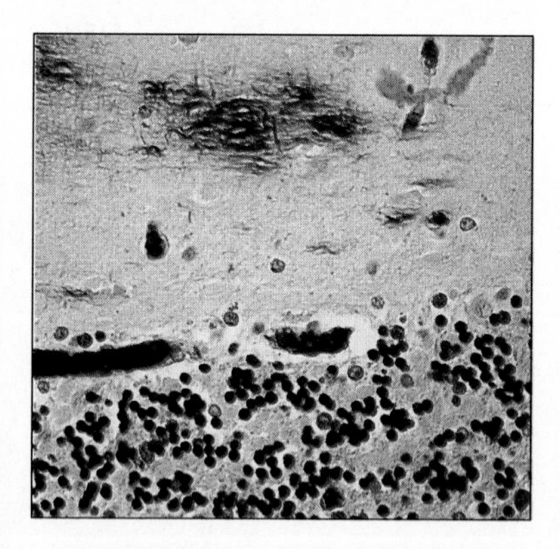

Figs 3.62–3.64 Diffuse amyloid deposits in the molecular layer of the cerebellum. These deposits either radiate perpendicularly to the pial surface (**Figs 3.62** (left) and **3.63** (middle)) or track linearly (**Fig. 3.64** (right)) along the molecular layer. *(Methenamine silver stain × 100.)*

(see **Fig. 3.64**). Sometimes, other large, coarse and irregular or more stellate deposits occur within the Purkinje cell and granule cell layers (**Figs 3.65–3.70**) or in the molecular layer (**Figs 3.71–3.73**), some existing as subpial deposits (**Fig. 3.74**).

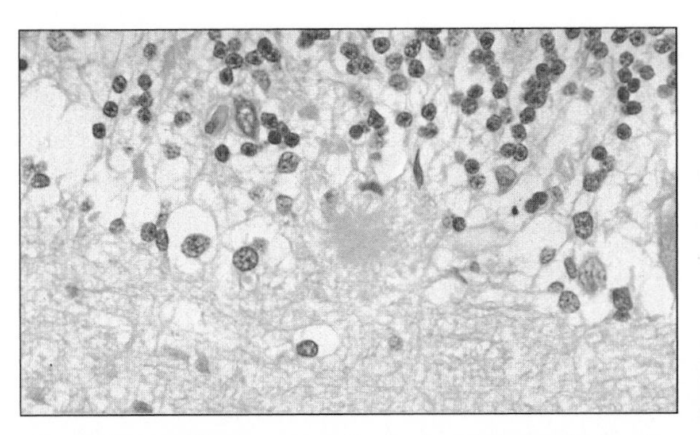

Fig. 3.65 Stellate type of amyloid deposit in the Purkinje cell layer of the cerebellum. *(Haematoxylin–eosin × 400.)*

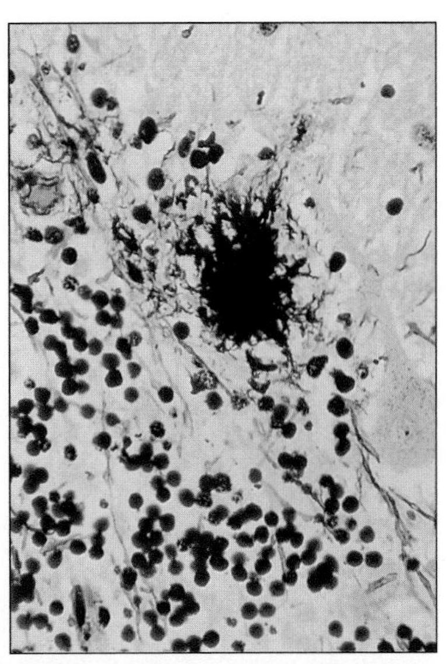

Fig. 3.66 (right) Stellate type of amyloid deposit in the Purkinje cell layer of the cerebellum. As **Fig. 3.65**, but methenamine silver stain. *(× 400.)*

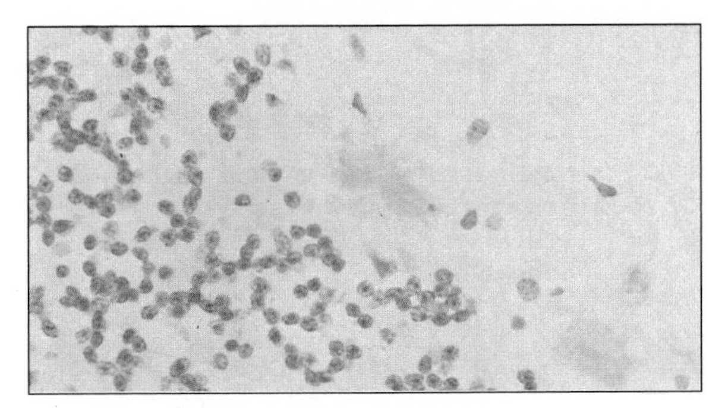

Fig. 3.67 Stellate type of amyloid deposit in the Purkinje cell layer of the cerebellum. As **Fig. 3.65**, but Congo red stain. *(× 400.)*

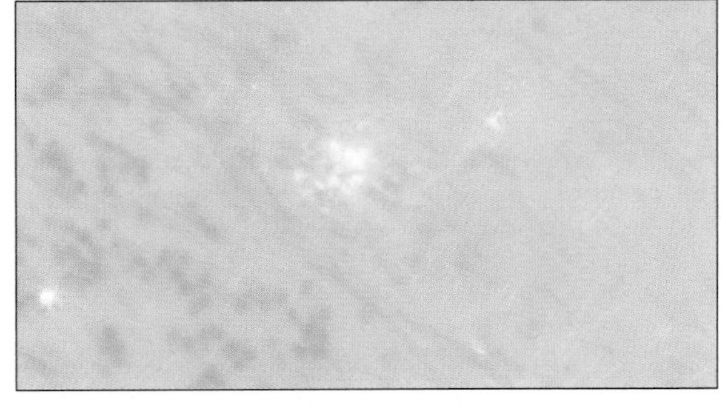

Fig. 3.68 Stellate type of amyloid deposit in the Purkinje cell layer of the cerebellum. As **Fig. 3.67**, but Congo red staining viewed through cross-polarised light. The amyloid deposit displays characteristic yellow-green birefringence. *(× 400.)*

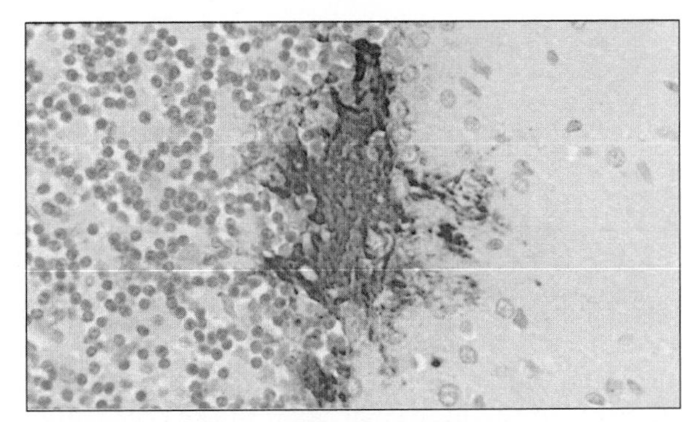

Fig. 3.69 Stellate type of amyloid deposit in the Purkinje cell layer of the cerebellum. As **Fig. 3.65**, but anti-β/A4 immunostaining. *(× 400.)*

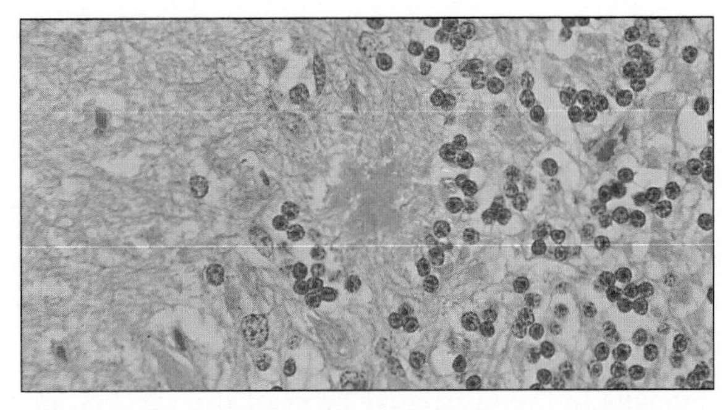

Fig. 3.70 An amyloid plaque in the Purkinje cell layer shows only little surrounding astrocytic reaction. *(Phosphotungstic acid–haematoxylin × 400.)*

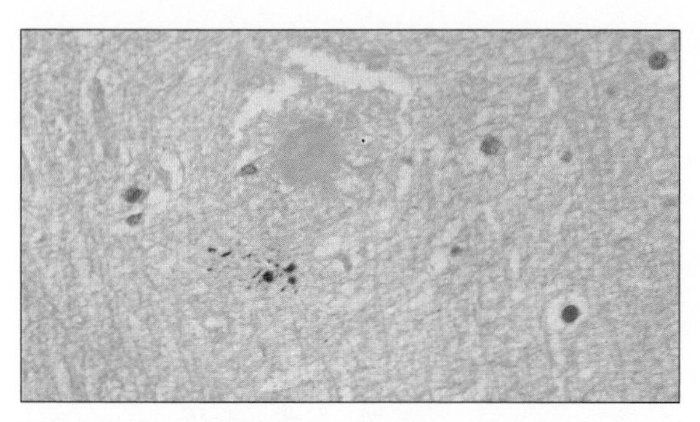

Fig. 3.71 Amyloid plaque in the molecular layer of the cerebellum. *(Haematoxylin–eosin × 400.)*

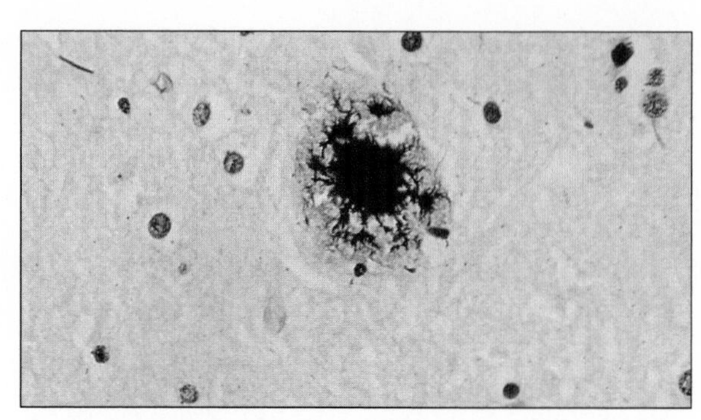

Fig. 3.72 Amyloid plaque in the molecular layer of the cerebellum. As **Fig. 3.71**, but methenamine silver stain. *(× 400.)*

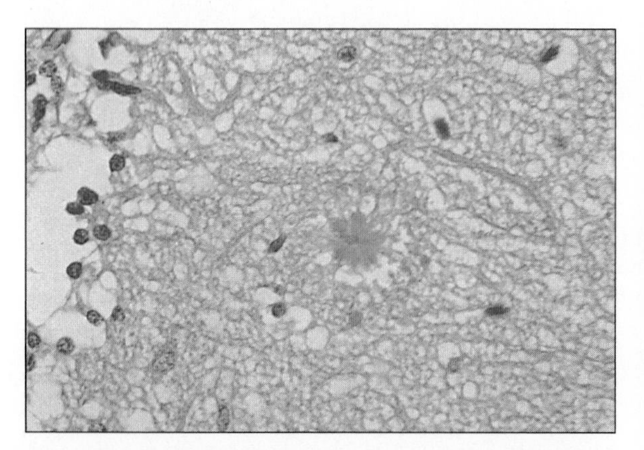

Fig. 3.73 Amyloid plaques in the molecular layer of the cerebellum. As **Fig. 3.71**, but phosphotungstic acid–haematoxylin. *(× 400.)*

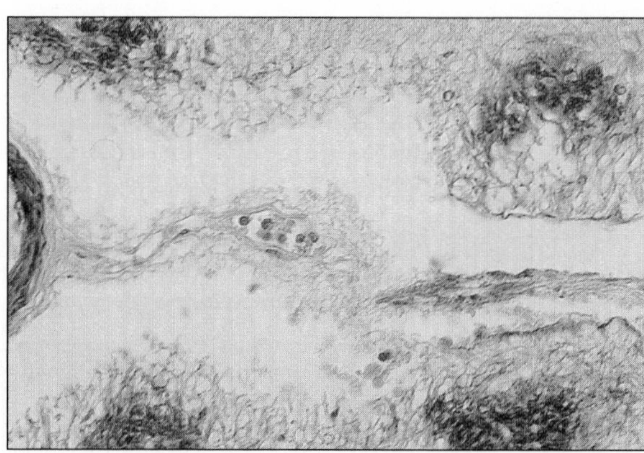

Fig. 3.74 Subpial deposits of amyloid protein in the cerebellar cortex. Note also the deposition of amyloid in the wall of a leptomeningeal artery. *(Anti-β/A4 immunostaining × 400.)*

Although cerebellar amyloid deposits are never associated with PHF-containing nerve terminals, and tangles are not seen in Purkinje or other cell perikarya, granular ubiquitinated deposits within nerve endings are widely present within parenchymal (**Fig. 3.75**) and subpial (**Fig. 3.76**) deposits.

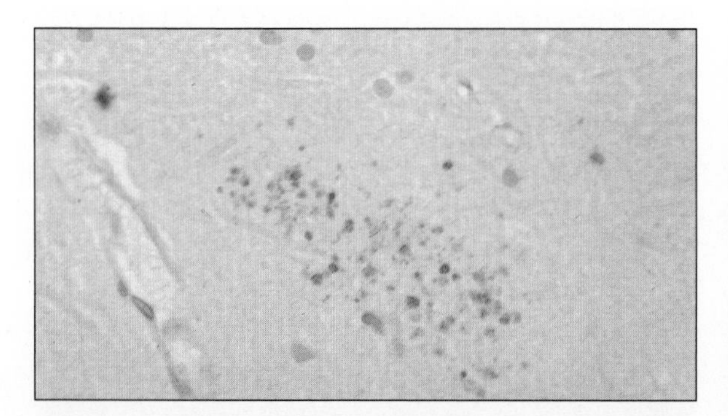

Fig. 3.75 Ubiquitinated material within amyloid deposits in the molecular layer of the cerebellum. Note these have a granular, rather than a filamentous, appearance. *(Anti-ubiquitin × 400.)*

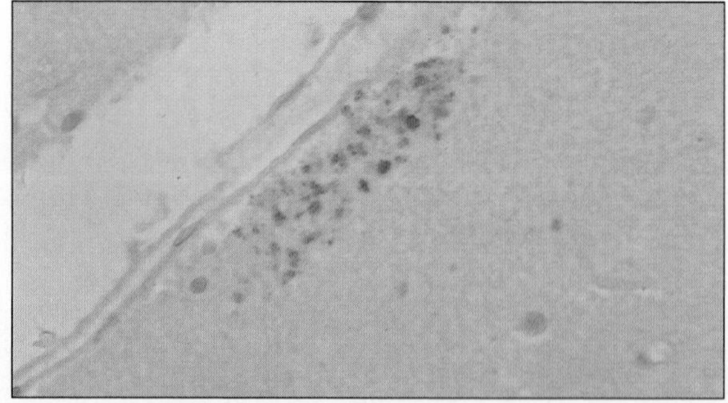

Fig. 3.76 Ubiquitinated material within amyloid deposits in the molecular layer of the cerebellum. As **Fig. 3.75**, but appearing within a subpial amyloid deposit. *(Anti-ubiquitin × 400.)*

Astrocytes are not usually (or are only minimally) present in or around these deposits (see **Fig. 3.70**, and **Fig. 3.73**) and there is merely a mild microglial involvement (**Fig. 3.77**). In contrast to amyloid plaques in the cerebral cortex, these cerebellar deposits do not contain excessive amounts of oligosaccharide or heparan sulphate proteoglycan.

The striatum and thalamus often contain amyloid plaques similar to the diffuse deposits in the cerebellum.

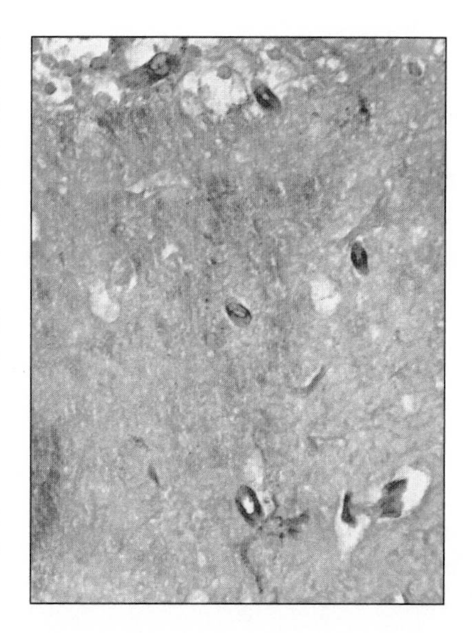

Fig. 3.77 Sparse microglial cell activity (brown) within amyloid deposits (red) in the molecular layer of the cerebellum. *(Double stain with anti-β/A4 immunostaining (red) and lectin histochemistry using Sambucus nigra as marker lectin (brown) × 400.)*

Neurofibrillary tangles

Appearance and distribution

Neurofibrillary tangles are bands of an abnormal filamentous material, which is formed and accumulated within the perikaryon of nerve cells and often extends into the dendrites and axon. As with plaques, tangles can be demonstrated with routine histological stains such as haematoxylin–eosin or phosphotungstic acid–haematoxylin, but this is not usually easy (see **Figs 3.104–3.107** later). They are, however, readily impregnated in paraffin sections by silver staining methods, such as Bodian, Bielschowsky and Palmgren (**Fig. 3.78**) techniques, or in frozen sections by the Von Braunmuhl method (**Fig. 3.79**).

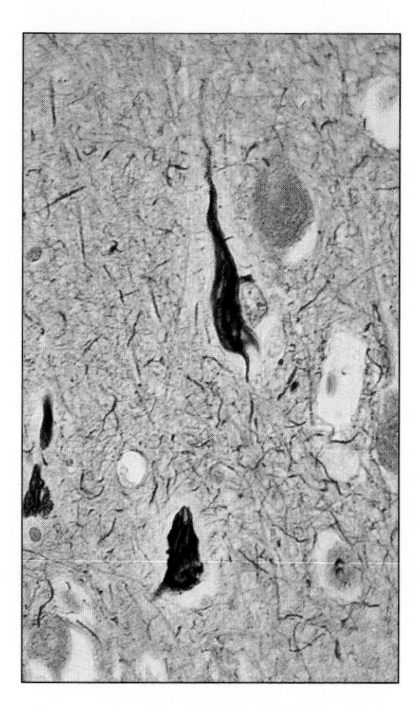

Fig. 3.78 'Flame-shaped' neurofibrillary tangle in a pyramidal cell of the temporal cortex. Note that the cytoplasm is packed with filamentous material, which also exists within the apical dendrite and proximal axon. 'Threads' of material, widely dispersed throughout the neuropil, are probably contained within dendrites and are continuous with tangle material within nearby affected cells. *(Palmgren silver stain × 400.)*

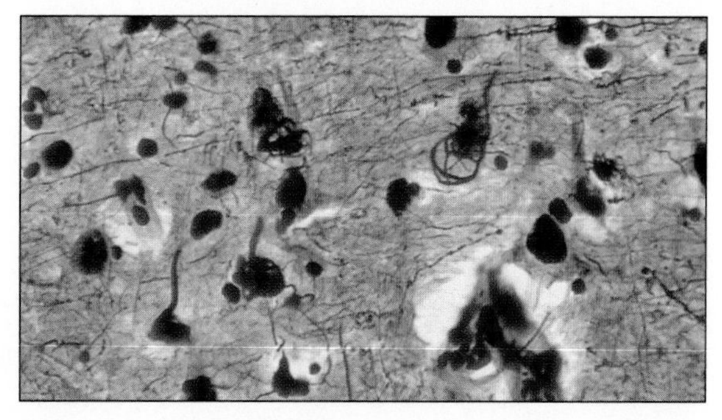

Fig. 3.79 Neurofibrillary tangles in the temporal cortex. *(Von Braunmuhl silver stain × 400.)*

When present in pyramidal cells of the cerebral cortex or hippocampus, tangles adopt a characteristic flame shape (see **Figs 3.78** and **3.79**), though in other brain regions, such as the amygdala, nucleus basalis of Meynert (**Fig. 3.80**), locus caeruleus, substantia nigra, and dorsal raphe (**Fig. 3.81**), a 'looser', more globose type of tangle is seen. Tangles are common within the granule cells of the dentate gyrus of the hippocampus and here assume a crescent or globular shape on silver staining (**Fig. 3.82**).

Tangles occur in most patients, though in variable numbers, in hypothalamic, striatal and thalamic (see **Fig. 3.90**) neurones, but rarely or never in cells of the pontine, olivary or dentate nuclei, and the cerebellar cortex, or in anterior horn cells or ganglion cells of the sympathetic or parasympathetic nuclei. They are, however, usually present in neurones of the olfactory nuclei and tracts (**Fig. 3.83**).

Tangle material occurs within the proximal dendrites and axonal processes of affected nerve cells

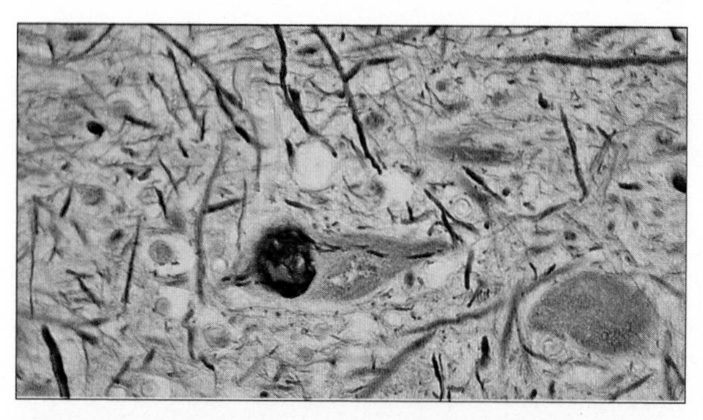

Fig. 3.80 Globose form of neurofibrillary tangle in the nucleus basalis of Meynert. *(Palmgren silver stain × 400.)*

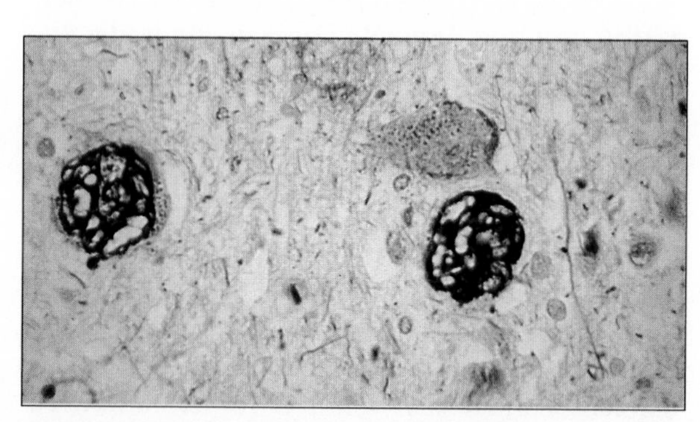

Fig. 3.81 As Fig. 3.80, but in the nucleus dorsalis raphe. *(Palmgren silver stain × 400.)*

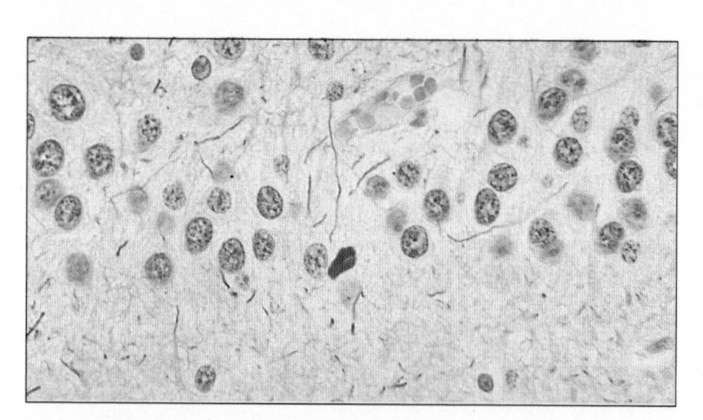

Fig. 3.82 Small tangle in a granule cell of the dentate gyrus of the hippocampus. *(Palmgren silver stain × 400.)*

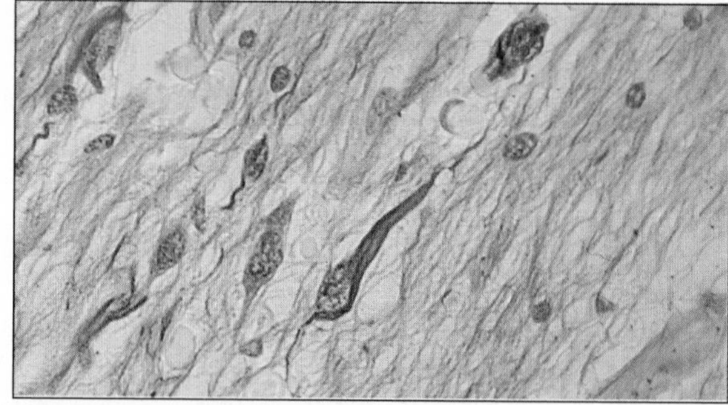

Fig. 3.83 Tangle in a nerve cell of the olfactory tract. *(Palmgren silver stain × 400.)*

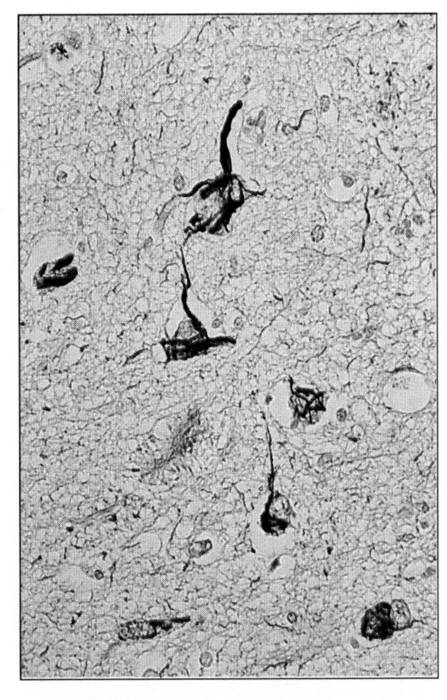

Fig. 3.84 Tangles in neurones of layer II of the entorhinal cortex. Note also the many neuropil threads. *(Palmgren silver stain × 400.)*

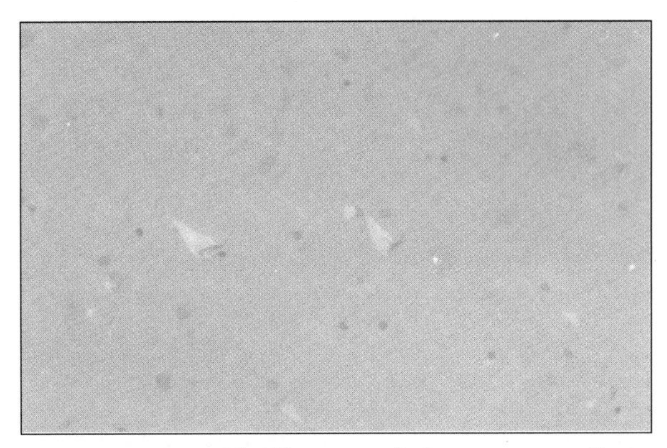

Fig. 3.85 Neurofibrillary tangle in a nerve cells in the entorhinal cortex. This displays characteristic green-yellow birefringence after Congo red staining and viewing through cross-polarised light. *(× 400.)*

(see **Fig. 3.78**) and also, more distally, as 'neuropil threads' (see **Figs 3.78** and **3.84**). Because the protein within tangle-bearing cells is present in a β-pleated configuration, like plaque cores, such perikaryal material can be detected using the dyes, Congo red (**Fig. 3.85**) and thioflavin S.

Structure of neurofibrillary tangles

Irrespective of site or morphological appearance, tangles adopt the same basic fine anatomical structure comprising of bundles of fibrils, each fibril being made from a pair of helically wound filaments (**Fig. 3.86**) with a periodicity of about 160 nm. The term 'paired helical filaments' (PHF) is used to describe such a structure. The filaments are thought to be 'stacked' from 'C-shaped' subunits, each domain within this subunit relating to part of the particular molecule from which it is derived.The tangle seems to consist of a dense 'central core' with a surrounding 'fuzzy coat'.

PHFs within tangles and neuropil threads are comprised of several molecular entities (**Fig. 3.87**).

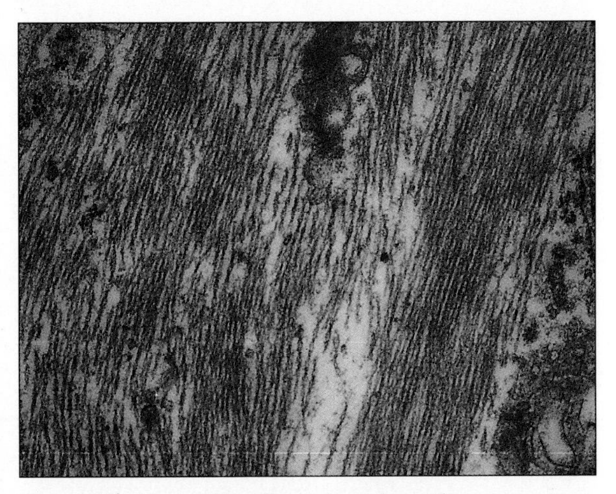

Fig. 3.86 Neurofibrillary tangles. These are comprised of bundles of parallel aligned paired helical filaments. *(Circa , 50,000.)*

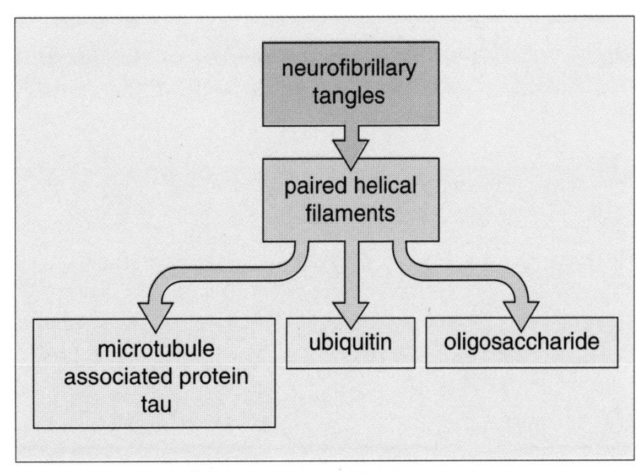

Fig. 3.87 Molecular structure of neurofibrillary tangles.

They have been shown by immunohistochemistry at both light (**Figs 3.88–3.91**) and electron microscopic (**Fig. 3.92**) levels, and by direct protein chemical analysis, to comprise (largely) of the microtubule-associated protein, tau along with a further protein, ubiquitin (**Figs 3.93** and **3.94**). Ubiquitin is a small (76 amino-acid) protein that is used by cells as an intracellular marker labelling effete or damaged proteins for proteolysis. Variable amounts of the proteoglycan HSPG and other oligosaccharides (**Fig. 3.96**), amyloid P component and Apolipoprotein E (**Fig. 3.95**) are also present.

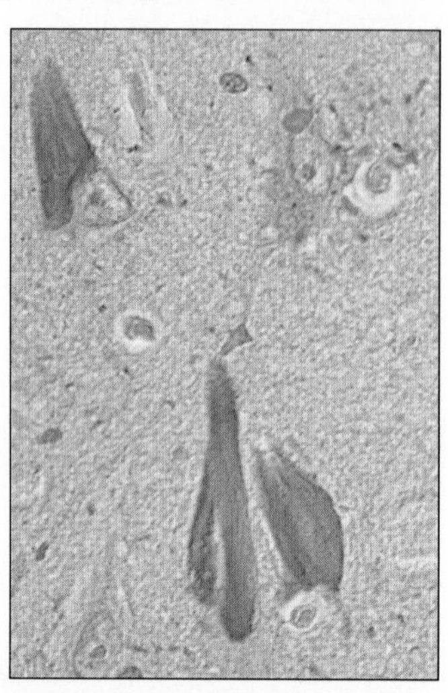

Fig. 3.88 Neurofibrillary tangle in a pyramidal cell of area CA1 of the hippocampus containing tau protein. Note that neuropil threads also contain tau. *(Anti-tau × 400.)*

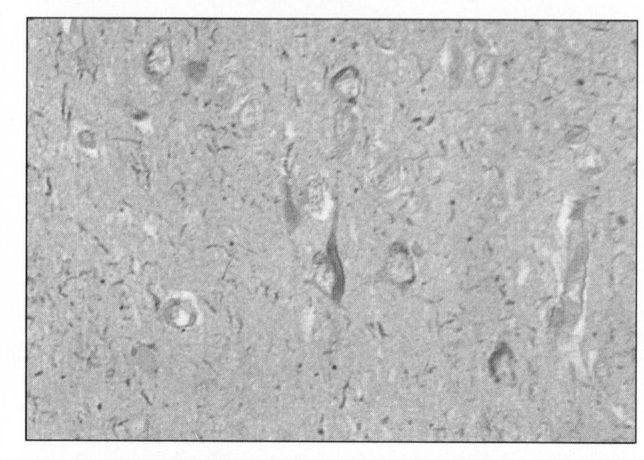

Fig. 3.89 As Fig. 3.88, but pyramidal cells of layer III of the temporal cortex. *(Anti-tau counterstained with periodic acid–Schiff × 200.)*

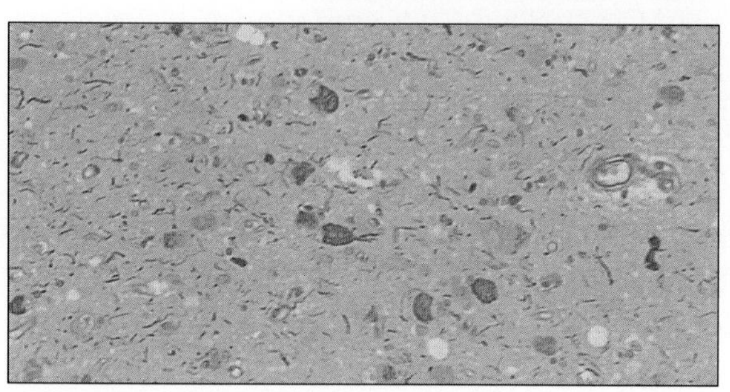

Fig. 3.90 As Fig. 3.89, but neurones of the medial thalamus. *(Anti-tau counterstained with periodic acid–Schiff × 100.)*

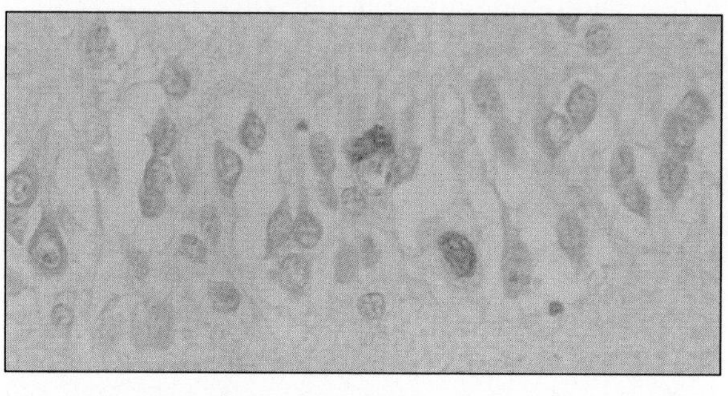

Fig. 3.91 Tangles in granule cells of the dentate gyrus of the hippocampus contain tau proteins. *(Anti-tau × 400.)*

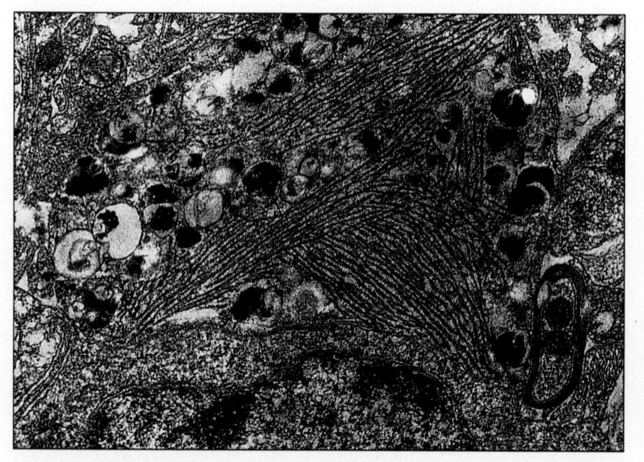

Fig. 3.92 PHFs of neurofibrillary tangles. These are gold-labelled following anti-tau immunostaining. *(× 15,000.)*

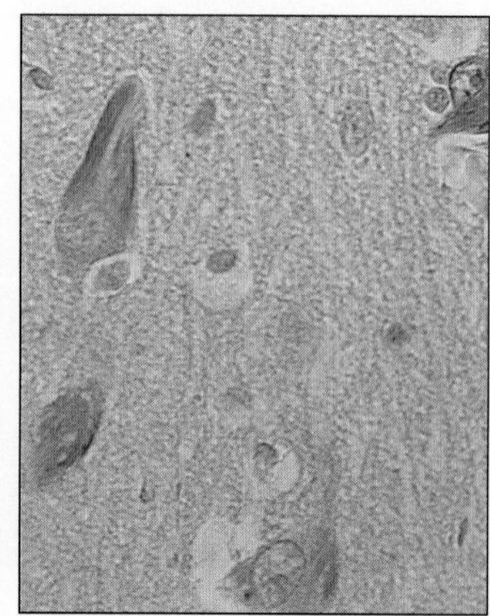

Fig. 3.93 Neurofibrillary tangles of pyramidal cells of area CA1 of the hippocampus. These contain ubiquitin. *(Anti- ubiquitin × 400.)*

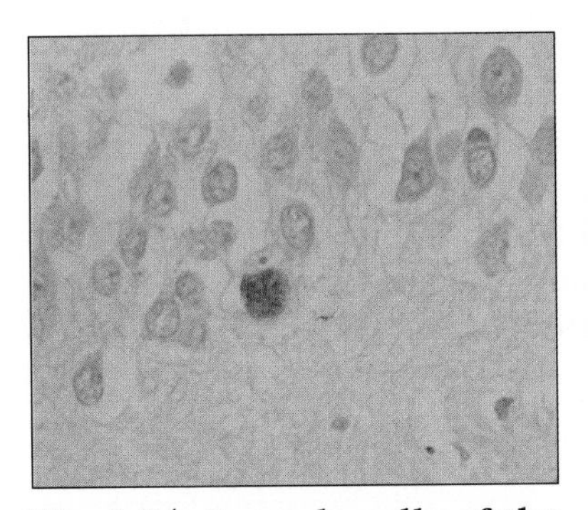

Fig. 3.94 Granule cells of the dentate gyrus of the hippocampus. These contain ubiquitinated tangles. *(Anti-ubiquitin × 400.)*

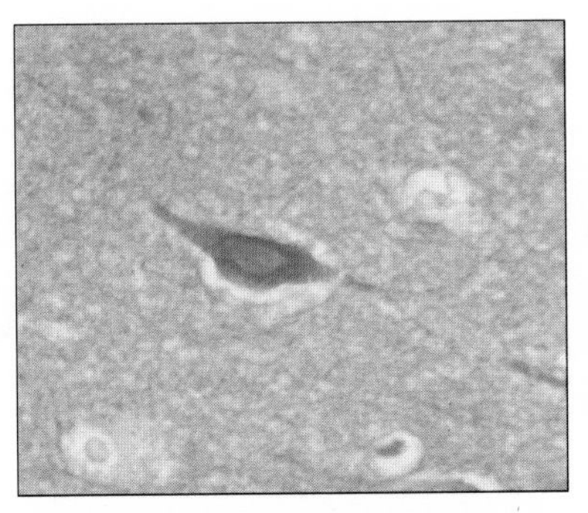

Fig. 3.95 Apolipoprotein E immunoreactivity within a neurofibrillary tangle-containing nerve cell. *(Anti-apolipoprotein E × 400.)*

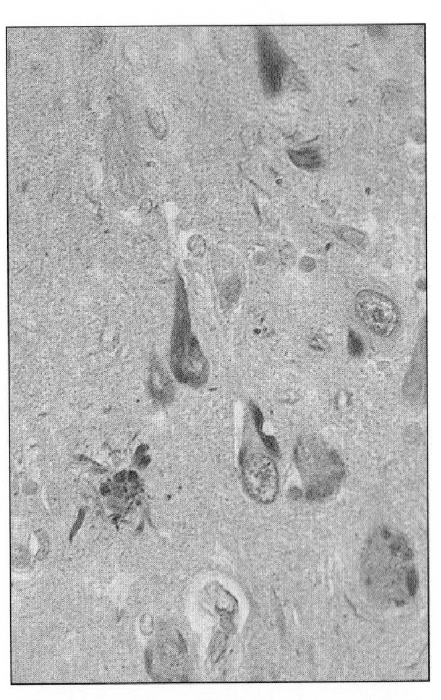

Fig. 3.96 Neurofibrillary tangles of pyramidal cells of the hippocampus. These contain oligosaccharides. *(Lectin (Arachis hypogea) histochemistry × 400.)*

The tau protein present in PHF is abnormally phosphorylated and this property may alter its tertiary structure in such a way that it can become 'stacked' into PHF. The whole of the tau molecule is incorporated into PHF by insertion of the microtubule-binding domain, which is present towards the carboxy terminus of the molecule. This gives tangles an extremely stable structure, and makes them easily extractable from brain tissue; antibodies produced against extracted PHF readily stain tangles by immunohistochemistry (**Fig. 3.97**). Moreover, neurones can be stained for tau protein even before PHF are detectable by silver staining (**Fig. 3.98**). Those molecules other than tau insert in tangles may be located in the outer 'fuzzy coat' being loosely attached to the abnormal tau, which comprises the 'central core'.

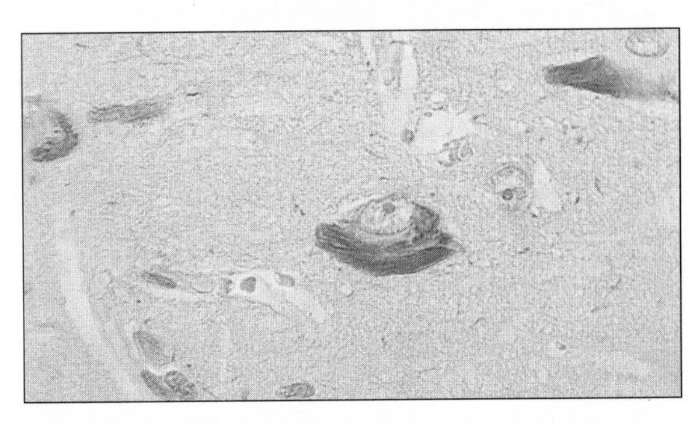

Fig. 3.97 Neurofibrillary tangles in the hippocampus. These are stained by an antibody produced following immunisation of an animal with purified paired helical filament protein. *(Anti-PHF × 400.)*

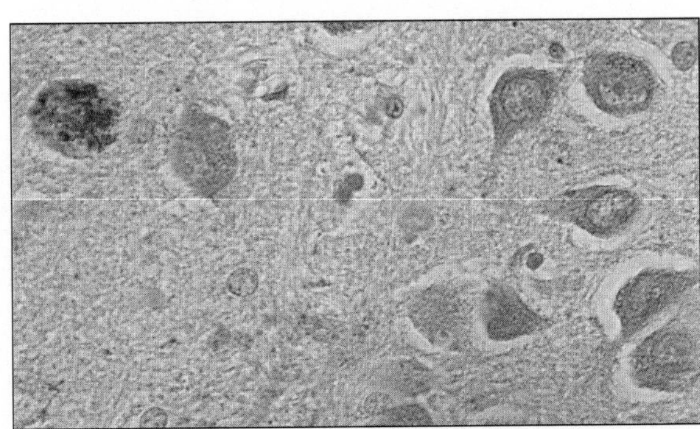

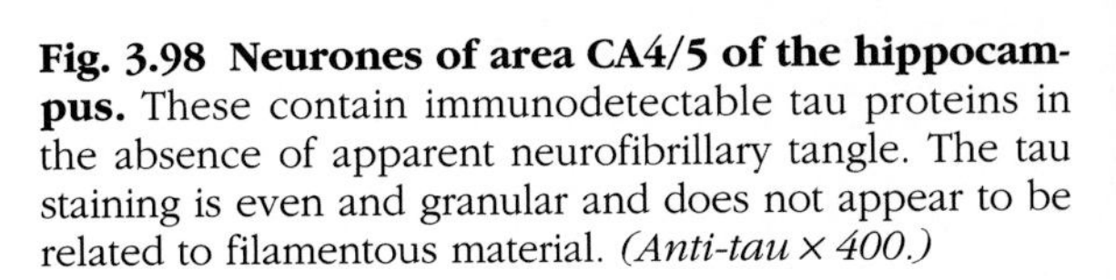

Fig. 3.98 Neurones of area CA4/5 of the hippocampus. These contain immunodetectable tau proteins in the absence of apparent neurofibrillary tangle. The tau staining is even and granular and does not appear to be related to filamentous material. *(Anti-tau × 400.)*

Effects of tangle accumulation

An excessive accumulation of PHF within the neuronal perikaryon and processes is undoubtedly detrimental to nerve cell function. As the amount of intracellular tangle increases the amount of 'useful' cytoplasm within the cell decreases (**Fig. 3.99**). With this there is a parallel loss of protein synthesis capacity (**Fig. 3.100**) and oxidative reserve. A 'mechanical' rather than a direct toxic metabolic effect is probably responsible. An interruption of intracellular transport mechanisms, due to disruption or dissolution of the cell's microtubular network, will also contribute towards its demise.

Following cell death and breakdown of the external cell membrane there is a limited proteolysis, probably by microglial cells, in which the tau (**Figs 3.101** and **3.102**) and ubiquitin (**Fig. 3.103**) epitopes are lost. These extracellular tangles then

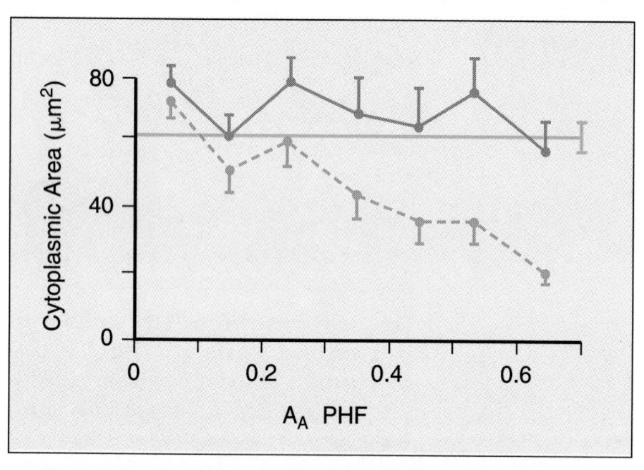

Fig. 3.99 The effects of accumulation of PHF on the amount of neuronal cytoplasm. Overall, the area of cytoplasm does not change as the proportion of cell occupied by PHF (A_A PHF) increases (solid line), remaining close to that in non-PHF containing cells (continuous line). However, as the proportion of cell occupied by PHF increases the amount of useful cytoplasm (i.e. total cytoplasmic area minus area occupied by PHF) falls (dotted line), so that in heavily tangled cells more than 75% of cytoplasm is occupied by 'useless' tangle material.

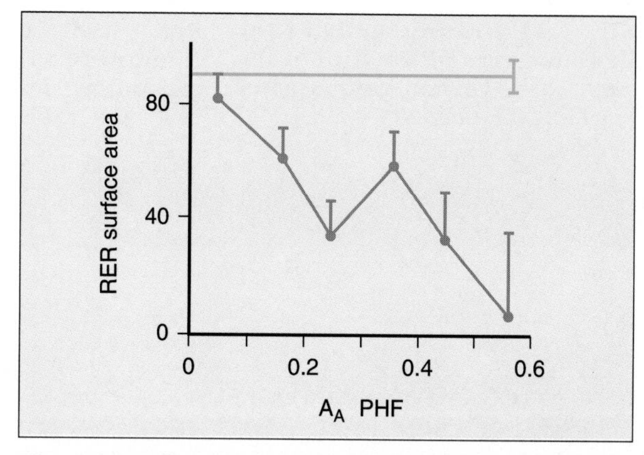

Fig. 3.100 The effects of accumulation of PHF on the amount of rough endoplasmic reticulum. Similarly, the surface area of rough endoplasmic reticulum decreases in proportion to the amount of cytoplasm occupied by PHF, so that in heavily tangled cells less than 50% of the original quantity of rough endoplasm reticulum remains. The continuous line represents the value for rough endoplasmic reticulum in non-tangled cells.

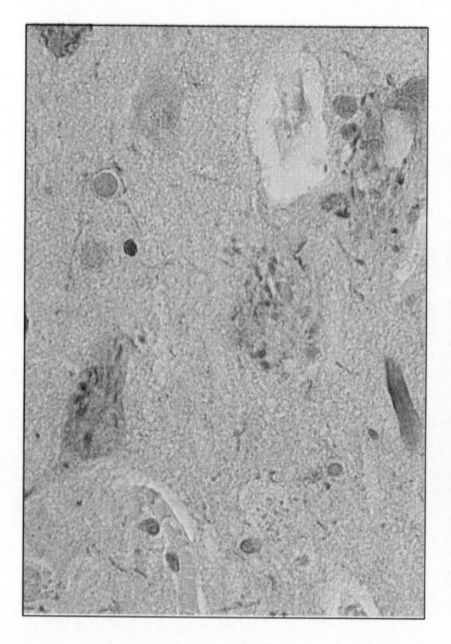

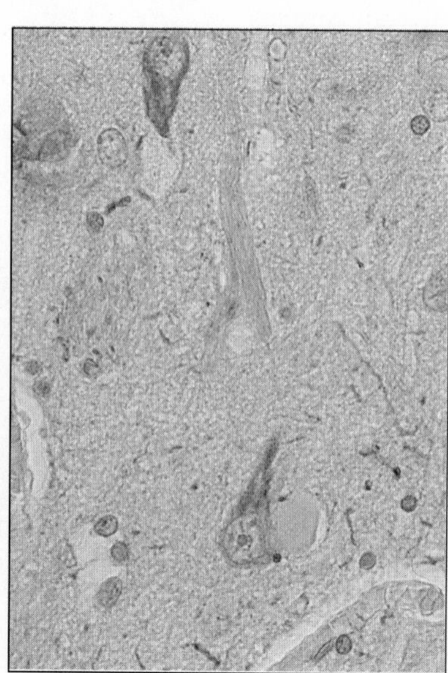

Fig. 3.101 (left) Extracellular neurofibrillary tangles containing less immunoreactive tau protein. The protein is patchy in distribution. *(Anti-tau × 400.)*

Fig. 3.102 (right) Some extracellular tangles show no tau immunoreactivity. *(Anti-tau × 400.)*

become weakly stainable with haematoxylin–eosin (**Figs 3.104** and **3.105**). They also become stainable with phosphotungstic acid–haematoxylin (**Figs 3.106** and **3.107**) and with antibodies against glial fibrillary acidic protein because they are infiltrated by the processes of reactive astrocytes. Despite the partial degradation, the 'skeleton' of the PHF remains detectable as a 'ghost tangle' by both silver

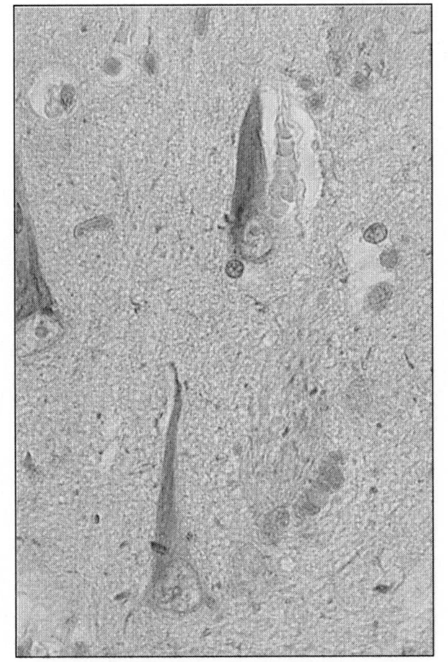

Fig. 3.103 Extracellular tangles lose ubiquitin immunoreactivity. *(Anti-ubiquitin × 400.)*

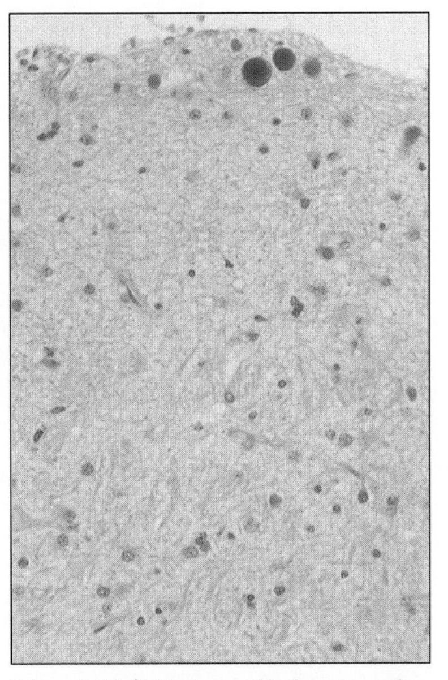

Fig. 3.104 Extracellular tangles in the entorhinal cortex. These become eosinophilic due to astrocytic infiltration. *(Haematoxylin–eosin × 100.)*

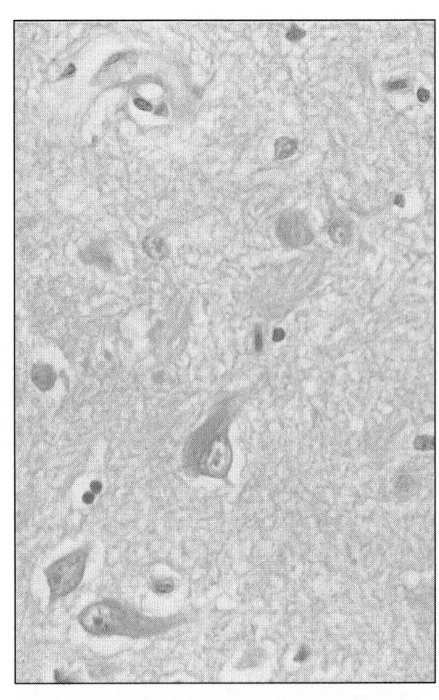

Fig. 3.105 As Fig. 3.104, but in area CA1 of the hippocampus. *(Haematoxylin–eosin × 400.)*

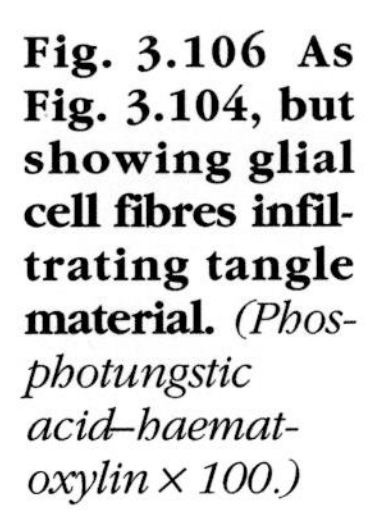

Fig. 3.106 As Fig. 3.104, but showing glial cell fibres infiltrating tangle material. *(Phosphotungstic acid–haematoxylin × 100.)*

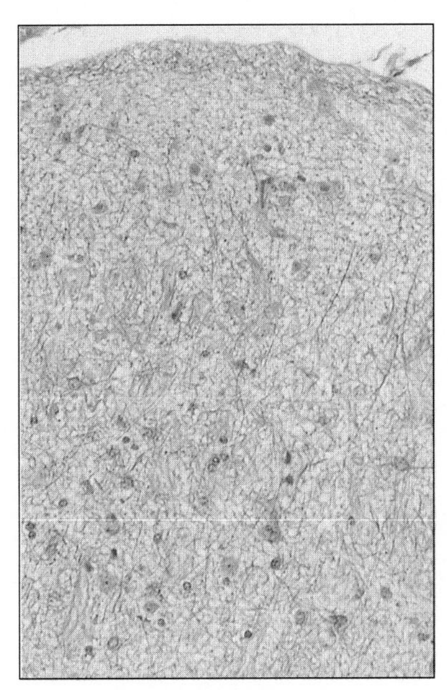

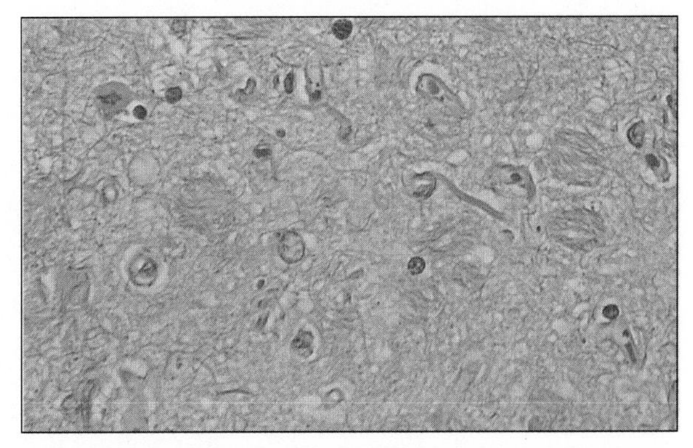

Fig. 3.107 As Fig. 3.106, but showing neurones in the subiculum of the hippocampus. *(Phosphotungstic acid–haematoxylin × 400.)*

staining (**Figs 3.108** and **3.109**) and anti-PHF antibodies (**Fig. 3.110**). However, comparative studies of tissues examined at autopsy and at previous biopsy show that, as neurones are lost (**Fig. 3.111**), some of the extracellular PHF skeletons are eventually removed (**Fig. 3.112**). This removal of PHF may be mediated by reactive astrocytes.

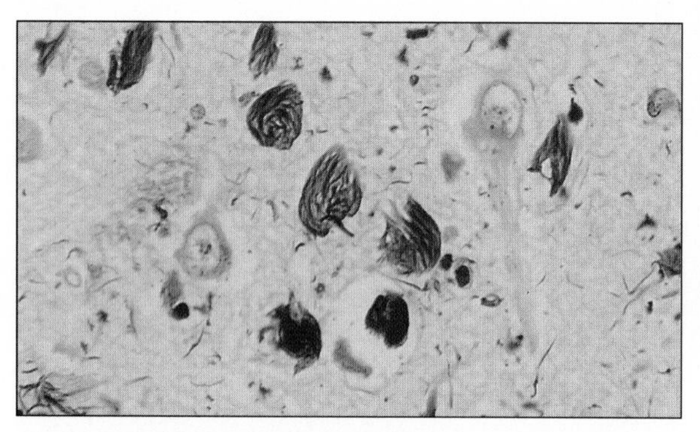

Fig. 3.108 Extracellular tangles in the subiculum of the hippocampus. *(Methenamine silver stain × 400.)*

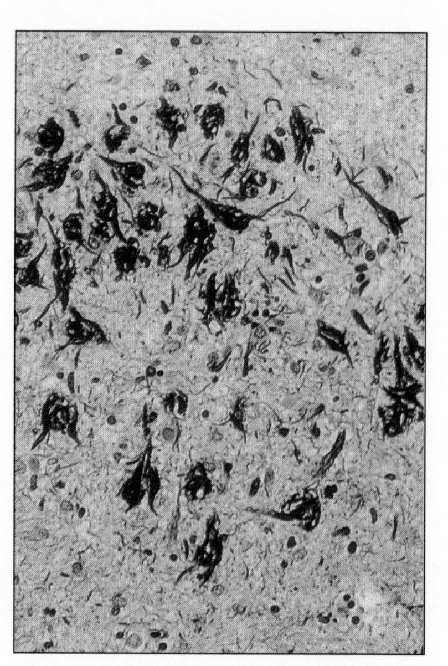

Fig. 3.109 As Fig. 3.108, in entorhinal cortex, layer II stellate cells. *(Methenamine silver stain × 400.)*

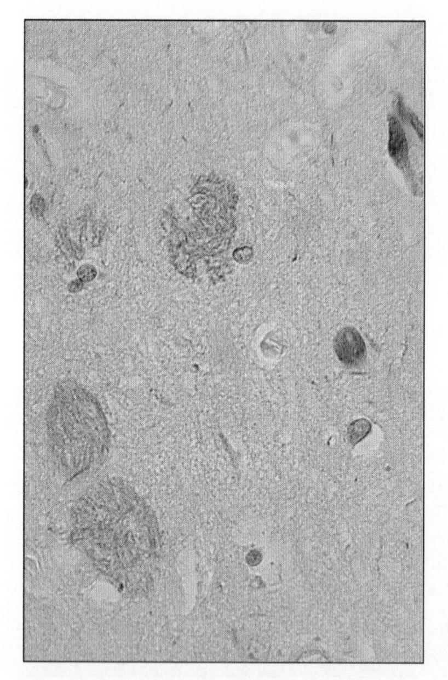

Fig. 3.110 Extracellular tangles in the subiculum of the hippocampus retain anti-PHF immunoreactivity. Note, however, that the filaments are less compact due to astrocytic infiltration. *(Anti-PHF × 400.)*

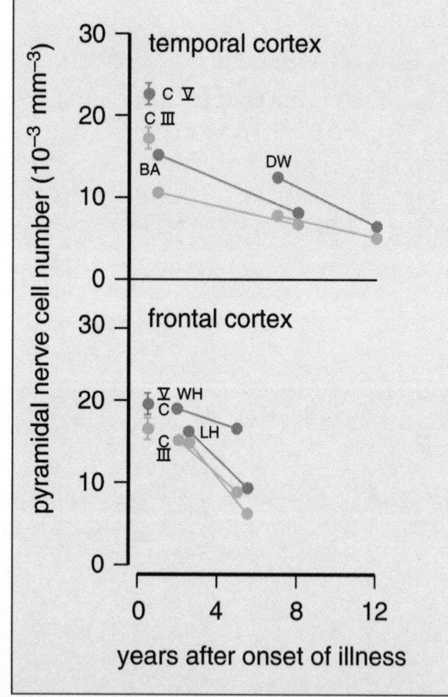

Fig. 3.111 Changes in the number of pyramidal cells of the frontal and temporal cortex between biopsy and autopsy in four patients. Cells of layer III are shown by (•), layer V by (○). Control (non-demented) values are indicated. Note the continuing loss of neurones throughout the illness.

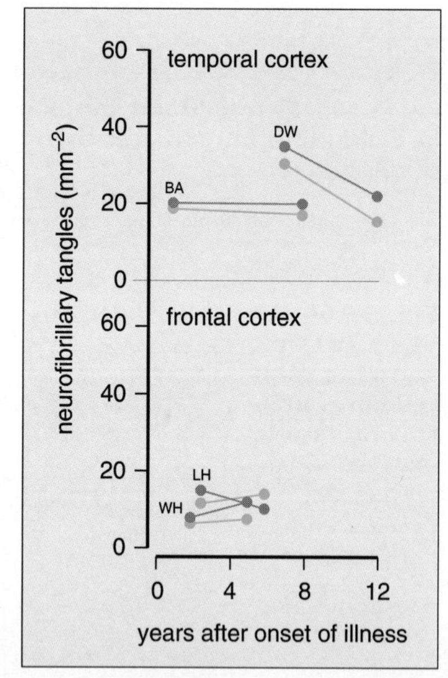

Fig. 3.112 Changes in neurofibrillary tangle density in frontal and temporal cortex between biopsy and autopsy in four patients. Note in the earlier and more severely affected temporal cortex, the density of tangles is less at autopsy than at biopsy, whereas in the less affected frontal cortex no such difference is seen.

Vascular changes

Many patients with Alzheimer's disease have some vascular pathology. In one type, which occurs in as many as 90% of patients, penetrating intraparenchymal (**Figs 3.113–3.120**) arteries and leptomeningeal arteries (**Figs 3.121–3.123**) are involved. Posterior hemisphere and cerebellar vessels are more affected than those supplying the anterior hemisphere and basal ganglia. The vessel walls contain a peptide similar to the β/A4 peptide within plaques; only a single amino acid difference has been recorded. Both peptides can therefore be recognized by the same antibodies (**Figs 3.118** and **3.123**). The vascular β/A4 peptide is also β-pleated and therefore Congophilic (see **Figs 3.115, 3.116, 3.121** and **3.122**) and thioflavin S positive (see **Fig. 3.117**). It additionally contains heparan sulphate proteoglycan, amyloid P and Apolipoprotein E. The

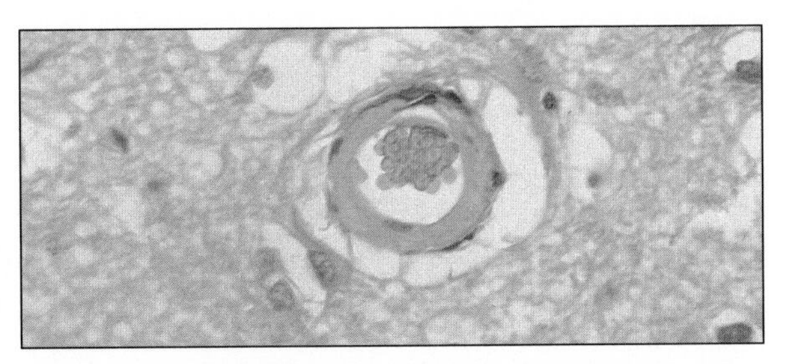

Fig. 3.113 Amyloidaceous artery within the occipital cortex grey matter. *(Haematoxylin–eosin × 400.)*

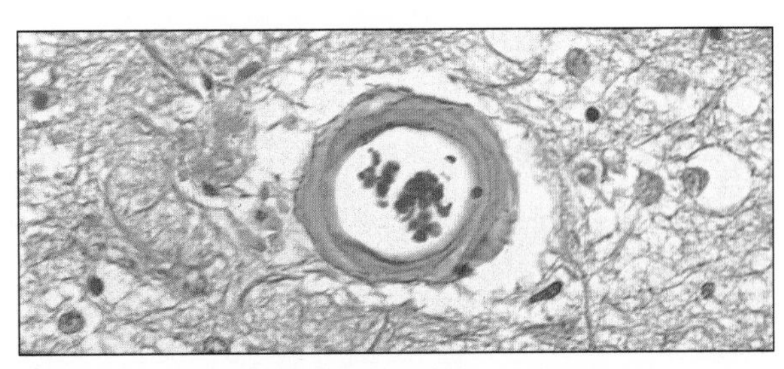

Fig. 3.114 Amyloidaceous artery within the occipital cortex grey matter. As **Fig. 3.112**, but showing mild astrocytosis within the grey matter around the affected vessel. *(Phosphotungstic acid–haematoxylin × 400.)*

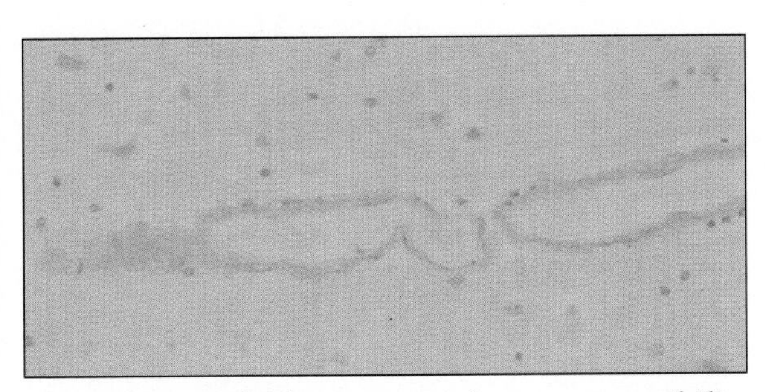

Fig. 3.115 Amyloidaceous arteries are congophilic. *(Congo red × 200.)*

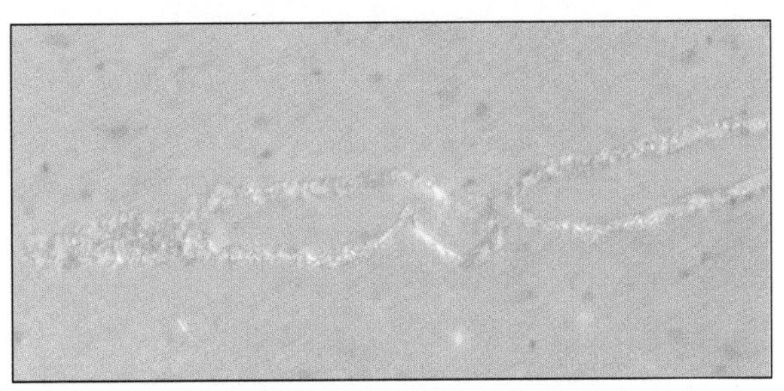

Fig. 3.116 Congo red stained arteries. These display yellow-green birefringence following viewing through cross-polarised light. *(Congo red × 200.)*

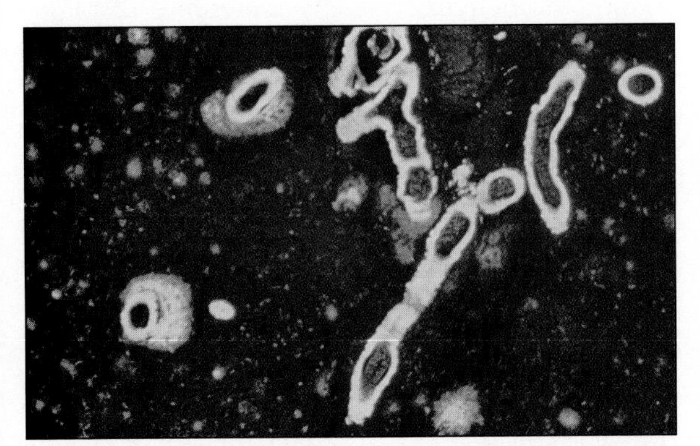

Fig. 3.117 Amyloidaceous arteries fluoresce strongly following staining with thioflavin S and excitation with ultraviolet light. *(Thioflavin S × 200.)*

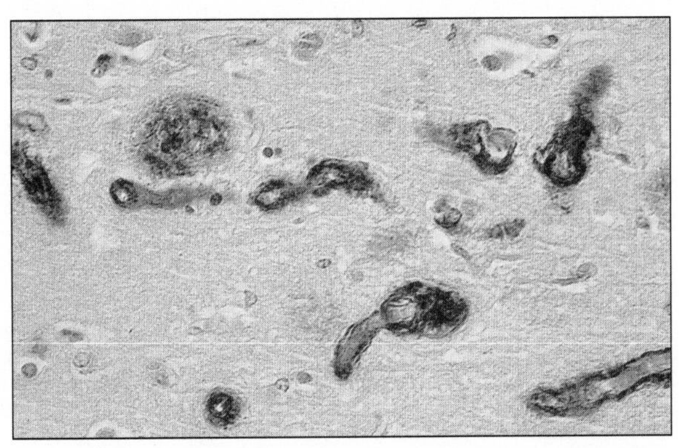

Fig. 3.118 Amyloidaceous arteries react strongly with antibodies to β/A4 protein. Note also the parenchymal deposition of β/A4 as plaques. *(Anti-β/A4 × 200.)*

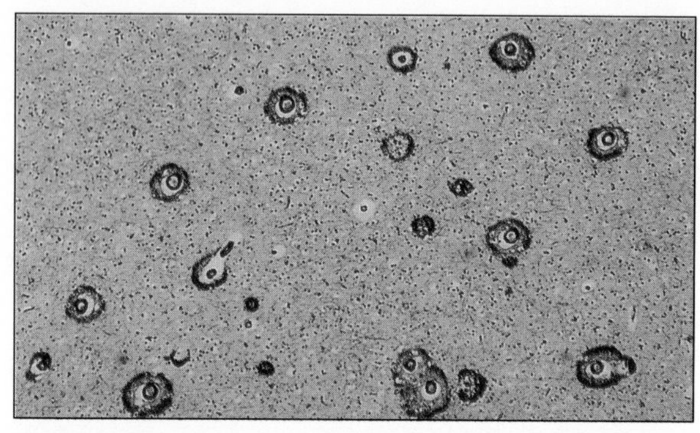

Fig. 3.119 Arteries within the occipital cortex (calcarine gyrus). Many contain β/A4 protein and are surrounded by a 'halo' of parenchymal β/A4 protein. *(Methenamine silver stain × 100.)*

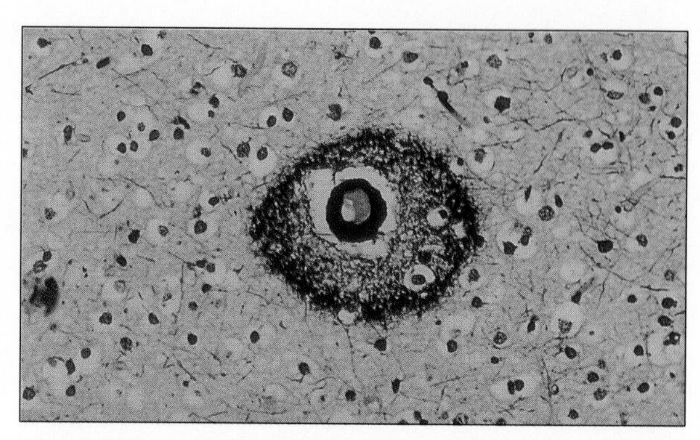

Fig. 3.120 Arteries within the occipital cortex (calcarine gyrus). As **Fig. 3.119**. *(× 400.)*

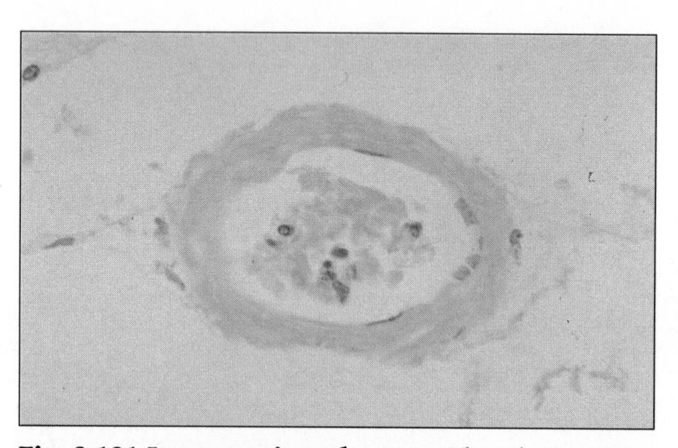

Fig. 3.121 Leptomeningeal artery. This also contains amyloid. *(Congo Red × 200.)*

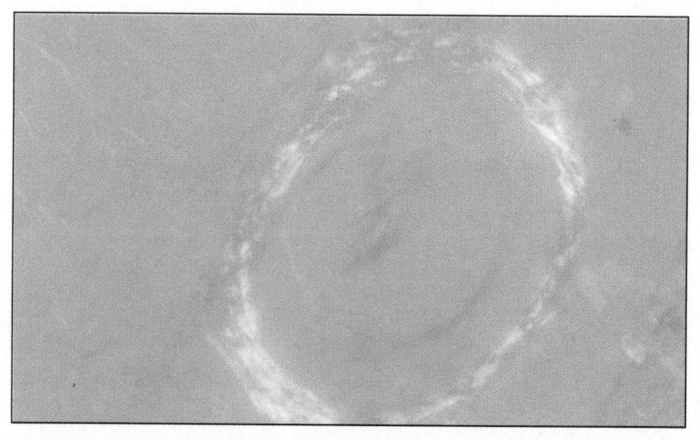

Fig. 3.122 Leptomeningeal artery. This Congo red-stained leptomeningeal artery displays characteristic yellow-green birefingence. *(× 200.)*

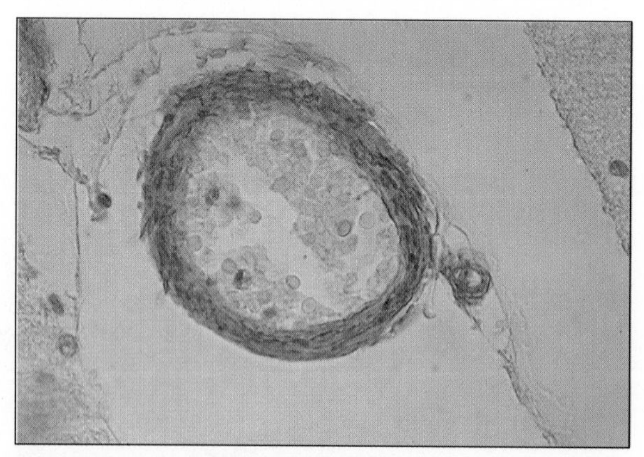

Fig. 3.123 Leptomeningeal artery. This contains β/A4 protein. *(Anti-β/A4 × 200.)*

β/A4 peptide is thought to be produced by the smooth muscle cells of these blood vessels and processed locally into amyloid fibrils by microglial cells or pericytes.

Intraparenchymal vessels sometimes display a change known as 'dyshoric angiopathy' in which the amyloid appears to 'stream' away from the vessel wall into the surrounding parenchyma (**Figs 3.124** and **3.125**). Surrounding such vessels there is often a 'neuritic' change (**Fig. 3.126**) similar to to that seen in neuritic plaques (**Fig. 3.127**). Although microinfarctions and microhaemorrhages can often accompany this angiopathy (**Figs 3.128–3.133**), gross cerebral haemorrhage is rare, except in the inherited condition of hereditary cerebral haemorrhage with amyloidosis (HCHWA) (see **Figs 3.158** and **3.175**) found in certain Dutch families, when it is a common cause of death (see page 59).

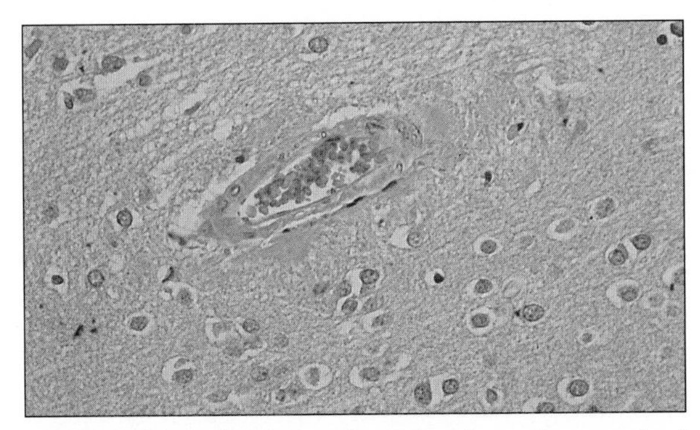

Fig. 3.124 Dyshoric angiopathy. Some intracerebral arteries affected by amyloid deposition display a 'streaming' of amyloid into the brain parenchyma (dyshoric angiopathy). *(Haematoxylin–eosin × 200.)*

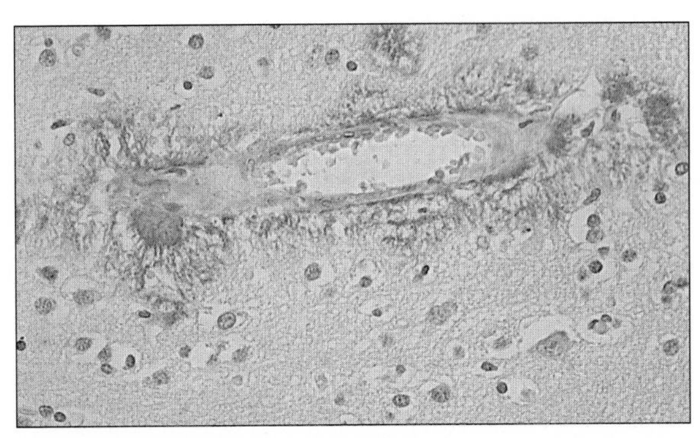

Fig. 3.125 Dyshoric angiopathy. Amyloid within and surrounding vessels affected by dyshoric angiopathy containing β/A4 protein. *(Anti-β/A4 × 200.)*

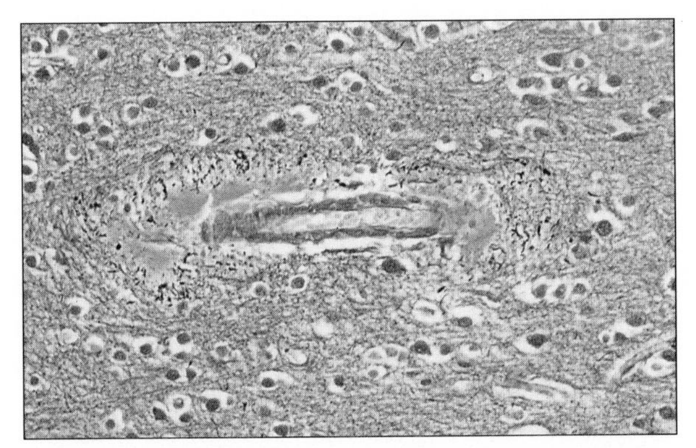

Fig. 3.126 Neuritic change within the parenchymal amyloid deposits surrounding blood vessels. The blood vessels are also affected by amyloid deposition. *(Palmgren silver stain × 200.)*

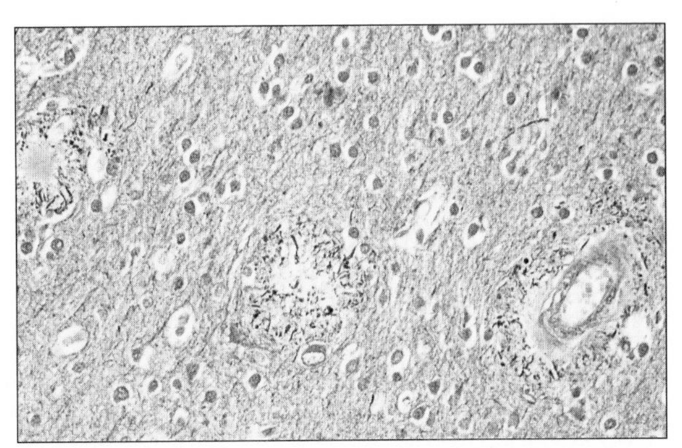

Fig. 3.127 Neuritic change within the parenchymal amyloid deposits surrounding blood vessels. As **Fig. 3.126** but note that other deposits do not seem to be associated with blood vessels and may represent parenchymal cored plaques. *(Palmgren silver stain × 200.)*

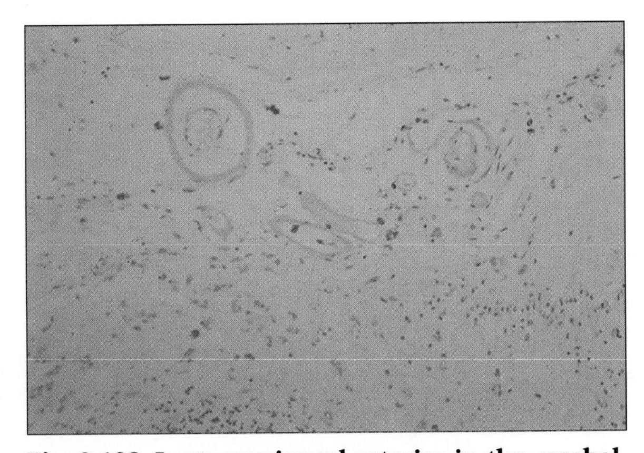

Fig. 3.128 Leptomeningeal arteries in the cerebellum. These are affected by amyloid deposition, show haemorrhage, and are associated with microinfarction of the cerebellar cortex. *(Congo red × 100.)*

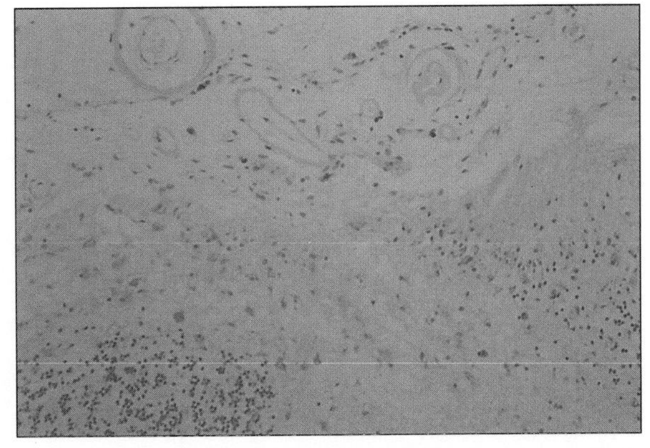

Fig. 3.129 Leptomeningeal arteries in the cerebellum. As **Fig. 3.128**, but note astrocytic proliferation in the area of infarction. *(Anti-GFAP × 200.)*

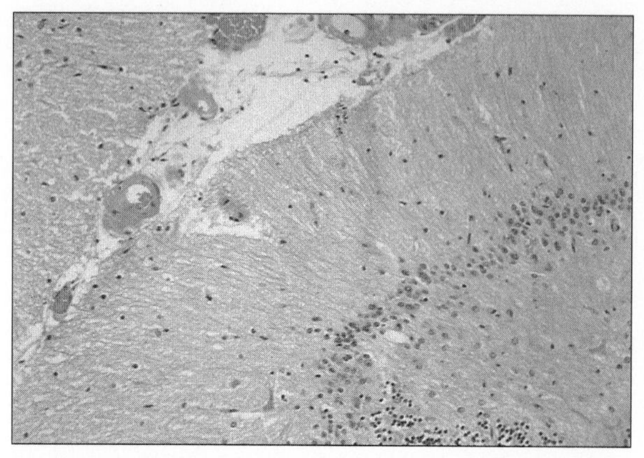

Fig. 3.130 Microinfarction in the cerebellar cortex associated with amyloidotic arteries. *(Haematoxylin–eosin × 100.)*

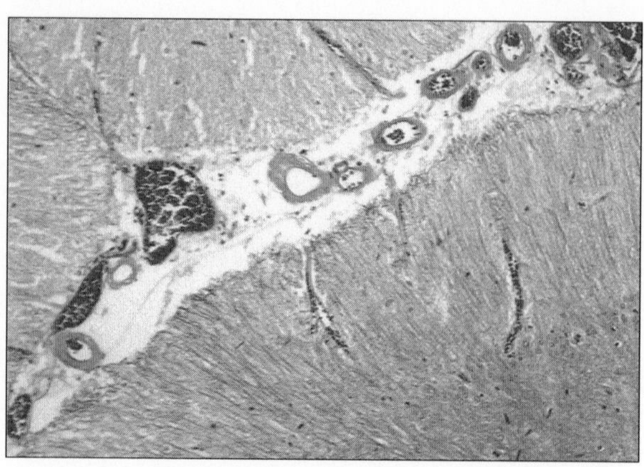

Fig. 3.131 Microinfarction in the cerebellar cortex associated with amyloidotic arteries. As **Fig. 3.130**, but showing reactive astrocytosis in areas of infarction. *(Phosphotungstic acid–haematoxylin × 100.)*

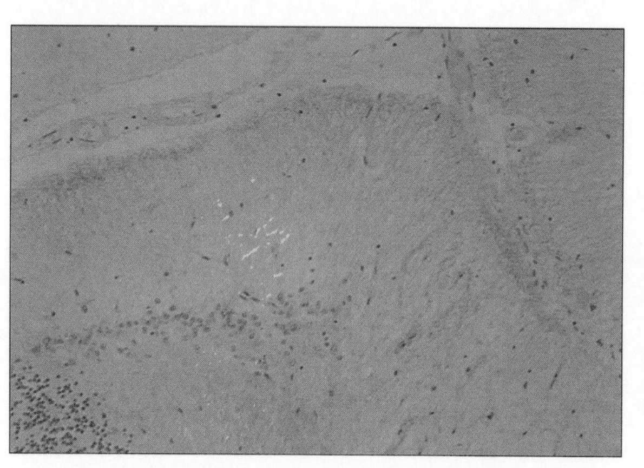

Fig. 3.132 Microinfarction in the cerebellar cortex associated with amyloidotic arteries. As **Fig. 3.133**, showing astrocytosis in the area of microinfarction. *(Anti-GFAP × 100.)*

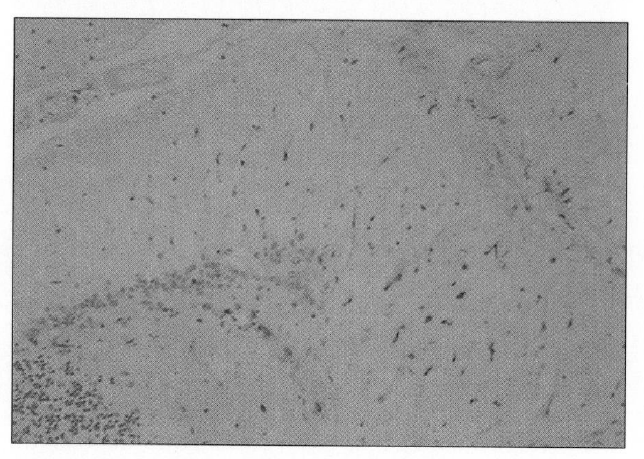

Fig. 3.133 Microglial cell activity in regions of microinfarction. *(Anti-ferritin × 100.)*

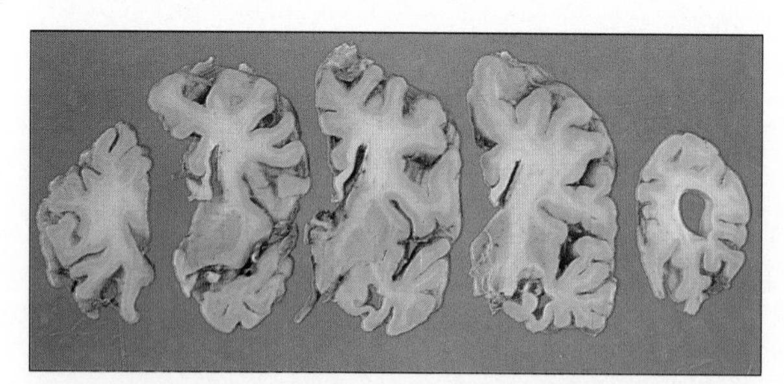

Fig. 3.134 Coronal sections of brain from a 74-year-old woman. These show a partial loss of myelin from the white matter, which appears brownish and less distinct than usual, especially within the frontal cortex.

Many other patients with Alzheimer's disease show a loss of myelin from the white matter, which in some instances, and particularly in the frontal lobes, can be severe (**Fig. 3.134**). The deeper white matter is lost more than the arcuate pathways (U-fibres) (**Figs 3.135** and **3.136**). This can be accompanied by a pronounced astrocytosis of a gemistocytic type. The walls of small arteries in these areas can be, but are not always, hyalinised (**Figs 3.137–3.139**) or show fibrous thickening with stenosis (**Fig. 3.140**). A local microcystic degeneration frequently surrounds such vessels (**Fig. 3.141**).

Fig. 3.135 (left) Section of frontal cortex. This shows loss of myelin from the deeper white matter, but there is some preservation of the arcuate fibres. *(Haematoxylin–eosin × 0.5.)*

Fig. 3.136 (right) Section of frontal cortex. As **Fig. 3.135**, but Luxol fast blue. *(× 0.5.)*

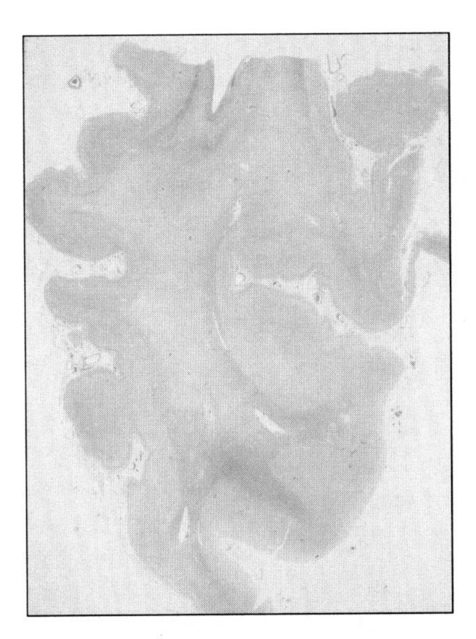

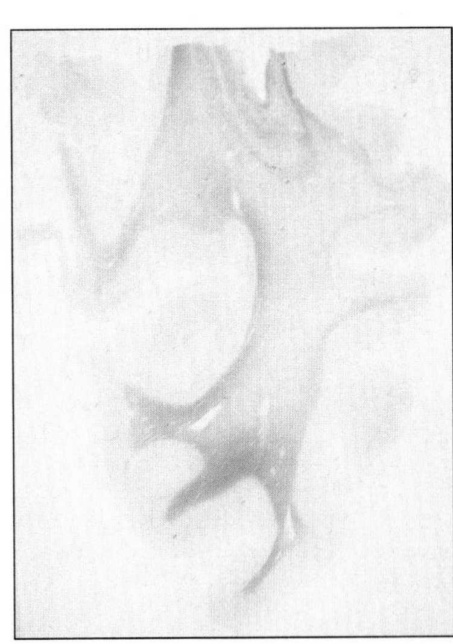

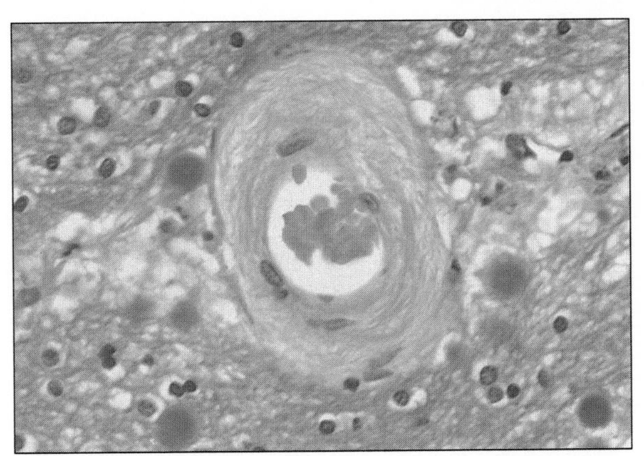

Fig. 3.137 Hyalinised fibrotic artery in frontal cortical white matter showing narrowing of the lumen. Note the presence of haemosiderin around the vessel, indicating some extravasation of red cells. *(Haematoxylin–eosin × 400.)*

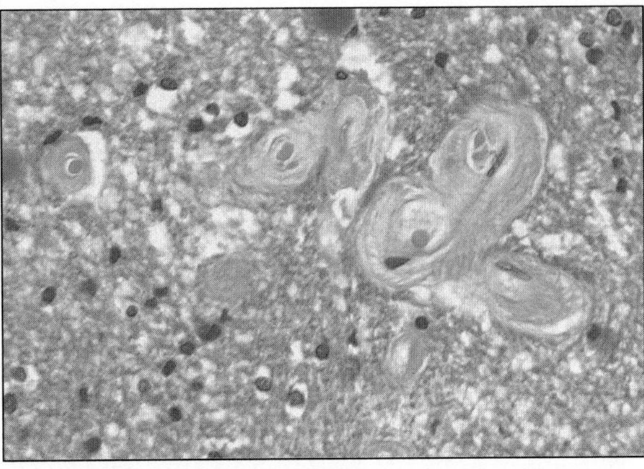

Figs 3.138 Hyalinised arteries and arterioles in the temporal cortical white matter. These show a reduction in lumen, with 'onion-skinning' of the vessel walls. *(Haematoxylin–eosin × 400.)*

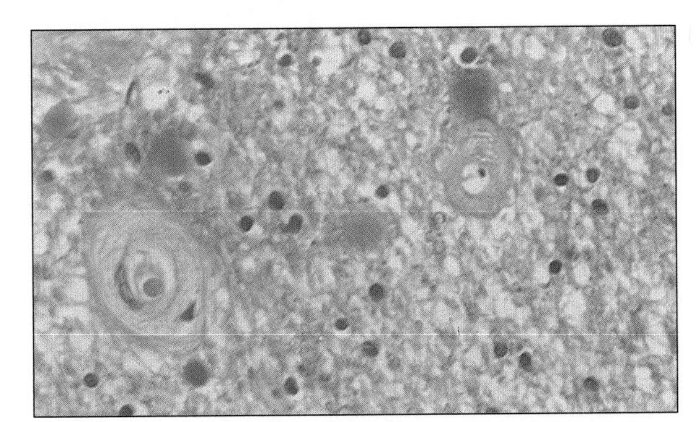

Figs 3.139 Hyalinised arteries and arterioles in the temporal cortical white matter. These show a reduction in lumen, with 'onion-skinning' of the vessel walls. *(Haematoxylin–eosin × 400.)*

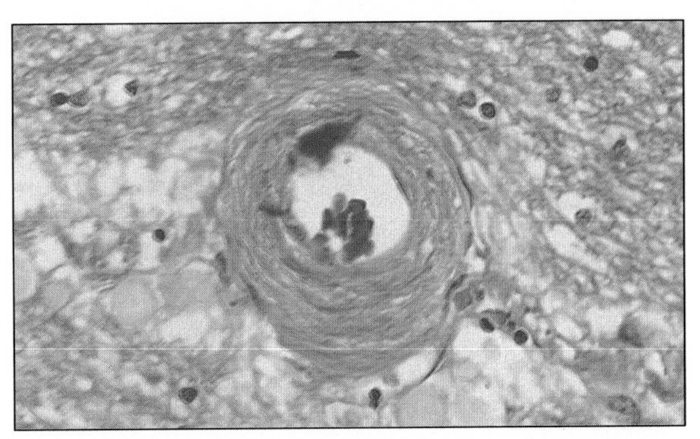

Fig. 3.140 As Fig. 3.137, but phosphotungstic acid–haematoxylin. *(× 400.)*

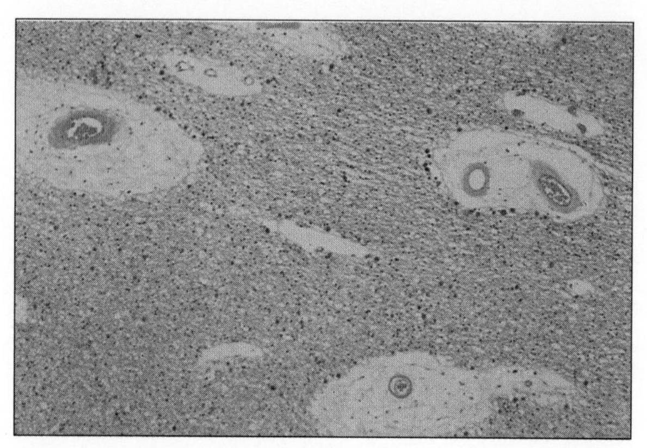

Fig. 3.141 Microcystic degeneration of white matter surrounding hyalinised arteries. *(Haematoxylin–eosin × 100.)*

Immunohistochemistry often reveals plasma proteins within vessel walls and enlarged astrocytes (**Fig. 3.142**), and sometimes in plaques surrounding 'leaky' vessels (**Fig. 3.143**). These changes probably relate to an incidental hypertension, which is particularly common in those (usually elderly) people who have Alzheimer's disease in conjunction with overt cerebrovascular disease (see page 137). The net effect of these vascular changes is an 'incomplete' infarction of the white matter (see **Figs 3.135** and **3.136**), which on CT or MRI scan appears as a region of 'leukoaraiosis'. This kind of damage undoubtedly adds to the dysfunction and destruction of the grey matter generated by plaque and tangle formation.

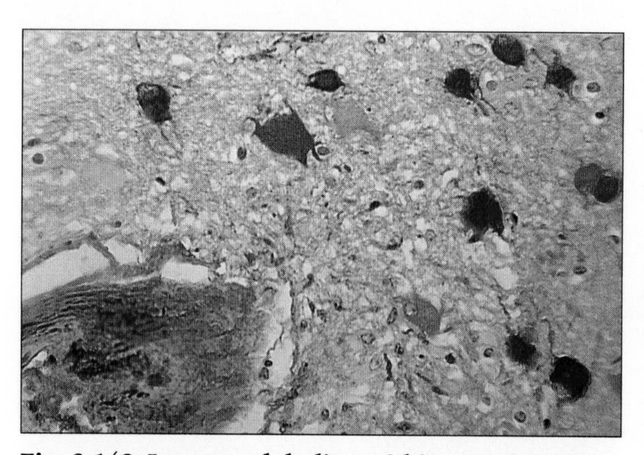

Fig. 3.142 Immunoglobulins within reactive astrocytes and within the wall of a hyalinised artery. *(Anti-*IgG × 200.)

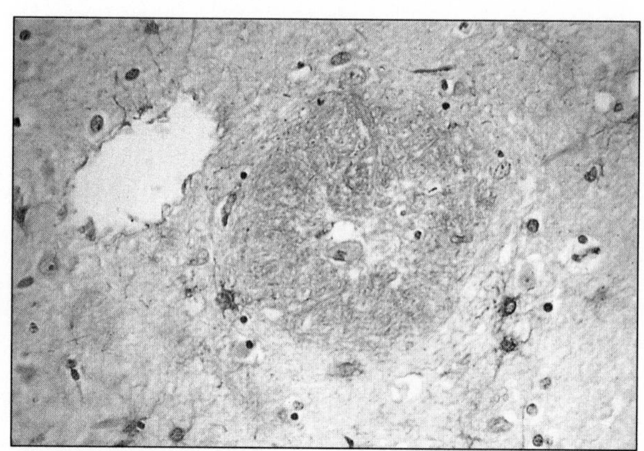

Fig. 3.143 Immunoglobulins within a senile plaque and reactive astrocytes. *(Anti-IgG × 200.)*

Other changes

The presence in the hippocampus of numerous 'Hirano bodies' and neurones showing 'granulovacuolar degeneration' is a further histopathological feature of Alzheimer's disease.

- Hirano bodies are intracellular and extracellular paracrystalline structures (**Fig. 3.144**) comprising parallel arrays of microfilaments (**Fig. 3.145**) immunoreactive to antisera against actin protein.
- Granulovacuoles (**Fig. 3.146**) are structures measuring about 3–5 μm in diameter, the granular component being 0.5–1.5 μm wide and argyrophilic (**Fig. 3.147**), but non-nucleic acid containing. Immunohistochemistry suggests the presence of tau and tubulin.

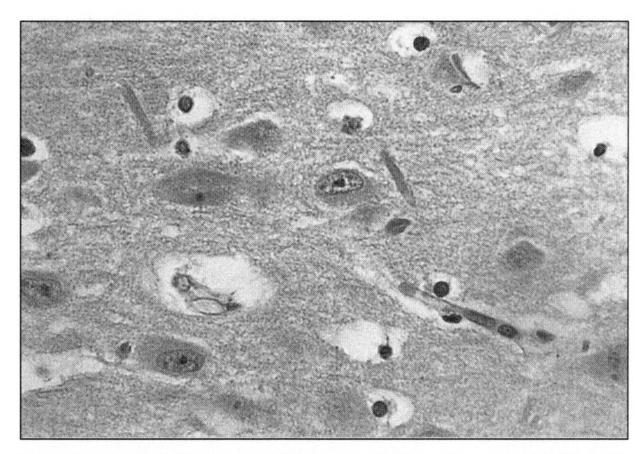

Fig. 3.144 Hirano bodies in the pyramidal cell layer of the hippocampus. *(Haematoxylin–eosin × 400.)*

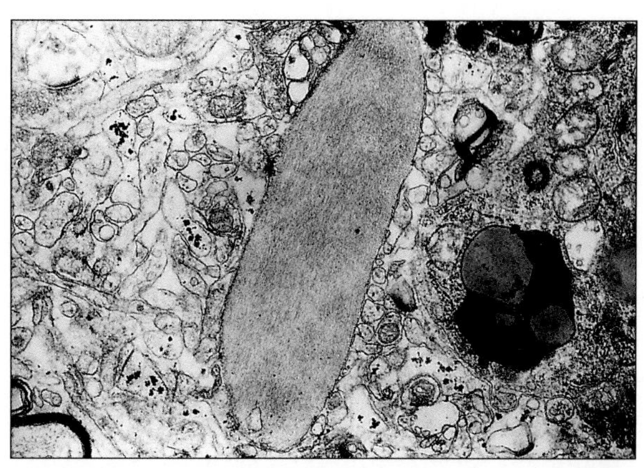

Fig. 3.145 Ultrastructural appearance of Hirano bodies. Note the paracrystalline array of filaments. The Hirano body is enclosed within the membrane of a cell, but whether this is neuronal or glial cannot be determined. *(Circa x 5,000.)*

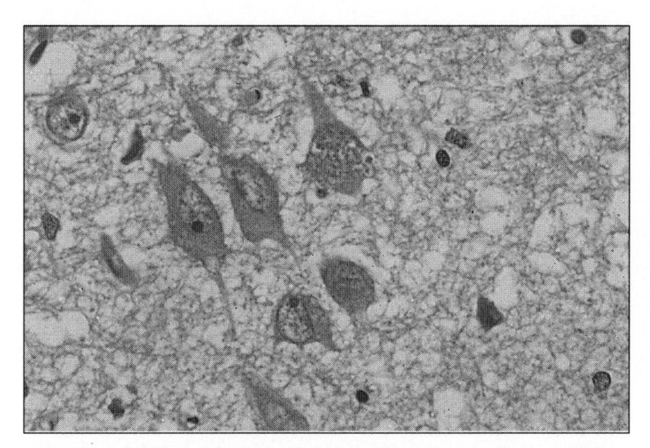

Fig. 3.146 Granulovacuolar degeneration of hippocampal pyramidal cells. *(Haematoxylin–eosin × 200.)*

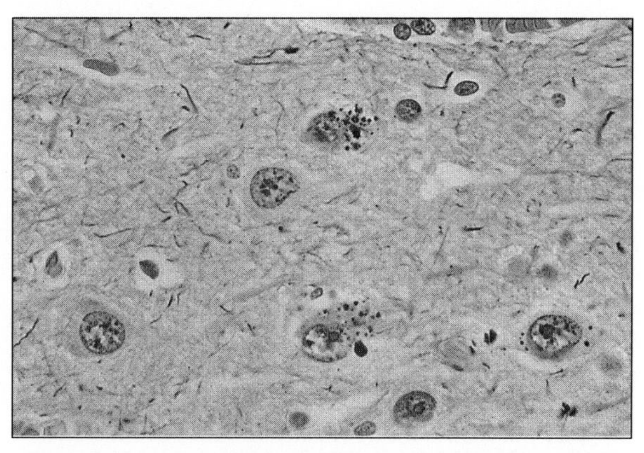

Fig. 3.147 Granulovacuolar degeneration of hippocampal pyramidal cells. As **Fig. 3.146** but Palmgren silver stain. *(× 200.)*

Both these changes occur to a lesser extent in the parahippocampal gyrus and amygdala. Like plaques and tangles they are also present, but again to a much lesser extent, in the hippocampus of non-demented elderly people. The origin and significance of these particular pathological changes are uncertain.

Excessive calcification of the walls of larger arteries (**Fig. 3.148**) and calcium deposition as calcospherites along the walls of smaller vessels in the globus pallidus (**Fig. 3.149**) are common changes in patients with Alzheimer's disease. Sometimes the end-folium region of the hippocampus is also affected (**Figs 3.150** and **3.151**). However, as

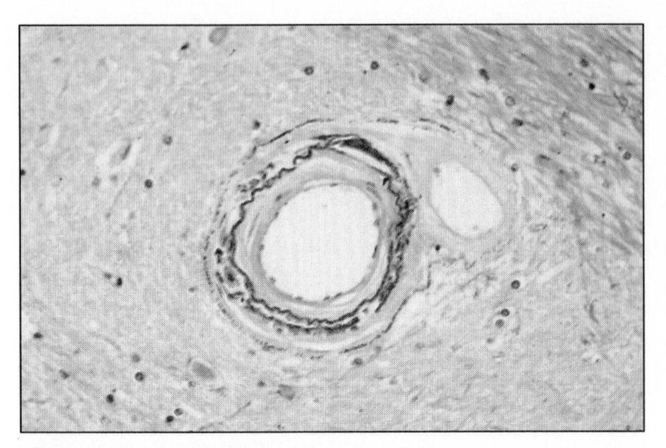

Fig. 3.148 Calcification of a large artery in the globus pallidus. *(Haematoxylin–eosin × 100.)*

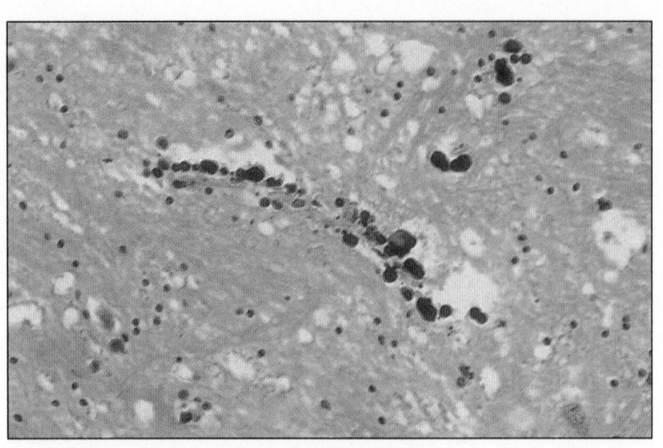

Fig. 3.149 Calcospherite deposition. Deposition of calcium, as calcospherites, along small arteries and capillaries of the globus pallidus. *(Haematoxylin–eosin × 200.)*

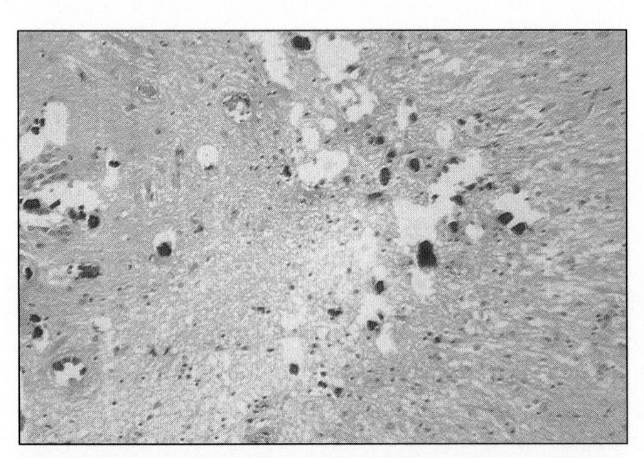

Fig. 3.150 Calcospherite deposition. This is associated with microinfarction within the end-folium (CA4/5) of the Ammon's horn region of the hippocampus. *(Haematoxylin–eosin × 100.)*

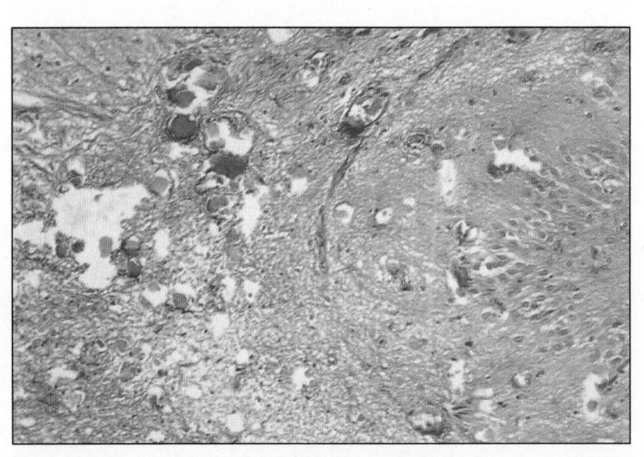

Fig. 3.151 Calcospherite deposition. As **Fig. 3.150**, but showing reactive astrocytosis in the area of microinfarction. *(Phosphotungstic acid–haematoxylin × 100.)*

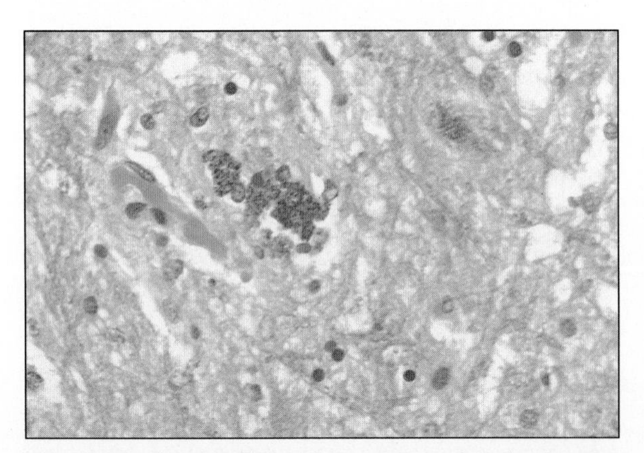

Fig. 3.152 Extracellular deposition of melanin pigment with microglial 'scar' in the substantia nigra. This is associated with a loss of nerve cells. *(Haematoxylin–eosin × 400.)*

these kinds of change also occur in many other neurodegenerative disorders and in mentally or neurologically normal elderly individuals, their relevance to disease and any possible effects on tissue function are not clear.

Many patients with Alzheimer's disease have a mild to moderate loss of cells from the substantia nigra (**Fig. 3.152**) and an occasional Lewy body may be present within surviving cells (**Figs 3.153** and **3.154**). This, in most instances, may be an age-associated rather than a disease-associated change, although occasionally nigral damage is severe and causes Parkinson-like features, which exist in conjunction with the typical Alzheimer-type pathology. The nosological status of such disease will be discussed later (see pages 118, 120 and 164).

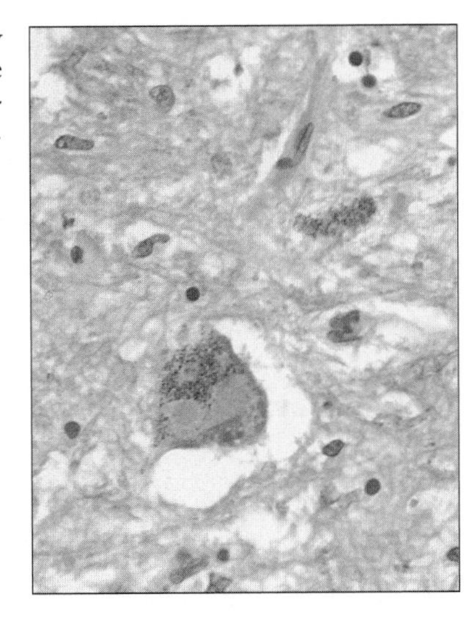

Fig. 3.153 Lewy body in a nerve cell of the substantia nigra. *(Haematoxylin–eosin × 400.)*

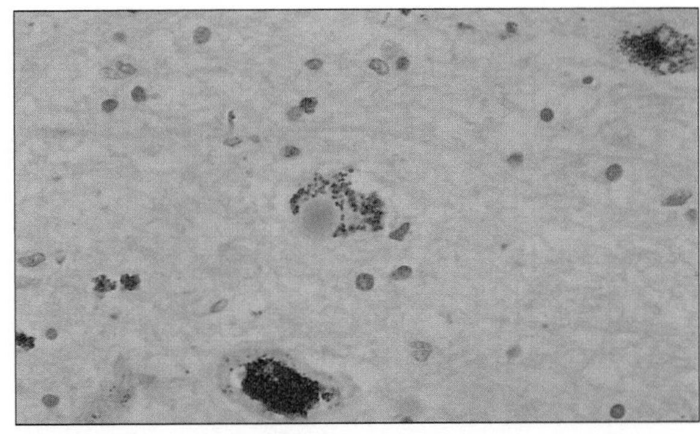

Fig. 3.154 Ubiquitinated Lewy body in a nerve cell of the substantia nigra. *(Anti-ubiquitin × 400.)*

Age and Alzheimer's disease

After 30 years of age, Alzheimer's disease can start at any time. It is perhaps only to be anticipated that the pathological changes described so far need not necessarily be present to the same extent in all persons regardless of their age. Consequently, the severity (but not the kind) of the pathology is greater in people who have an early onset of disease than in those who have a later onset, with the changes lying along an age-dependent continuum. This applies not only to the loss of brain weight and the extent and distribution of atrophy, but also to the histopathological changes of (neuritic) plaques and tangles (**Fig. 3.155**) and loss of nerve cells (**Figs 3.156** and **3.157**). Why this age-depen-

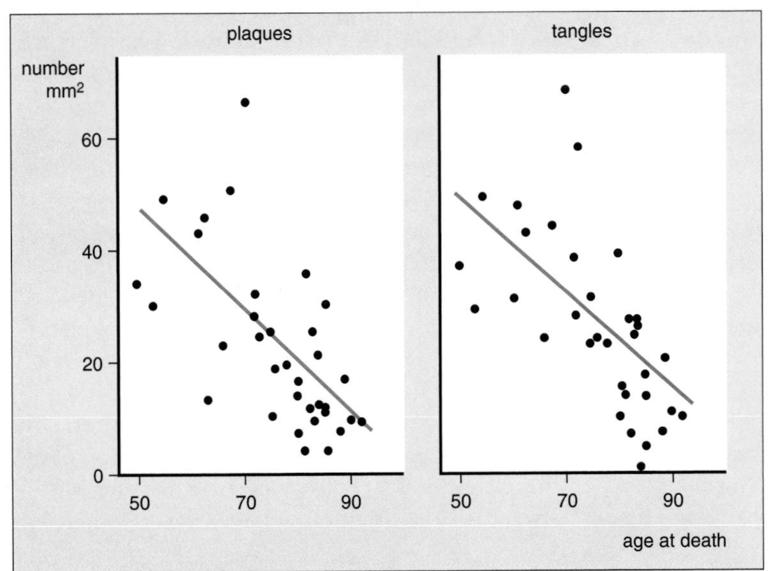

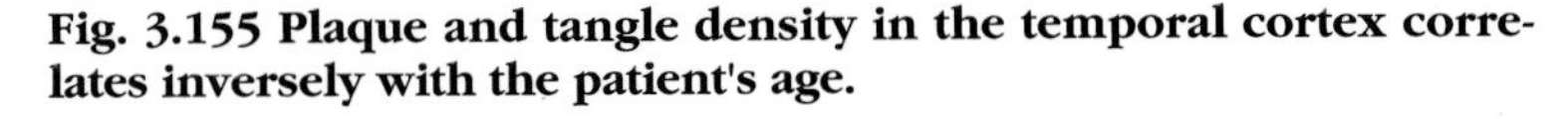

Fig. 3.155 Plaque and tangle density in the temporal cortex correlates inversely with the patient's age.

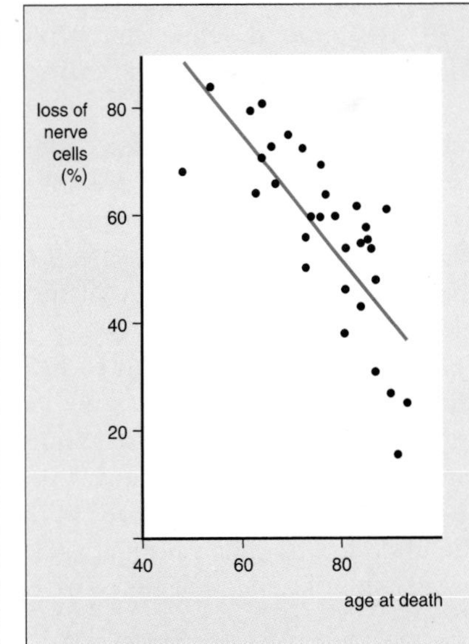

Fig. 3.156 Percentage loss of nerve cells from the temporal cortex due to Alzheimer's disease becomes less in older patients.

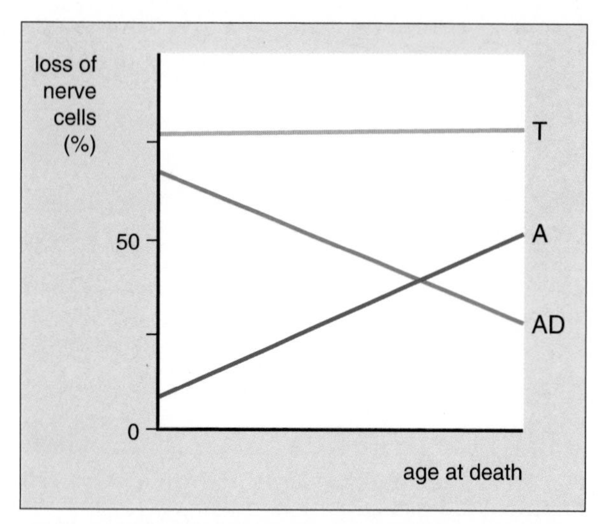

Fig. 3.157 Effects of ageing and Alzheimer's disease on nerve cell loss from the temporal cortex. The total (T) nerve cell loss is constant, irrespective of age, but the component parts of that loss due to age (A) and Alzheimer's disease (AD) differ, as illustrated, according to patient age. The cell loss of young individuals almost exclusively results from disease, whereas in older people an increasing proportion of cell loss is the result of age alone and less because of the additional presence of Alzheimer's disease.

dency exists is not clear, but an individual's pre-morbid state of physical well-being may play a part. Younger, fitter people who have less intercurrent systemic disease may live longer with Alzheimer's disease than frailer older people. Nonetheless, aetiological factors may also contribute, dictating a 'dose-effect', with genetic influences in younger persons possibly having a more pronounced action that the (presumed) non-genetic and genetic factors that are thought to play a major role in the aetiology of the disease in the elderly.

If older individuals tend to have less specific Alzheimer-type damage in their brains than their younger counterparts, why should the extent of clinical derangement (dementia) be similar in both regardless of age? The answer to this may lie with the effects of so-called normal ageing, this taking a greater toll of nerve cells in older people (see **Figs 3.156** and **3.157**). Therefore, in elderly people with dementia part of the total damage to the brain that manifests as dementia is due to ageing and part due to superadded Alzheimer's disease, but in younger individuals with dementia ageing plays a minimal part, if at all, and the damage is entirely due to the presence of Alzheimer's disease.

Diagnostic criteria

Although convention requires the presence of *numerous* plaques and tangles within the brain for the diagnosis of Alzheimer's disease, there is as yet no consistent or acceptable 'benchmark' as to how the term *numerous* should be applied. The reasons for this failure to produce such a 'gold-standard' for diagnosis are multiple and include problems concerned with lesion morphology, lesion distribution, and lesion specificity, as follows:

- **There is no general agreement about what constitutes, for diagnostic purposes, a plaque.** Clearly, methods such as β-immunostaining and certain silver techniques (modified Bielschowsky, methenamine silver) detect many more plaques (as amyloid deposits) than other methods that rely on the presence of PHF within the amyloid deposits (neuritic plaques) for their efficiency (e.g. Bodian and Palmgren silver methods, and anti-tau and anti-ubiquitin immunostaining).
- **The term *numerous* is without an intrinsic definition.** To avoid potential inconsistencies in its use a working definition based on cortical plaque and tangle densities has been devised. Furthermore, because plaques and tangles are increasingly common with age in non-demented individuals, threshold values have been defined, so that higher plaque and tangle densities are required to satisfy minimal criteria in older people than in younger ones. However, this scheme was introduced before the widespread use of β-immunostaining and other sil-

ver techniques for detecting amyloid plaques and was based on the earlier 'conventional' staining methods. It has not yet been possible to take these newer methods and the findings resulting from their use (see page 34) into account and produce a revised protocol that satisfies all (morphological) definitions of a 'plaque'.

- **It is not clear to which parts of the brain such diagnostic criteria should be applied.** Usually, plaques and tangles (by any morphological criteria) are numerous in the hippocampus, amygdala and neocortex, yet amyloid deposition *alone* is much more widespread, being common in the basal ganglia and cerebellum, and in the periventricular and periaqueductal grey matter. In addition, tangles may be rare in the neocortex of many elderly demented patients, though plaques are numerous, with both being common in the hippocampus.
- **Many elderly, but non-demented, patients have many plaques and tangles in the hippocampus alone.** Although some of these individuals may have early Alzheimer's disease, this is not a safe assumption for all such people.
- **Many diffuse amyloid deposits (but not usually neuritic plaques) occur in the brains of other non-demented elderly persons.** They also occur in many elderly people with dementing and non-dementing neurodegenerative diseases other than Alzheimer's disease (and Down's syndrome).
- **With time, extracellular tangles, and possibly plaques, are removed from the tissue.** The density of each at any particular point in time during the course of the illness might reflect the 'aggressiveness' of the disease process. This changes and consequently the number of lesions decreases as the tissue reaches a pathological end-stage after a long duration.

As with gross anatomy, there is therefore no precise histopathological marker of the disease or any feature whose size or quantity can act as a simple mathematical predictor. It is not clear how these controversies can be easily resolved. Amyloid deposition *per se* and tangles are not specific to Alzheimer's disease, and the number of neuritic plaques (and tangles) may change with prolonged disease.

There is clearly a need to develop more relevant (molecular) markers for diagnosis. Some success has been achieved when the disease is inherited as a point mutation of the APP gene, but individuals with this form of the disease represent only a tiny minority of the total number of people with Alzheimer's disease.

Meanwhile, it is necessary to use what morphological markers are available; neuritic plaques seem more specific to the disease than amyloid deposits and no other situations exist where neuritic plaques *and* tangles exist together. A practical definition of the disease working within the limitations discussed above that probably accounts for the majority of cases is to take the presence of numerous *neuritic* plaques *and* tangles in the *neocortex* and hippocampus as discriminating factors. However, it is recognised that within this definition the term *numerous* will still be subject to varying interpretations according to the observer's range of personal experience and sense of intuition.

Amyloid precursor protein

The β/A4 Amyloid precursor protein (APP) is a transmembrane protein (**Fig. 3.158**). It occurs in both neural and non-neural tissues as a family of at least five alternatively spliced products of a single gene transcript of which APP_{695}, APP_{751} and APP_{770} are the major molecular forms. These have a molecular weight of 110–135 kDa. APP_{751} and APP_{770} (especially), are produced largely in extraneural tissues and although showing the same basic peptide sequence as APP_{695} they also contain inserts corresponding to a Kunitz-type protease inhibitor, the APP_{770} variant also having a further insert similar to the MRC OX2 antigen. The major brain-associated forms are APP_{695} (mostly) and APP_{751} these being produced mainly by neurones (**Fig. 3.159**).

The function of APP is unknown, although roles as a receptor, cell adhesion molecule, growth factor or protease inhibitor have been proposed. The mol-

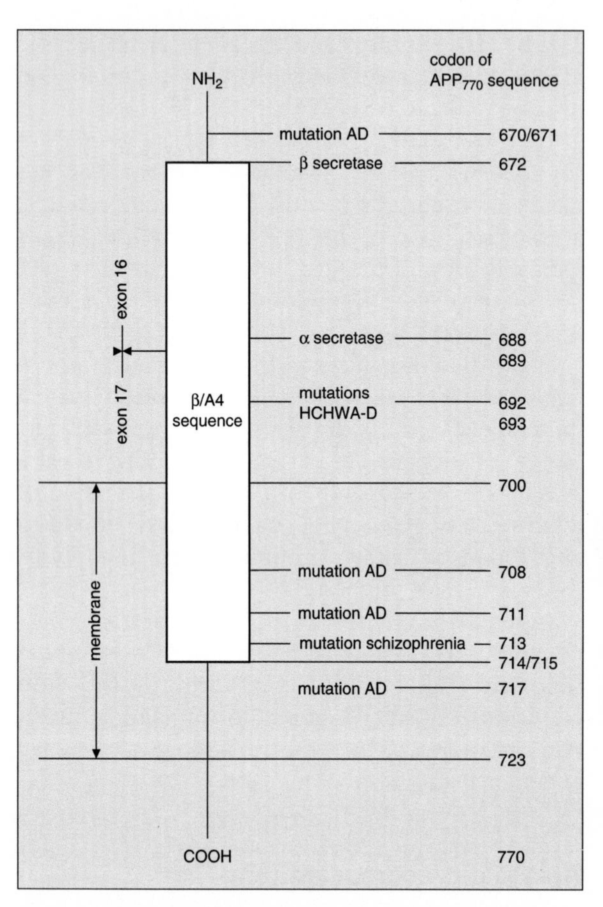

Fig. 3.158 Diagram of the APP gene. This shows the boundary between exons 16 and 17 and the points within these exons where mutations have been identified. The part of the gene corresponding to the β/A4 sequence is 'blocked'.

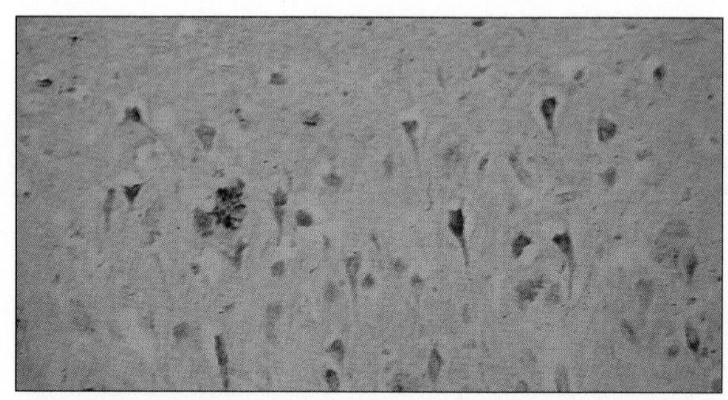

Fig. 3.159 Neurones of the pyramidal cell layer of the hippocampus. These contain much amyloid precursor protein. Note the presence of APP in dystrophic neurites within a plaque region. *(Anti-APP × 200.) (Courtesy of Dr G W Roberts.)*

ecule may take part in cellular repair processes or in the modulation of cell growth. The gene for APP is 300–400 kilobases in length and the open reading frame (coding region) is contained within 19 exons.

As the sequence for β/A4 peptide lies across two neighbouring exons (exons 16 and 17) in the APP gene (see **Fig. 3.158**), its production and deposition in Alzheimer's disease cannot be due to an unusual splicing mechanism. Because of the linkage of Alzheimer's disease to point mutations in the APP gene, it has therefore been postulated (see page 63) that an 'aberrant' metabolism of normally formed APP leads to deposition of β/A4 peptide and that this causes the full constellation of pathological changes to follow. This is the so-called 'amyloid hypothesis' of Alzheimer's disease (see **Fig. 3.175**).

The ways in which APP can be metabolised are now becoming clearer. A secretory pathway cleaves the APP across the β/A4 sequence, at residue 16 producing an N-terminal portion, which is apparently released into the circulation, and a carboxy-terminal fragment (CTF), which is degraded internally. Neither of these products contain the full β/A4 sequence and neither can therefore produce the amyloid fibrils that accumulate in the brain. However, alternative pathways, both secretory and lysosomal, also exist in which the APP is cleaved N-terminally to the β/A4 sequence, leaving CTFs that are potentially amyloidogenic.

The finding of a soluble form of β/A4 in human cerebrospinal fluid, and in cell cultures expressing much APP, leads to the conclusion that the CTFs are further degraded. Their release into the extracellular space could then result in the formation of fibrillary β/A4 (amyloid).

As these degradative pathways exist normally production of β/A4 does not require an 'abberrant' metabolic process or cellular damage to take place. An overexpression of APP, the production of missense variants, a failure to remove newly formed β/A4 from the extracellular space adequately, or an enhanced fibrillogenesis could all be factors playing a part in driving the end-result (i.e. the extracellular accumulation of β/A4 in brain parenchyma and in blood vessel walls).

APP can be present within the dystrophic neurites of many, but not all, plaques (see **Fig. 3.159**). Its presence within such well-formed plaques probably reflects a 'damming up' of newly formed APP delivered by axonal flow from the perikayon to the altered (damaged) nerve endings. APP also accumulates within the neurites of prion plaques (see page 154) and in axon dystrophies close to cerebral infarcts or in the retraction bulbs of severed axons (see page 69, **Fig 3.188**) for similar reasons.

Genetic factors

There is a genetic link between Alzheimer's disease and chromosome 21 in some families,in whom abnormalities within the APP gene have been identified (see **Fig. 3.158**).

- Three (separate) point mutations, all occurring at codon 717 of the APP sequence and involving a valine→isoleucine (mainly), valine→glycine and valine→phenylalanine change, have been identified in European, North American and Japanese families.
- A double mutation at codons 670/671 involving a lysine/methionine→asparginine/leucine change, respectively, has been identified in a Swedish pedigree, though in this the 671 base change is critical.
- Other 'silent' (non-pathogenic) mutations at codons 708 and 711 have also been found in some patients with Alzheimer's disease, and one at codon 713 in a patient with schizophrenia; these are all considered incidental and are not thought to play a role in the pathogenesis of the disease.
- Mutations at codons 692 and 693 (see **Fig. 3.158**) relate to a (pathologically) similar disorder of cerebral haemorrhage with amyloidosis (see **Fig. 3.175**).

The precise loci on chromosomes 14 and 22 responsible for Alzheimer's disease have yet to be identified; patients showing chromosome 14 linkage have an identical pathology, although disease onset is unusually early, at 30 to 40 years of age. The locus on chromosome 19, linked to Alzheimer's disease, is very close to and may be

Table 3.1 Prevalence according to age of senile plaques and neurofibrillary tangles in the brains of people with Down's syndrome.

Age range (years)	Total number of persons	Number showing plaques and tangles	Percentage
0–9	38	0	0
10–19	81	6	7.4
20–29	59	10	16.9
30–39	45	36	80.0
All <39	**223**	**52**	**23.3**
40–49	62	61	98.4
50–59	.98	96	98.0
60–69	.48	48	100.0
70–79	3	3	100.0
All >40	**211**	**208**	**98.6**
All 0–79	**434**	**260**	**59.9**

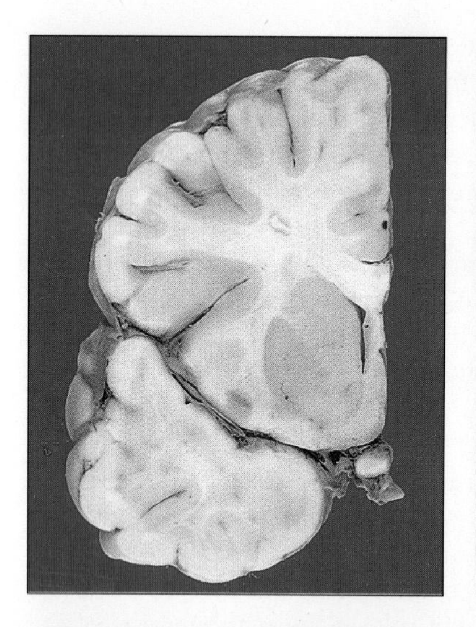

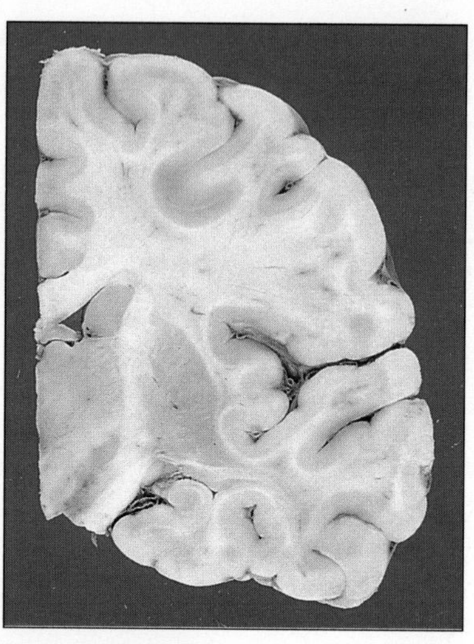

Figs 3.160 and 3.161 Down's syndrome. Coronal sections of the brain of a 37-year-old woman with Down's syndrome. Note the incomplete development of the superior temporal gyrus.

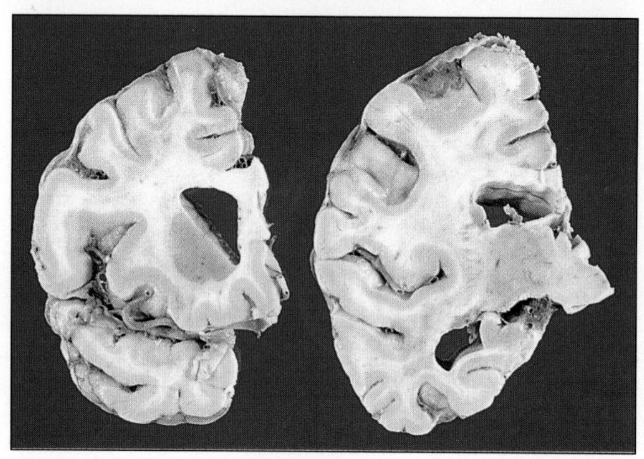

Fig. 3.162 Down's syndrome. Coronal sections of the brain showing cerebral atrophy and ventricular dilatation in a 56-year-old woman with Down's syndrome .

identical to that coding for the cholesterol carrying protein Apolipoprotein E. There are 3 particular normal allelic variants of this gene, E2, E3 and E4. The E3 allele is the ancestral form and occurs in 90% of the general population. E3 has a cysteine at position 112 and arginine at position 158; in E4 arginine is present at both sites whereas in E2 cysteine is present at both. The particular risk factor associated with Alzheimer's disease seems to be the possession of an E4 allele with persons homozygous for E4 having a more than eight times the risk of developing the disease over those with no E4 copies. Patients with Alzheimer's disease associated with point mutations in the APP gene or a chromosome 14 linkage have the normal population frequency distribution of E4 alleles, as indeed do individuals with Down's syndrome.

Hence in at least one form of late onset (inherited and sporadic) Alzheimer's disease an E4 allele seems to be a major determining factor whereas in other forms of early and late onset inherited disease a mutated APP gene is the driving force. Nonetheless, despite this clear association between E4 and the development of Alzheimer's disease other factors (apart from the above mentioned mutations) must be involved in order to explain why there are persons in the general population who possess E4 yet live long and healthy lives and why also there are many other elderly persons who develop Alzheimer's disease yet lack an E4 allele. It remains possible that E4 simply represents a disease marker in tight linkage with an alternative locus on chromosome 19, the latter being the key player in determining the onset of disease.

Down's syndrome and Alzheimer's disease

Probably everyone with Down's syndrome due to trisomy of chromosome 21 who lives beyond 50 years of age will exhibit all the pathological features of Alzheimer's disease (**Table 3.1**).

These pathological changes appear to be 'acquired' during later life (**Figs 3.160–3.162**); such changes are not present before 10–15 years of age or later (up to 30 years) in some individuals. It is possible that the genetic abnormality causing the mental retardation of Down's syndrome also predisposes to, or accelerates, the development of Alzheimer's disease in later life.

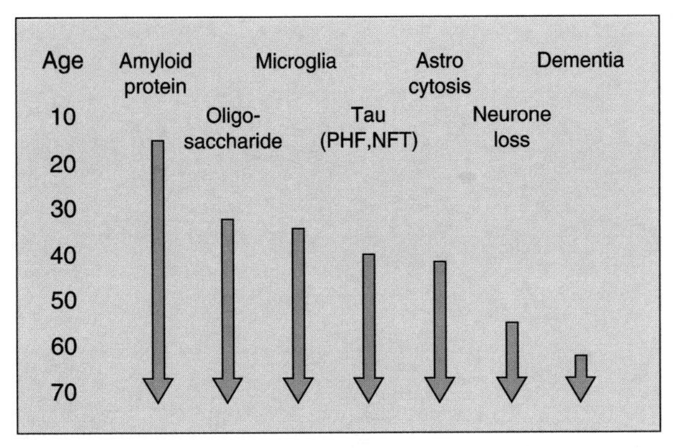

Fig. 3.163 Down's syndrome. Diagram showing the time of onset and progression of the various pathological changes associated with Alzheimer's disease in Down's syndrome.

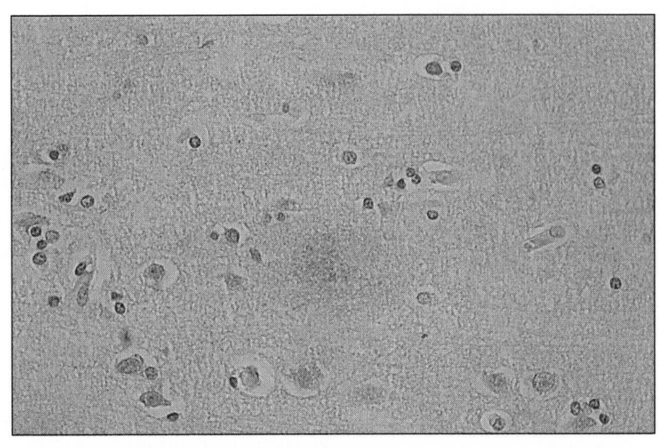

Fig. 3.164 Down's syndrome. Fine diffuse deposits of β/A4 protein in the temporal cortex of a 31-year-old man with Down's syndrome. *(Anti-β/A4 × 400.)*

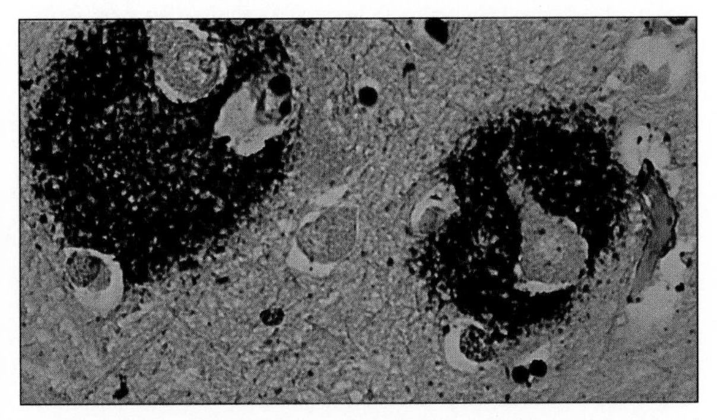

Fig. 3.165 Down's syndrome. Diffuse amyloid deposits surrounding hippocampal pyramidal cells in a 37-year-old woman with Down's syndrome. *(Methenamine silver stain × 400.)*

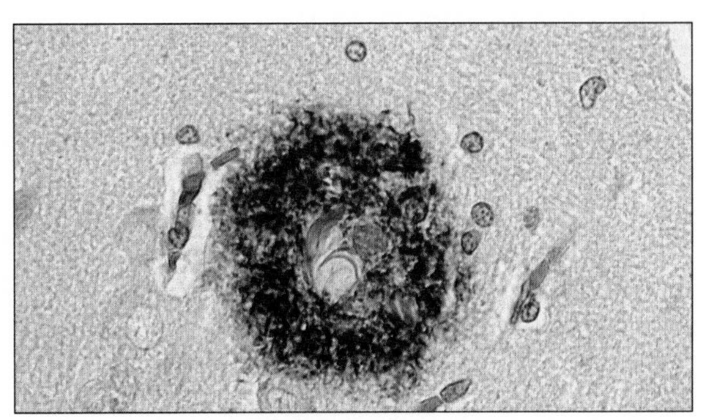

Fig. 3.166 Down's syndrome.Diffuse amyloid deposits enclosing a blood vessel in a 37-year-old woman with Down's syndrome. *(Methenamine silver stain × 400.)*

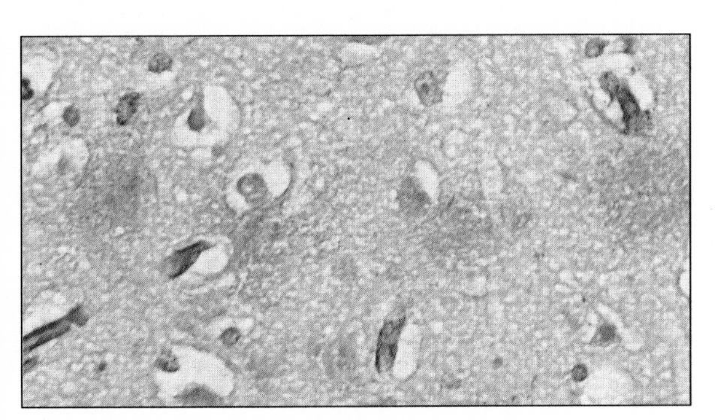

Fig. 3.167 Down's syndrome. Diffuse deposits of β/A4 protein in the temporal cortex of a 31-year-old man with Down's syndrome do not contain microglial cells. *(Double stain, anti-β/A4 (red) and lectin (*Sambucus nigra*) histochemistry (brown) × 400.)*

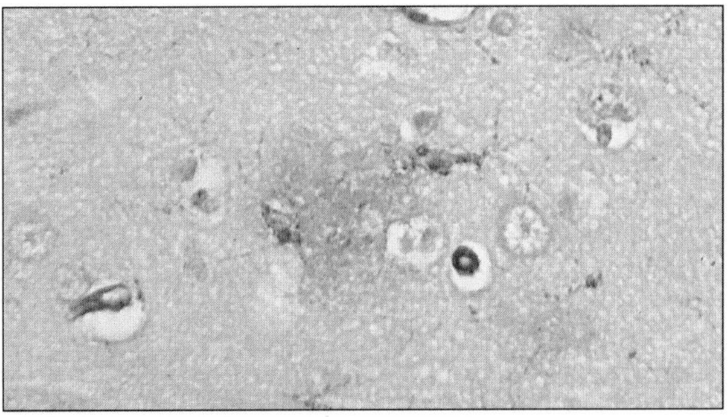

Fig. 3.168 Down's syndrome.Diffuse deposits of β/A4 protein in the temporal cortex of a 37-year-old woman contain a few microglial cells. *(Double stain, anti-β/A4 (red) and lectin (*Sambucus nigra*) histochemistry (brown) × 400.)*

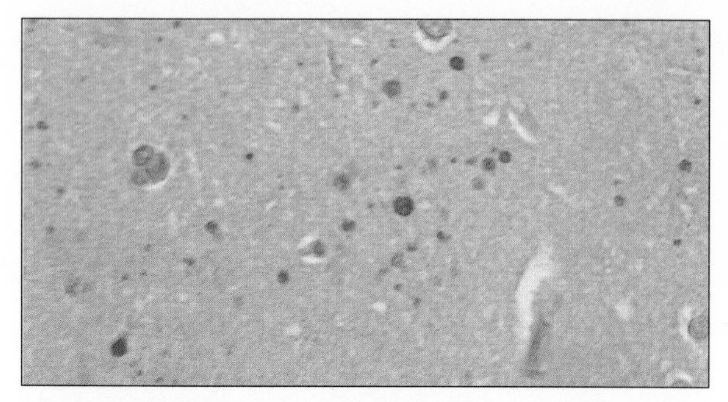

Fig. 3.169 Down's syndrome. Scattered granular ubiquitin immunoreactive material within diffuse amyloid plaques in a 37-year-old woman with Down's syndrome. *(Anti-ubiquitin × 400.)*

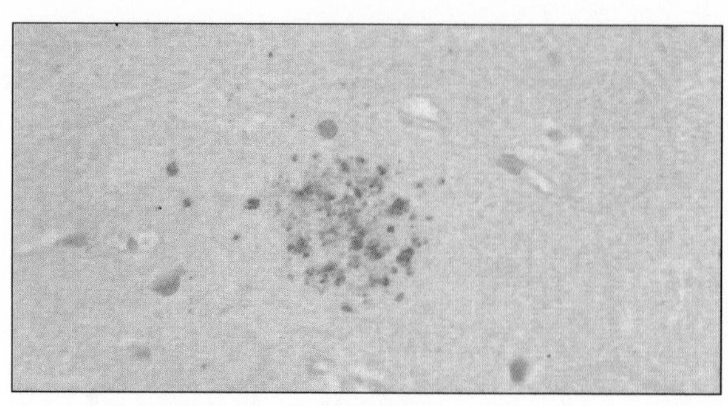

Fig. 3.170 Down's syndrome. More concentrated granular ubiquitin immunoreactive material within diffuse amyloid plaques in a 37-year-old womanwith Down's syndrome. *(Anti-ubiquitin × 400.)*

Time course of pathological events in Alzheimer's disease

In Down's syndrome there is a variable transitional period of about 20–40 years during which the complete absence of Alzheimer-related pathology changes into a universal and entirely typical presence of such features. The predictability of this association means that a longitudinal time course of pathological events associated with the onset and progress of Alzheimer's disease in such individuals can be 'reconstructed' from cross-sectional data obtained from patients dying at different ages. A clear order to the acquisition of Alzheimer-type changes in Down's syndrome is then evident (**Fig. 3.163**).

- First, it seems to start during the second or third decade with the deposition of β/A4 protein as diffuse plaques (**Figs 3.164–3.166**). These early deposits can occur widely throughout the cerebral cortex, sometimes with an emphasis in the hippocampus and amygdala. They often appear to enclose neuronal perikarya (**Fig. 3.165**), but only occasionally blood vessels (**Fig. 3.166**). The β/A4 is probably produced by local neu-

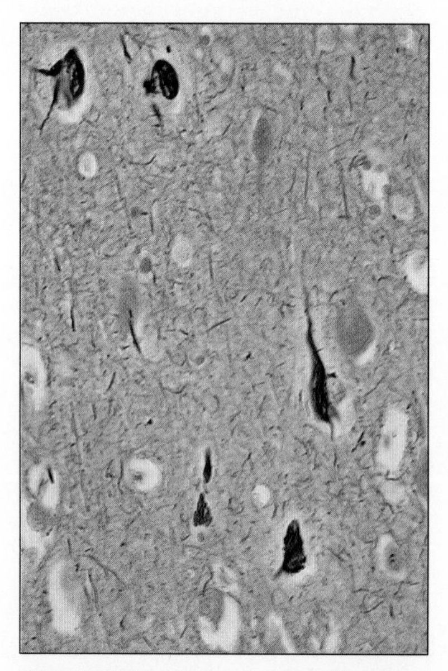

Fig. 3.171 Down's syndrome. Neurofibrillary tangles in the entorhinal cortex of a 37-year-old woman with Down's syndrome. *(Palmgren silver stain × 200.)*

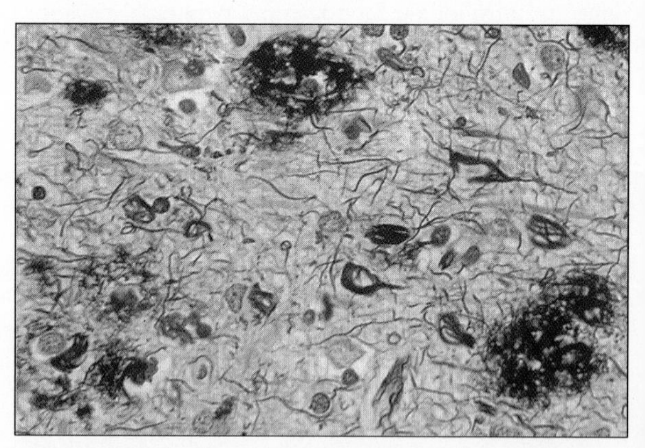

Fig. 3.172 Down's syndrome. Typical Alzheimer-type changes in the subiculum of the hippocampus in a 56-year-old man with Down's syndrome. *(Methenamine silver × 200.)*

rones. Initially, these deposits do not seem to be associated with other pathological changes (**Fig. 3.167**) other than Apolipoprotein E immunoreactivity and proteoglycan though many soon contain microglial cells (**Fig. 3.168**) and granular ubiquitinated deposits (**Figs 3.169** and **3.170**), the latter probably within enlarged neuronal terminals. The presence of both these features increases with time (see **Fig. 3.163**).

- Next, 'neuritic' amyloid deposits with cores and silver-, tau-, or PHF-positive neurites appear, but only after 40–50 years of age. Such plaques also contain GFAP positive astrocyctes and their processes. At this same time tangles can be seen within nerve cell perikarya, initially within the hippocampus (area CA1), and particularly the parahippocampal gyrus (entorhinal cortex) (**Fig. 3.171**), and amygdala.
- Later, in people over 50 years of age, tangles become widespread throughout the neocortex and subcortex, and at this time the full pathological picture of Alzheimer's disease is usually firmly established (**Fig. 3.172**).

Amyloid deposits usually occur in the cerebellum of most, but not all, patients after 40 years of age, although, as in Alzheimer's disease itself, these are never associated with a neuritic change. By 50 years of age there is nothing in pathological terms to differentiate fully developed Down's syndrome from Alzheimer's disease. In addition, many people with pathologically early Alzheimer's disease, as well as other mentally alert and/or mildly impaired elderly persons, show a pathology identical to that seen in younger Down's individuals. It therefore seems safe to conclude that the pattern of development of the pathological changes of Alzheimer's disease in people with Down's syndrome closely mirrors that occurring in the general population. However, there are notable time differences.

- In Down's syndrome there is a prolonged 'prodromal' period of diffuse amyloid deposition followed by a more 'aggressive' neurofibrillary degeneration with the whole process taking some 30–40 years to complete.
- In the general population the time scale is compressed into 10–15 years or much less.

This difference is probably a reflection of the varying aetiologies underlying and driving the common pathogenetic mechanism behind each clinical setting.

Spread of disease

Analysis of the distribution of pathological changes in the brains of younger individuals with Down's syndrome and in non-demented or mildly demented people in the general population points towards several conclusions about the sites of formation of the lesions.

- Deposition of β/A4 can occur in any part of the cerebral cortex, although the first appearance is in greatest quantities usually in the temporal lobe, and sometimes in the amygdala and parts of the hippocampus in particular.
- Such amyloid deposits clearly predate the appearance of neurofibrillary tangles and neuritic plaques.
- Neurofibrillary tangles are initially and invariably present within layer II stellate neurones of the entorhinal cortex and within area CA1 of the hippocampus. Neocortical tangles appear later and then become numerous.
- Neuritic plaques parallel the presence of neurofibrillary tangles, being present first in the hippocampus and amygdala, and later in the neocortex.

These observations strongly suggest that there is an ordered 'spread' of disease, possibly along connecting pathways, starting in the temporal lobe, perhaps in the medial structures of the hippocampus, parahippocampus and amygdala. Why such areas should be preferentially affected is not clear. At one time it was widely suggested that it was due to the connections of these particular regions with the outside world, via the olfactory tract, allowing an early access of pathogens to these brain areas; the presence of tangles and abnormal tau proteins in olfactory nuclei and nasal mucosa provided strong evidence for this view. However, recent observations of a particularly high expression of APP by neurones in these medial temporal lobe regions may provide an alternative explanation, when using the 'amyloid hypothesis' of the disease.

The net effect of the early hippocampal lesions is to disrupt the influx and outflow of information to and from this part of the brain, thereby isolating it and precipitating the disruption of memory processes central to the development and clinical progression of the disease.

Pathogenetic considerations

In Down's syndrome it is clear that a deposition of β/A4 protein is probably the first (so far)

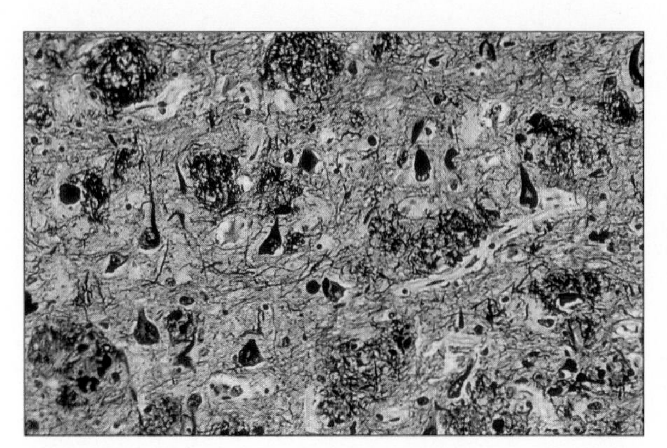

Fig. 3.173 Missense mutation. Typical pathology of Alzheimer's disease in the hippocampus of a 61-year-old woman with a missense mutation (valine→glycine) at codon 717 of the APP gene. *(Methenamine silver stain × 200.)*

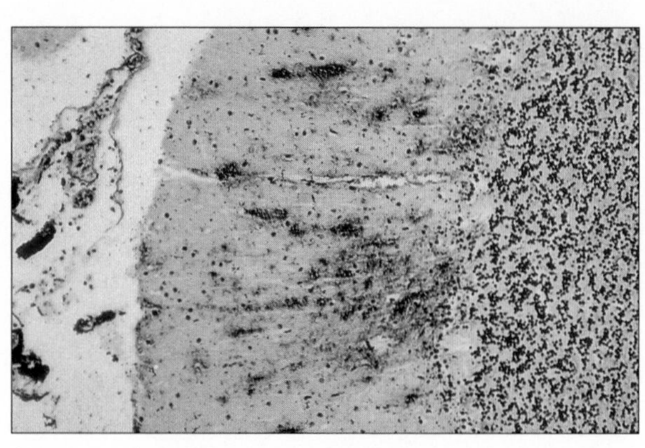

Fig. 3.174 Missense mutation. Typical amyloid deposits in the cerebellum of the patient featured in **Fig.3.173**. *(Methenamine silver stain × 200.)*

detectable histopathological change associated with the onset and progress of Alzheimer's disease. How this is brought about is not clear, but is presumably related to the duplication of the APP gene in such trisomic individuals. The overexpression of this gene may lead to a small, but prolonged, excess of APP, this ultimately being catabolized into β/A4.

In Alzheimer's disease, as in the general population, there is no duplication of the APP gene. It is also unlikely that any major overexpression of APP takes place in those families where mutations, in the APP gene on chromosome 21 have been identified (i.e. at codons 670/671 and 717). However, it is possible that there may be a faulty APP species that is overproduced or preferentially metabolized along pathways leading to β/A4 deposition and typical subsequent histopathology (**Figs 3.173** and **3.174**). Other families with Alzheimer's disease who do not apparently display any defect in the APP gene, may have an (as yet unidentified) affected locus on chromosome 14 or 22 that could interplay with the APP gene or regulate APP metabolism and where alterations may again impair normal APP function.

How the allelic variation on chromosome 19 for Apolipoprotein E might fit into the pathogenetic process is not clear. The E4 allele binds to βA4 protein much more avidly than the E3 allele. Moreover, in persons with Alzheimer's disease possessing two copies of the E4 allele there seems to be more βA4 deposited in the brain than in those persons homozygous for E3. Hence Apolipoprotein E4 may bind more vigorously to the *normally produced* and *soluble* form of βA4 rendering it *insoluble* and capable of becoming 'organized' into amyloid deposits. The cysteine→arginine change at position 112 producing a change in charge in the Apo E4 molecule may facilitate this. Apolipoprotein E immunoreactivity is always present in amyloid deposits, even in the youngest cases of Down's syndrome where βA4 deposition is the only histopathological change (see page 60). Subsequent binding to the amyloid/Apo E complex by amyloid P and proteoglycan may further stabilize the structure by a β-pleating mechanism, although whether such an interaction can influence the appearance of neuritic and neurofibrillary changes is not known. The relative lack of E2 (especially) and E3 alleles may contribute by promoting a 'destabilization' of tau thereby favouring neurofibrillary degeneration; E2 and E3 forms can bind to the microtubule binding domain of tau whereas E4 cannot.

Although the cause of Alzheimer's disease is apparently non-genetic (or at least no genetic defect has as yet been detected) for most patients, it cannot be assumed that an environmental or external cause is wholly responsible, although this may be the case. Cases of late onset *sporadic* disease, like late onset inherited disease show increased Apolipoprotein E4 allele frequency and in both these situations a similar pathogenic mechanism may operate. Nonetheless, it is well known that some of the pathological changes of Alzheimer's disease can be induced through head trauma due to sporting (boxing) injuries or an

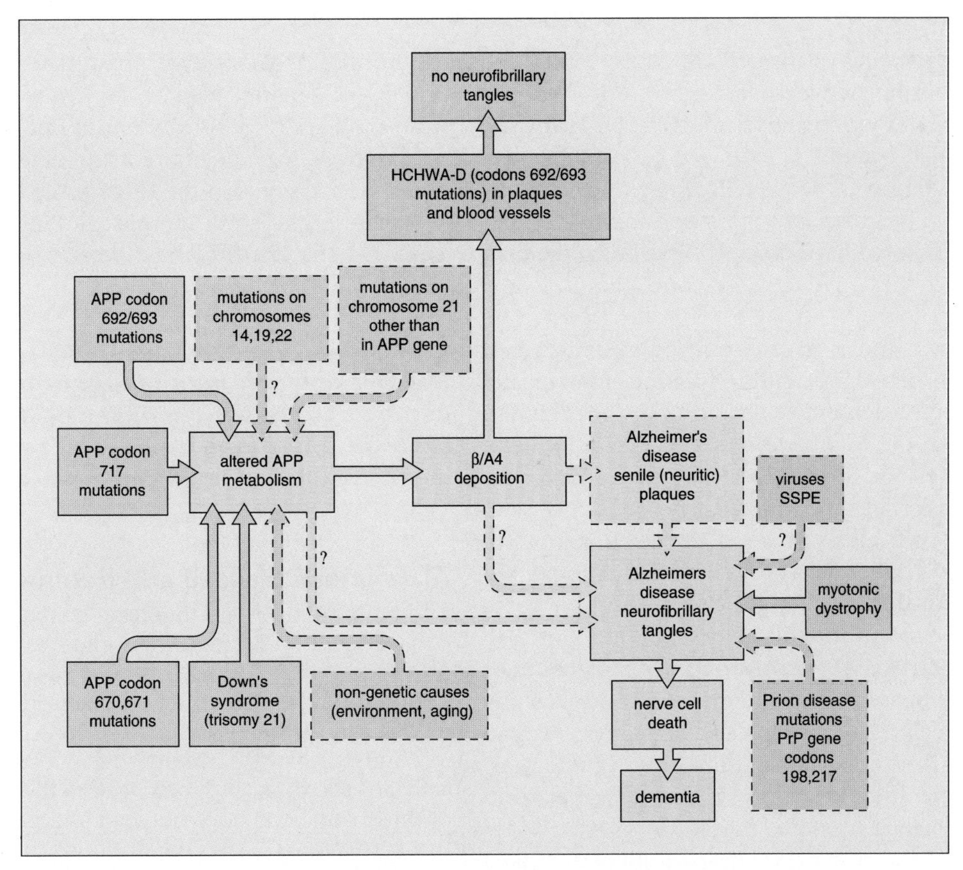

Fig. 3.175 Pathogenetic pathways in Alzheimer's disease. Diagram of possible pathogenetic pathways in Alzheimer's disease associated with the 'amyloid hypothesis'.

accident (i.e. closed head injury). Indeed, there are people with post-traumatic amnesia resembling typical Alzheimer's disease (see page 66). Metabolic stress, for example, due to chronic renal dialysis, can also induce β/A4 deposition (see page 70).

The so-called 'amyloid hypothesis' of Alzheimer's disease reconciles the pathological changes of the disease and Down's syndrome (**Fig. 3.175**), and postulates that a 'mismetabolism' of APP may be the crucial unifying event driving a common pathological process in all the aetiological variants (see **Fig. 3.158**). Although tangle formation is linked temporally to β/A4 amyloid deposition in both Alzheimer's disease and Down's syndrome, it is still not clear whether the two events are causally related with β/A4 deposition directly driving changes that culminate in tangle formation. The fact that both pathologies can occur widely and separately in other situations (see **Fig. 3.175**) implies that both may reflect the end-products of separate neurodegenerative events. Extensive amyloid deposition in the absence of tangles can occur in the cerebellum (especially) and striatum, and that the same β/A4 associated with Alzheimer's disease can occur widely in the cortex in the absence of tangles in disorders other than Alzheimer's disease and Down's syndrome, arguing strongly against a direct toxic action of β/A4 upon nerve cells. In Alzheimer's disease and Down's syndrome the primary aetiological events may predispose towards both pathologies, an apparent temporal progression from one stage into another perhaps reflecting differing 'time lags' in the induction of each change.

Clinico-pathological correlations

Although the presence of many neuritic plaques and neurofibrillary tangles in the cerebral cortex can be regarded as the tissue hallmark of Alzheimer's disease, the relevance of these features to the underlying pathophysiological production of dementia is less certain.

The early studies of Blessed and Roth emphasised the relationship between senile (neuritic) plaques and the degree of cognitive impairment. However, mentally able controls with few or no plaques were included along with demented persons with numerous lesions. It is therefore not surprising that such a correlation should have emerged. Excluding the controls, in this study, reduced the correlation to below significance level.

Many later studies have also failed to draw a firm correlation between (neuritic) plaque number and the degree of dementia. In addition, the 'amyloid load' within the brain, expressed either in terms of (amyloid) plaque density or in the proportion of tissue occupied, fails to correlate. The density of neurofibrillary tangles has been shown to correlate (weakly) with the degree of dementia in some, but not all, studies. Investigations of human cerebrospinal fluid to identify excess amounts of PHF protein, β/A4 or APP in patients with Alzheimer's disease compared to non-demented controls show group differences, but individual variation is marked and there is no clear relationship between the presence or the amount of any of these markers and clinical dementia.

Probably the best correlations between clinical change and any pathological markers have emerged when the density of cortical pyramidal neurones or synapses have been considered. This is clearly not an unreasonable expectation because it is possible to measure these features reliably and to estimate their cumulative loss from the tissue over the duration of the disease with reasonable accuracy. There is some 'turnover' of plaques and tangles, albeit slow, and so the actual density of each at any one time changes according to the balance struck between the rate of formation and removal. It is not possible, therefore, to estimate reliably the total number of plaques or tangles that may have accrued over the whole course of the illness.

Since the site of production of dementia probably lies at the synapse, more direct measures of synaptic failure (density of remaining synapses or neurones) would (as is the case) relate better to clinical dementia. Most neurotransmitter markers as indices of synaptic activity show a weak correlation with increasing dementia, but—given the widespread involvement of many different though integrated systems in the disease (i.e. cholinergic, noradrenergic, serotonergic, glutamatergic systems)— there is no 'best way' to predict the extent of dementia.

The *presence of many plaques and tangles* can be a *diagnostic marker of Alzheimer's disease*, but *quantity does not predict the degree* of clinical impairment.

Alzheimer's disease and trauma

The brain may sustain traumatic damage either as a consequence of a single episodic event (e.g. a fall or a road traffic accident) or as a result of multiple periodic blows, which may be self-inflicted, as in mental illness 'head-bashing', or inflicted by others in connection with criminal behaviour or sporting activities (boxing). If the damage to the brain in any of these situations does not lead to a prompt fatality the patient will survive, but often with some residual functional or cognitive deficiency, depending on the localisation and extent of the damage and the likelihood of continuing trauma. Alzheimer's disease has been linked epidemiologically with a single previous traumatic event. Post-traumatic amnesia with the pathology of Alzheimer's disease is well documented: the characteristic senile plaques and neurofibrillary tangles of Alzheimer's disease are present, in form, number, and distribution similar to those seen in Alzheimer's disease not associated with a history of head trauma. Such cases are, however, rare. While it is not proven that the original traumatic event caused the Alzheimer's disease, it may 'trigger' its onset at an earlier age in an individual in whom Alzheimer's disease might have developed spontaneously later in life.

Deposits of β/A4 protein, which are sometimes massive, in the form of diffuse plaques can commonly appear in the brain following survival after

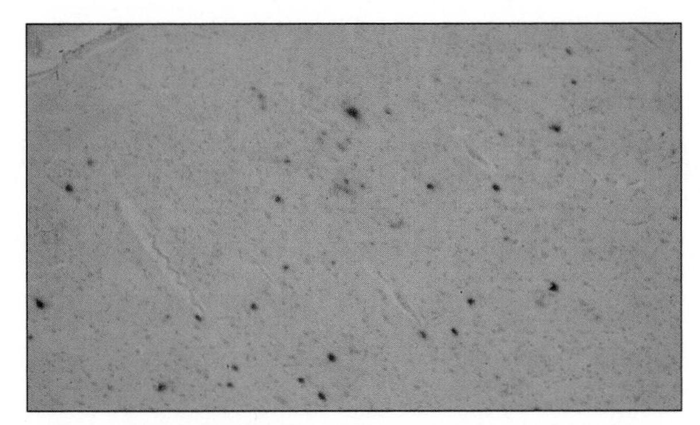

Fig. 3.176 Head injury. Diffuse deposits of β/A4 protein in the cerebral cortex of a patient who survived 10 days after a head injury. *(Anti-β/A4 × 40.) (Courtesy of Dr G. W. Roberts.)*

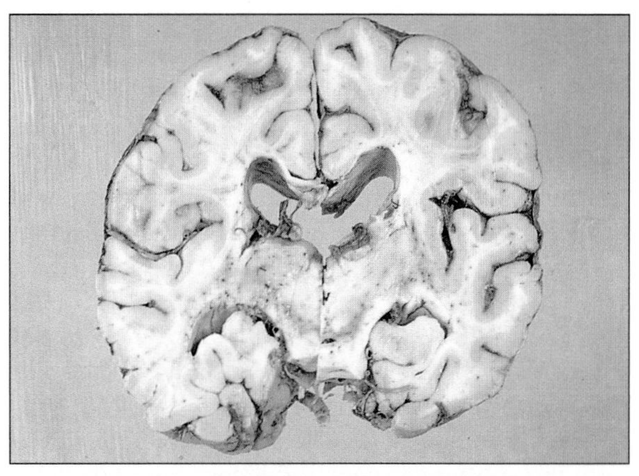

Fig. 3.177 Chronic traumatic encephalopathy. In chronic traumatic encephalopathy (due to boxing) the brain shows enlargement of the lateral ventricles, thinning of the corpus callosum, and tearing of the septum pellucidum.

a head injury (**Fig. 3.176**). These occasionally present within days or weeks of the event. Like the diffuse plaques of Alzheimer's disease, these deposits are not associated with a neuritic change and cannot be detected by routine histological procedures; isolated neurofibrillary tangles are only occasionally present.

Multiple and repeated sublethal blows to the head, as in boxing, lead to a different pathological picture and the clinical entity of dementia pugilistica –the 'punch-drunk' syndrome. This is, essentially, a subcortical dementia with dysarthria, ataxia and Parkinsonism, and a characteristic pattern of brain damage.

The principal macroscopic features are an enlargement of the lateral ventricles and the cavum of the septum pellucidum, often with fenestration (**Figs 3.177** and **3.178**). The fornices and the corpus callosum may be thinned (see **Fig. 3.178**), the cerebellum may be atrophied, and the locus caeruleus (**Fig. 3.179**) and substantia nigra may be grossly underpigmented. There is dilatation of the IV ventricle (see **Fig. 3.179**).

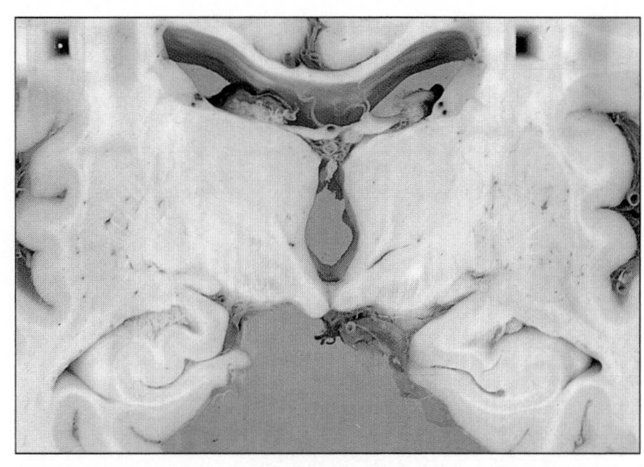

Fig. 3.178 Chronic traumatic encephalopathy. Enlargement of the cavum of the septum pellucidum in chronic traumatic encephalopathy. There is also enlargement of the III ventricle.

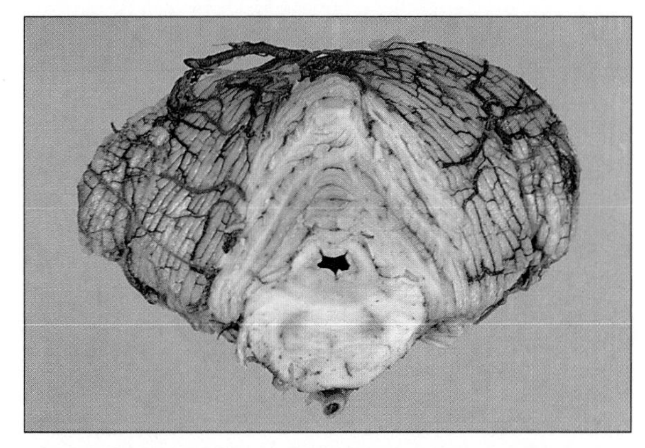

Fig. 3.179 Chronic traumatic encephalopathy. Depigmentation of the locus caeruleus with dilatation of the IV ventricle.

Again, massive diffuse deposits of β/A4 protein may be present in the cortex, often with a patchy distribution favouring the crowns of the gyri (**Figs 3.180** and **3.181**). Few, if any, of these deposits have a neuritic component and although numerous neurofibrillary tangles are usually widespread in the brain, especially in medial temporal (**Fig. 3.182**) and entorhinal cortex (**Fig. 3.183**), these are not necessarily always in the areas of β/A4 deposition. Tangle-bearing cells are also widespread outside the cortex, particularly in the midbrain and brainstem regions (**Figs 3.184–3.186**) where there is a severe loss of cells, especially from the substantia nigra and locus caeruleus.

The tangles are ultrastructurally identical to those in Alzheimer's disease, consisting of PHF, and are similarly immunoreactive with tau antisera (**Fig. 3.187**). Axonal spheroids are widespread in white matter tracts and contain large amounts of APP (**Fig. 3.188**). Deposition of β/A4 protein may be part of a 'stress' reaction in neurones and induced by trauma and other aetiological insults. Neurofibrillary tangle formation and axonal spheroids may result from the damage imposed by the stretching and shearing of nerve fibres generated by rotational forces set up by the blow to the head. It is notable that the 'dementia' of dementia pugilistica is progressive and continues in retired boxers where there is no exposure to further trauma. This contrasts with episodic (i.e. acute with partial recovery) trauma (**Fig. 3.189**) in which there is a non-progressive deficit.It is clear that both of the unusual proteins (βA4 and tau) that accumulate in the brain in Alzheimer's disease can also appear relatively quickly in the brain following trauma and other damage (e.g. ischaemia and infarction). The appearance of βA4 may relate to an upregulation of APP expression due to tissue injury (since APP is postulated to play a role in cellular repair). However, whether there is a definite aetiological linkage between such a short-term increase in APP expression and a chronic damage to the brain sustained many years later is uncertain.

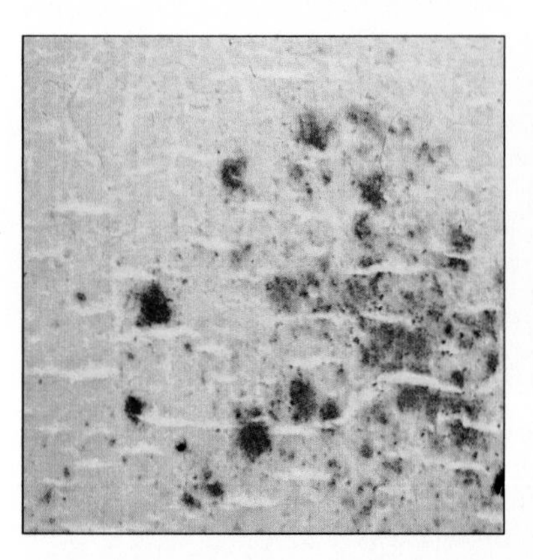

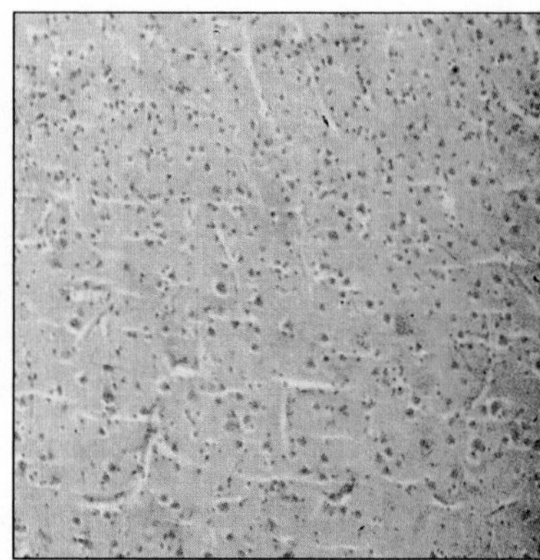

Fig. 3.180 (left) Chronic traumatic encephalopathy. Deposition of β/A4 protein as diffuse plaques. *(Anti-β/A4 × 100.) (Courtesy of Dr G. W. Roberts.)*

Fig. 3.181 Chronic traumatic encephalopathy. Deposition of β/A4 protein as diffuse plaques. These do not stain with Congo red. *(Congo red × 100.) (Courtesy of Dr G. W. Roberts.)*

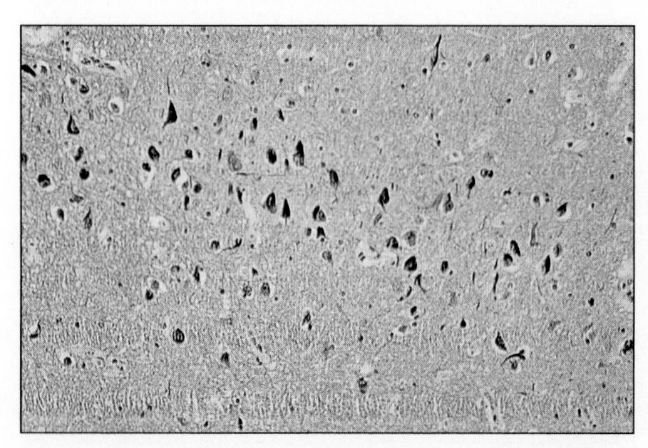

Fig. 3.182 Chronic traumatic encephalopathy. Neurofibrillary tangles in pyramidal neurones of the temporal cortex. *(Bielschowsky silver stain × 100.)*

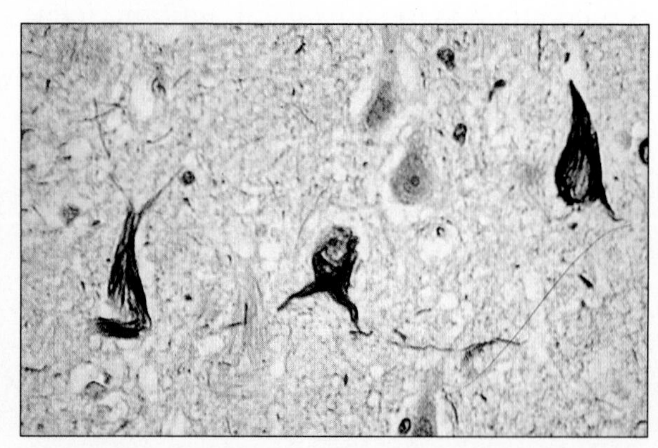

Fig. 3.183 Chronic traumatic encephalopathy. Neurofibrillary tangles in pyramidal cells in the entorhinal cortex. *(Bielschowsky silver stain × 400.)*

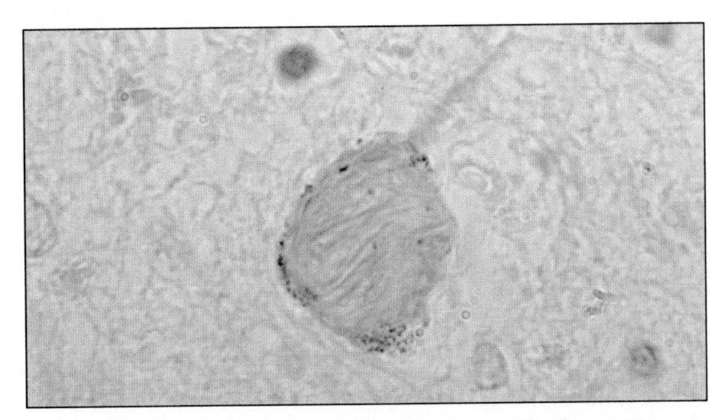

Fig. 3.184 Chronic traumatic encephalopathy. A neurofibrillary tangle in the substantia nigra. *(Nissl stain × 400.)*

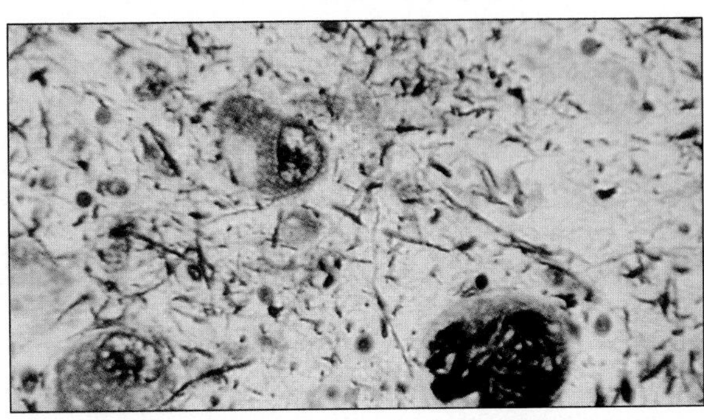

Fig. 3.185 Chronic traumatic encephalopathy. A neurofibrillary tangle in the locus caeruleus. *(Bielschowsky silver stain × 400.)*

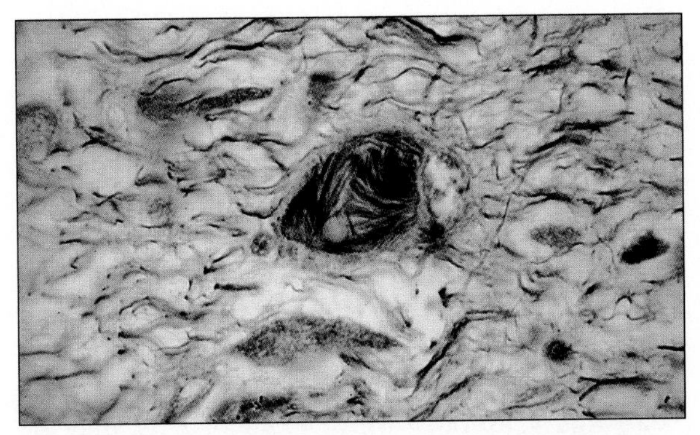

Fig. 3.186 Chronic traumatic encephalopathy. A neurofibrillary tangle in the pontine nuclei. *(Bielschowsky silver stain × 400.)*

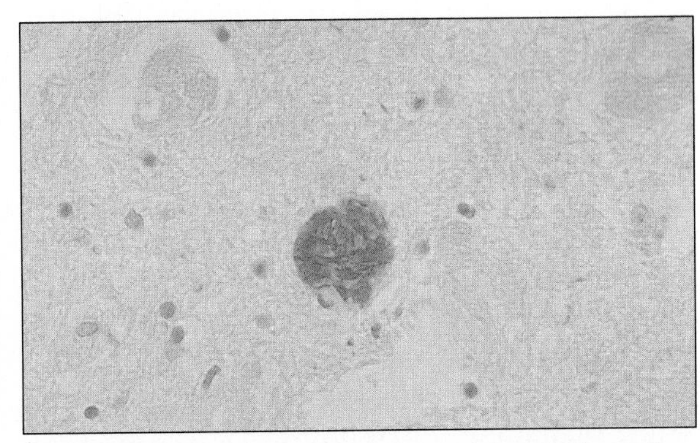

Fig. 3.187 Chronic traumatic encephalopathy. Neurofibrillary tangles containing tau protein. *(Anti-tau × 400.)*

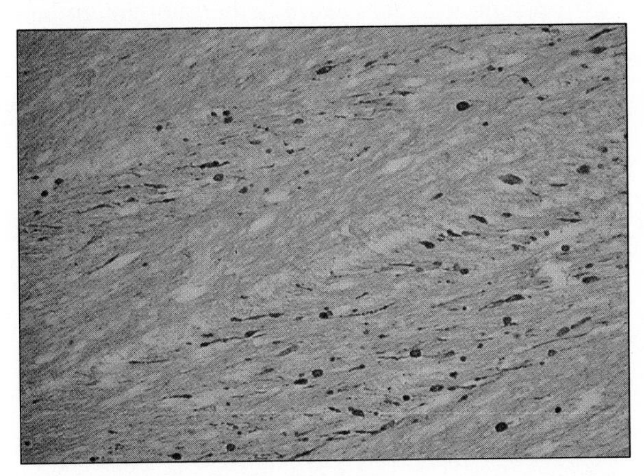

Fig. 3.188 Chronic traumatic encephalopathy. Axonal spheroids in white matter tracts containing large amounts of APP. *(Anti-APP × 200.) (Courtesy of Dr G. W. Roberts.)*

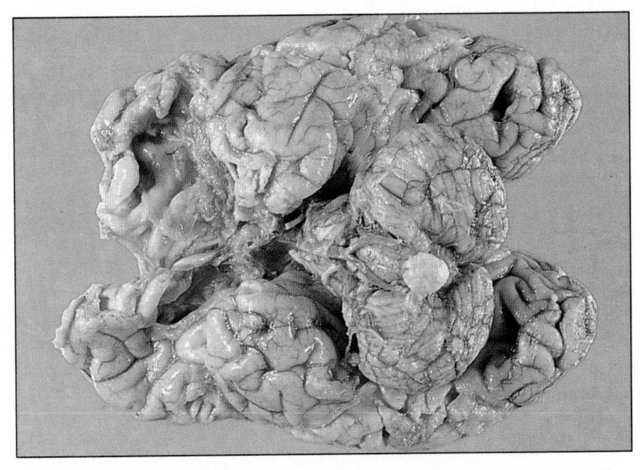

Fig. 3.189 Trauma. An old traumatic injury to the frontal lobes of a 34-year-old man after a fall 15 years previously. No amyloid deposits or tangles were present in the surviving brain tissue.

Alzheimer's disease and aluminium

A role for aluminium in the aetiology of Alzheimer's disease has long been postulated. The finding of excessive aluminium within the cores of senile plaques (see **Fig. 3.32**) in Alzheimer's disease and Down's syndrome lends weight to this hypothesis. Perhaps the best known neurotoxic action of aluminium in humans relates to its effects on patients undergoing prolonged dialysis for chronic renal disease, some of whom developed a dementing condition known as 'dialysis dementia' or 'dialysis encephalopathy'.

Dialysis encephalopathy is a progressive form of dementia in patients undergoing chronic renal dialysis. It is characterised by speech difficulty, myoclonus and epilepsy and is caused by high circulating levels of aluminium with high brain concentrations brought about by the use of aluminium hydroxide in the dialysate; recognition now precludes such use. Nonetheless, many people were exposed to the neurotoxic effects of aluminium in this way and many still survive to live with the consequences. Discontinued exposure leads to a (partial) reversal of the symptoms.

No specific pathological changes, particularly senile plaques and neurofibrillary tangles, have been detected in the brains of patients dying with dialysis encephalopathy, which in Alzheimer's disease have been associated with an increased aluminium content. It has been observed recently that many, but not all, patients have numerous deposits of β/A4 protein in the form of diffuse plaques within the cerebral cortex (**Fig. 3.190**).

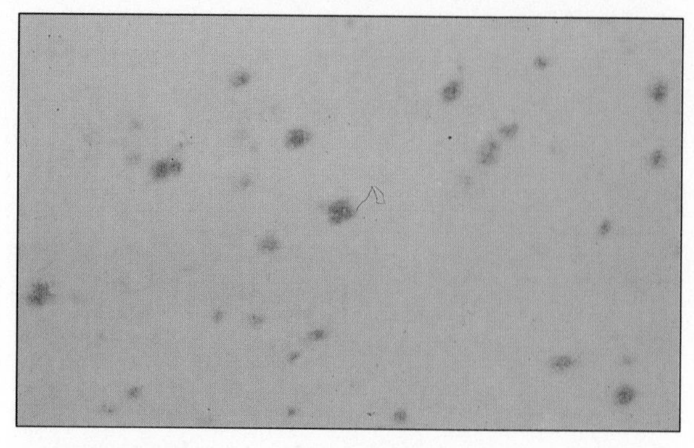

Fig. 3.190 Chronic renal dialysis. Diffuse deposits of β/A4 amyloid protein in the cerebral cortex in chronic renal dialysis. *(Anti-β/A4 × 100.) (Courtesy of Professor J. A. Edwardson.)*

Such deposits occur in the absence of neuritic changes, and neurofibrillary tangles in neurones are not seen. Although the numbers of diffuse deposits exceed the numbers that might be expected to occur through 'ageing' alone, their relevance to the clinical picture of the disorder and their relationship to the high (if transient) brain levels of aluminium are not known. As in acute head injury, deposition of β/A4 protein may be part of a 'stress reaction' within the tissue in which the amyloid precursor APP is upregulated and ultimately catabolized into β/A4 protein.

At present, it is not clear whether aluminium has a causative role in the pathogenesis of Alzheimer's disease or whether its presence (in plaques) is epiphenomenal.

LOBAR ATROPHY

Fronto-temporal atrophy of non-Alzheimer type

Cerebral atrophy of the fronto-temporal lobes is a highly familial disorder. It shows a range of histopathological features distinct from those of Alzheimer's disease, and manifests as three major clinical syndromes (see **Fig. 1.3**), these being determined by the anatomical distribution of the pathology.

- Symmetrical involvement, predominantly of the frontal lobes, leads to the syndrome of fronto-temporal dementia.
- Asymmetrical disease of the dominant cerebral hemisphere or temporal lobes produces the syndrome of progressive aphasia.
- The amyotrophic form of motor neurone disease is associated with fronto-temporal atrophy and can complicate both these clinical syndromes.

Demographic features of fronto-temporal dementia

Fronto-temporal dementia is probably the second most common form of early onset dementia after Alzheimer's disease, the ratio of occurrence between the two being 1:4–1:10.

The onset of fronto-temporal dementia nearly always occurs before 65 years of age (usually 45–65) and men and women are affected equally. Its duration is often protracted and is commonly 10–15 years.

About 50% of patients have a family history of a similar disorder in a first degree relative, and the condition is probably inherited in an autosomal dominant fashion. Because of survival effects and clinical unawareness of the disorder apparently sporadic cases may be familial.

Linkage studies within extended families proven to be affected by fronto-temporal dementia have only just begun. As yet, no genes have been identified in its aetiology.

Presenile presentation
Familial

Psychological symptoms
Personal and social misconduct (early)
Mutism (late)

Neurological signs
Frontal release signs (early)
Akinesia and rigidity (late)

Investigations
EEG: normal
SPET: fronto-temporal lobe abnormality

Gross changes of lobar atrophy in fronto-temporal dementia

On CT imaging prototypical patients with fronto-temporal dementia show a bilateral generalised atrophy with fronto-temporal emphasis and dilatation of the lateral ventricles anteriorly (**Fig. 3.191**). The temporal lobes are atrophic and the temporal horns of the lateral ventricles are enlarged (see **Fig. 3.191**).

SPET imaging demonstrates a reduced tracer uptake bilaterally within the frontal lobes (**Fig. 3.192**), although sometimes there may be a greater involvement on the left side.

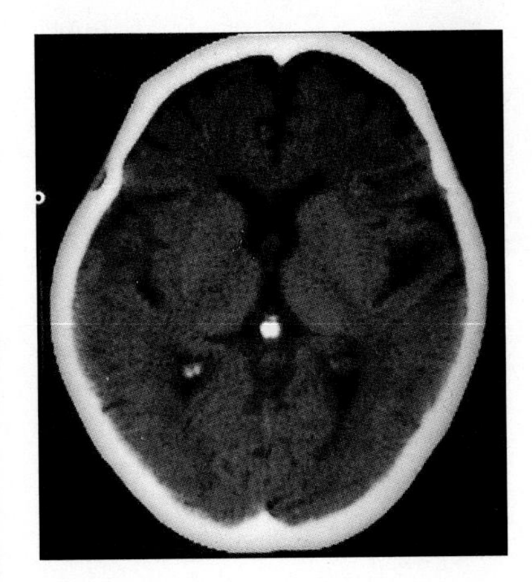

Fig. 3.191 (left) Bilateral atrophy of the frontal and anterior temporal lobes with dilatation of the lateral ventricles. CT scan of a 58-year-old woman. Note the preservation of the basal ganglia and the posterior hemisphere.

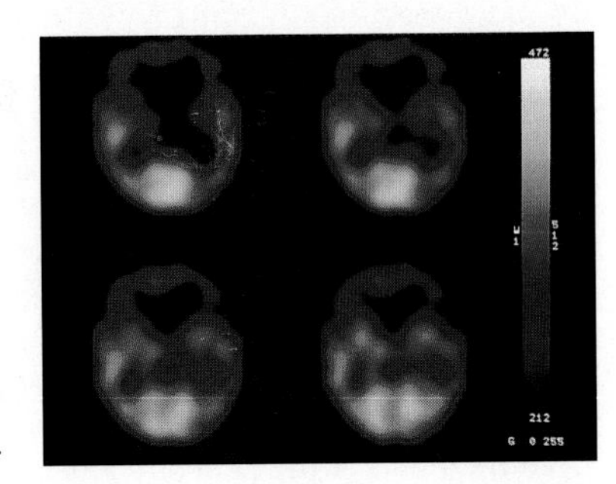

Fig. 3.192 (right) Characteristic bilateral frontal hypometabolism. SPET imaging of the brain of a 73-year-old woman.

At autopsy the brain shows a gross weight loss, often being reduced to less than 1000 g. Atrophy is severe within the frontal lobes (**Fig. 3.193**), the fronto-parietal cortex, cingulate gyrus (**Fig. 3.194**) and the temporal pole (see **Fig. 3.193**), where the gyri frequently adopt a narrow 'knife-edge' appearance. Characteristically, in comparison to the other temporal gyri, the superior temporal gyrus is conspicuously spared (see **Fig. 3.193**). Other cortical regions are less affected and the brain stem and cerebellum often appear normal or are only mildly shrunken.

When the brain is sliced coronally (**Figs 3.195** and **3.196**), there is obvious cortical atrophy within the frontal and temporal lobes. The anterior two-thirds of the temporal lobe are more atrophied than the posterior one-third, and there is relative sparing of the superior temporal gyrus, especially posteriorly (see **Figs 3.195** and **3.196**). The white matter often, but not always, loses much myelin and becomes brown and softened, and the anatomical distinction between grey and white matter, especially in severely atrophic regions, becomes less distinct (see **Fig. 3.195**). Usually, the amygdaloid nucleus is severely atrophied (see **Figs 3.195** and **3.196**), although the hippocampus is variably affected, often apparently being spared (see **Figs 3.195** and **3.196**). The temporal horn extension of the lateral ventricle is much enlarged, as is the lateral ventricle itself (see **Figs 3.195** and **3.196**). The corpus striatum and other basal structures appear smaller than usual (see **Fig. 3.195**), but without any major conformational change. The corpus callosum is thinned at all levels (see **Figs 3.195** and **3.196**), but especially anteriorly, as is the anterior commissure.

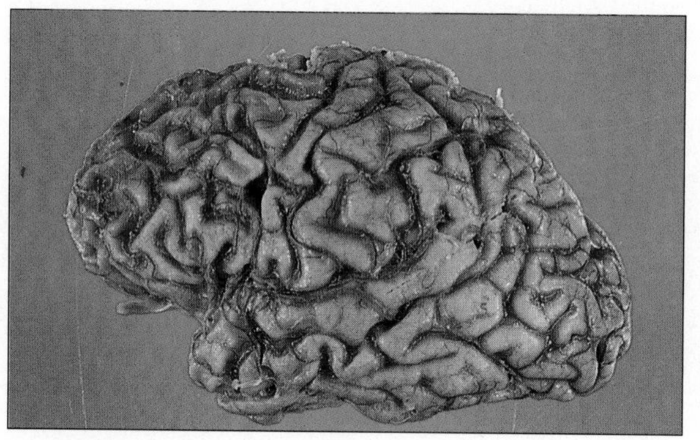

Fig. 3.193 Marked atrophy of frontal and anterior temporal lobes. Lateral view of the brain of a 69-year-old woman. This patient showed a Pick's disease type of histology.

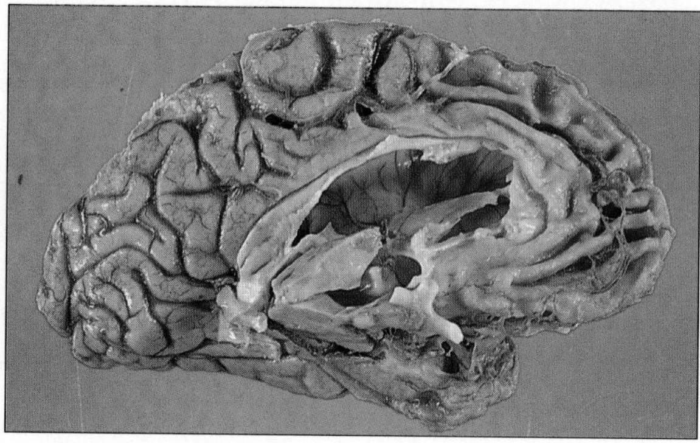

Fig. 3.194 Medial view of the brain of the patient featured in Fig. 3.193

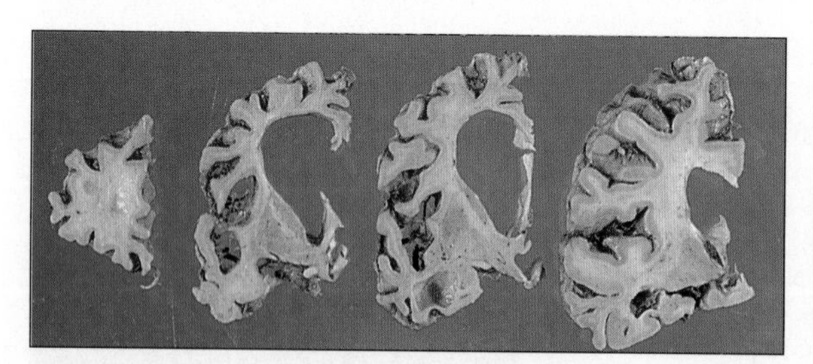

Fig. 3.195 Gross fronto-temporal atrophy involving the amygdala, but relatively sparing the hippocampus and superior temporal gyrus. Coronal slices taken from the brain of the patient featured in **Figs 3.193** and **3.194**. There is gross ventricular dilatation, thinning of the corpus callosum, and striatal atrophy.

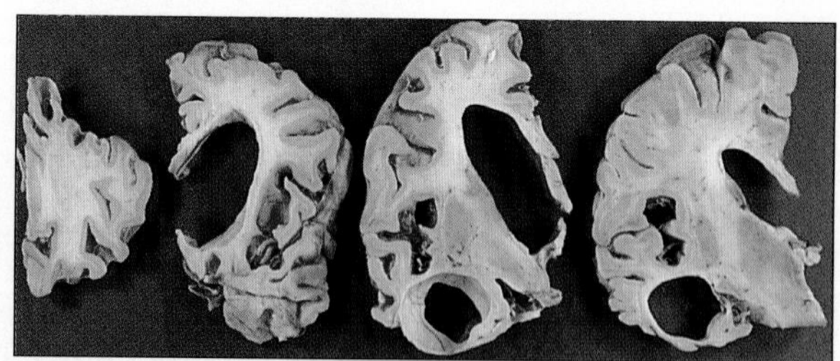

Fig. 3.196 Gross involvement of the temporal lobe. Coronal slices of the brain of a 62-year-old woman. Again the hippocampus and superior temporal gyrus are relatively spared.

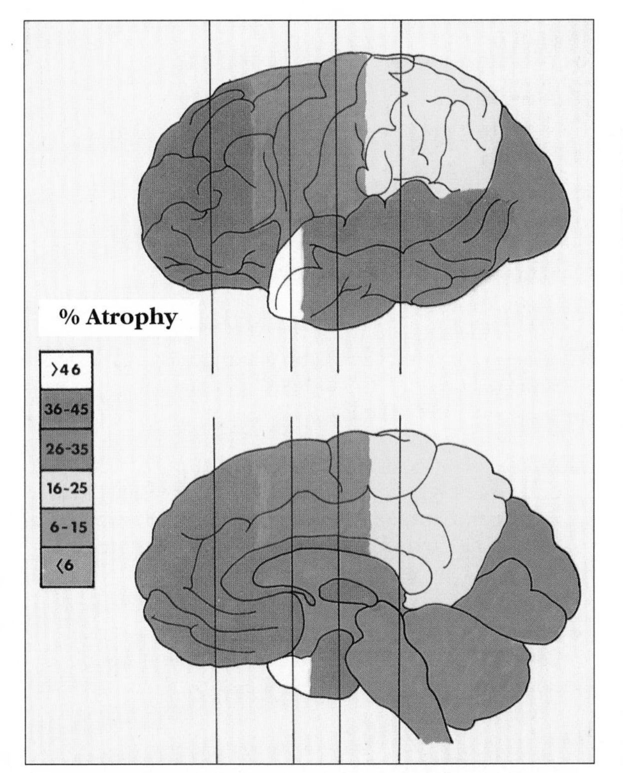

Fig. 3.197 Morphometric analysis of regional brain atrophy. Note the severe involvement of the fronto-temporal cortex.

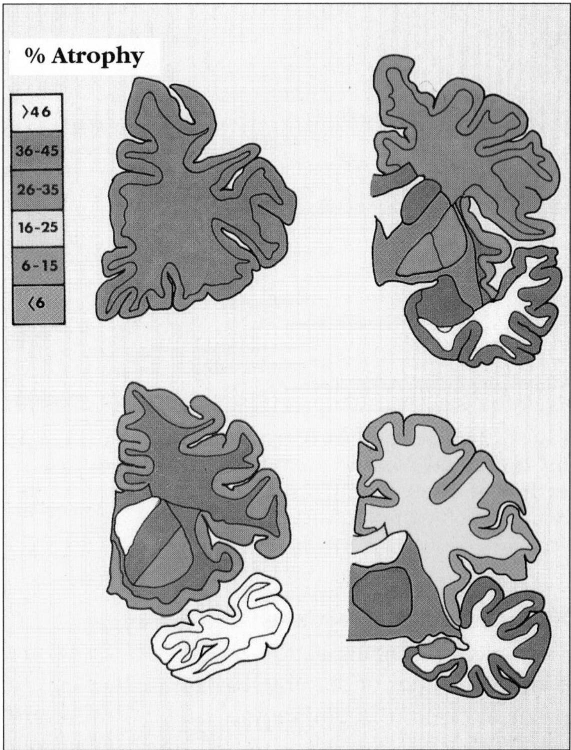

Fig. 3.198 Morphometric analysis of regional brain atrophy. The amygdala and thalamus are severely affected.

Morphometric measurements of regional brain atrophy confirm this pattern, with severely affected areas of cortex and amygdala being reduced in size by nearly 50% (**Figs 3.197** and **3.198**). In cortical regions grey and white matter are lost proportionately, leading to no major changes in the ratio between grey and white matter.

In other instances, the overall degree of atrophy is less, the brain weighing 1000–1250 g. Atrophy is then more restricted, often being confined to frontal and anterior parietal regions, with less involvement of the temporal cortex (**Figs 3.199** and **3.200**). Sometimes, there is a preferential involvement of the temporal pole and orbitofrontal cortex with relative sparing of the frontal convexity (**Fig. 3.201**).

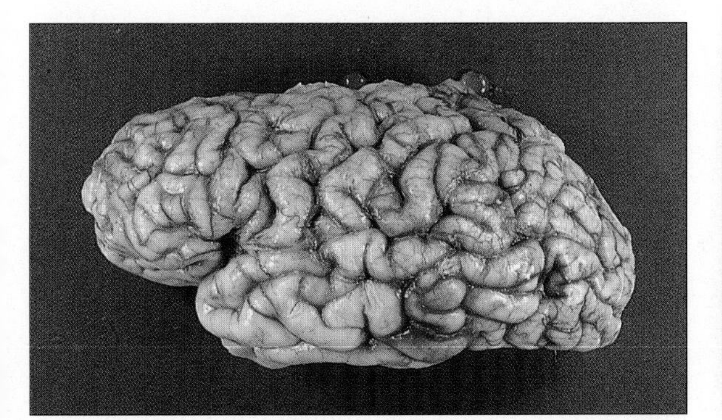

Fig. 3.199 Less pronounced atrophy of the frontal and anterior temporal regions. Lateral view of the brain of a 58-year-old man showing a microvacuolar type of cortical degeneration.

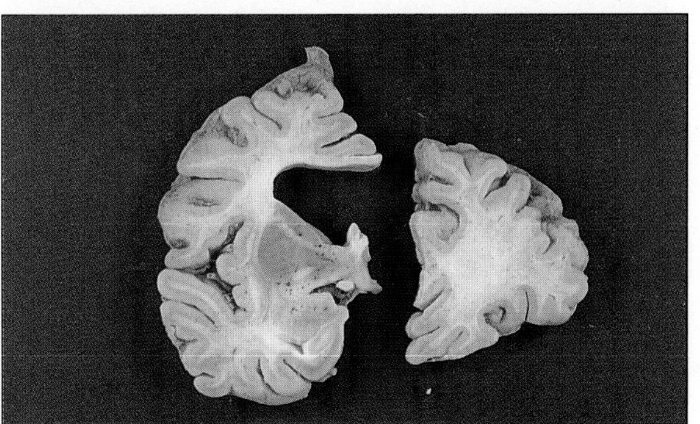

Fig. 3.200 Superior frontal and fronto-parietal atrophy, but preservation of the orbitofrontal cortex and temporal lobe. Coronal sections of the brain of the patient featured in **Fig. 3.199**.

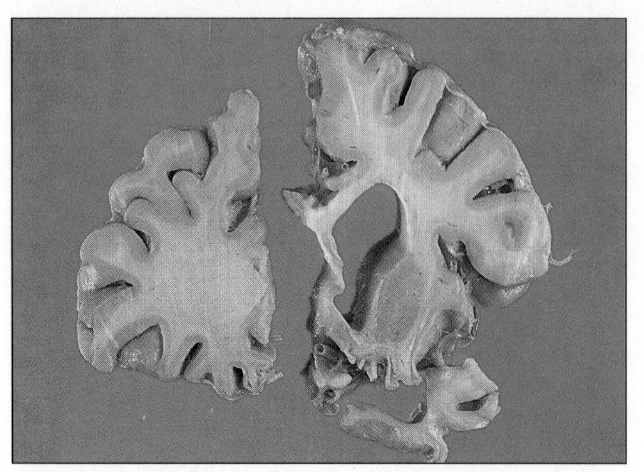

Fig. 3.201 Severe anterior temporal lobe and orbitofrontal cortical atrophy with relative preservation of other frontal areas. Coronal section of the brain of a 68-year-old man.

Age of onset
Usually 40–65 years
Sex incidence
Males and females equally affected
Duration
Usually long, often over 10 years
Gross features
Severe atrophy of frontal and anterior-temporal lobes
Ventricular dilatation anteriorly
Histopathology
- Affected cortex shows severe loss of pyramidal nerve cells, microvacuolation of outer cortical laminae and mild astrocytosis. No inclusion bodies or swollen nerve cells

Or
- Affected cortex shows severe loss of pyramidal nerve cells, severe astrocytosis with inclusion (Pick) bodies and swollen (Pick) neurones. Inclusions contain tau and ubiquitin proteins. Swollen cells react strongly with αB crystallin antibodies

Genetics
- In 50% of cases, a clear family history of a similar disorder exists, inherited probably in an autosomal dominant manner, but the genetic locus has not yet been established

Histopathological features

Two major histopathological profiles are associated with this pattern of atrophy, though neither can be predicted from the gross appearance of the brain, nor from comparisons of morphometric estimation of the degree and distribution of the atrophy. In addition, clinical assessment and neuropsychological profiling fail to discriminate between either type of pathology. Both familial and (apparently) non-familial cases are associated with either type of pathological change, though within families only a single pattern of pathology is observed.

Histological type associated with gliosis, Pick cells, and Pick bodies

In one histological type, the major changes within the neocortex consist of a severe, and often nearly complete, loss of nerve cells, especially the large pyramidal cells of layer III and the small pyramidal and non-pyramidal cells of layer II (**Fig. 3.202**). With this there is a loss of myelinated axons from the cortex (**Fig. 3.203**). Surviving nerve cells display two distinctive features.

- In one, the nerve cell (usually a pyramidal cell of layer III or V) is swollen (**Fig. 3.204**), rounded and argyrophilic (**Fig. 3.205**), and shows loss of basophilia, becoming the so-called 'ballooned' or 'Pick cell'.
- In the other, a rounded inclusion is present within the perikaryon (**Fig. 3.206**), and is well stained by silver impregnation methods (**Fig. 3.207**). These inclusions can occur in any cell in the cortex, but are often most prevalent in layer II, where nearly all cells can be affected. This change is termed the 'Pick body'.

The presence of Pick cells and Pick bodies together with a florid astrocytosis involving all cortical laminae (**Fig. 3.208**) is indicative of *Pick's disease.*

In other patients there is a similar level of astrocytosis, but without Pick cells or Pick bodies (**Fig. 3.209**).

While these histopathological changes are most prevalent within the frontal, fronto-parietal, cingulate, inferior and middle temporal gyri and the insular cortex, there is a distinctive histological sparing of the superior temporal gyrus (**Figs 3.210** and **3.211**).

Similar inclusions are present in the hippocampus, chiefly within the granular neurones of the dentate gyrus (**Fig. 3.212**), which may also exhibit a pronounced astrocytosis (**Fig. 3.213**).

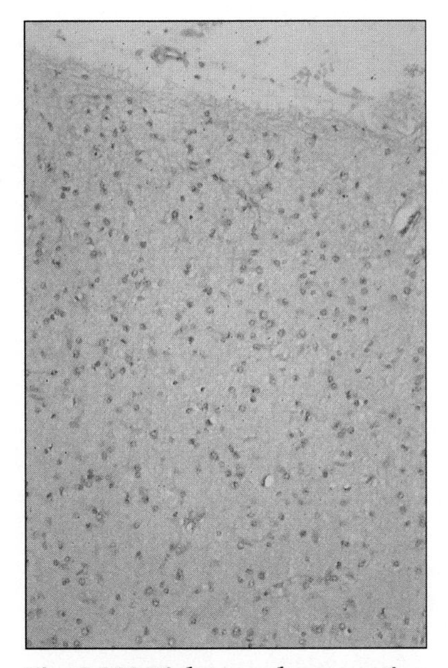

Fig. 3.202 Pick-type degeneration in the frontal cortex. There is a severe loss of nerve cells with heavy astrocytosis. *(Haematoxylin–eosin × 100.)*

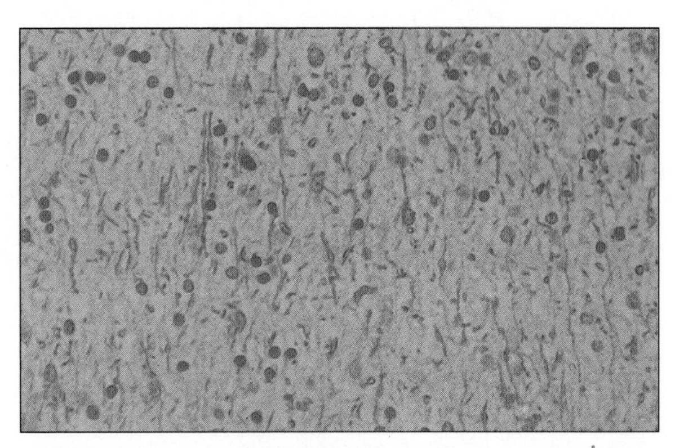

Fig. 3.203 Loss of myelinated axons from the white matter. *(Luxol fast blue × 200.)*

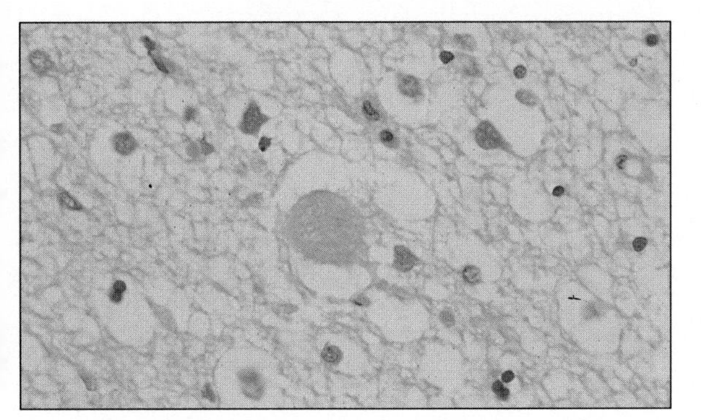

Fig. 3.204 'Ballooned' nerve cell (Pick cell) in the temporal cortex. *(Haematoxylin–eosin × 400.)*

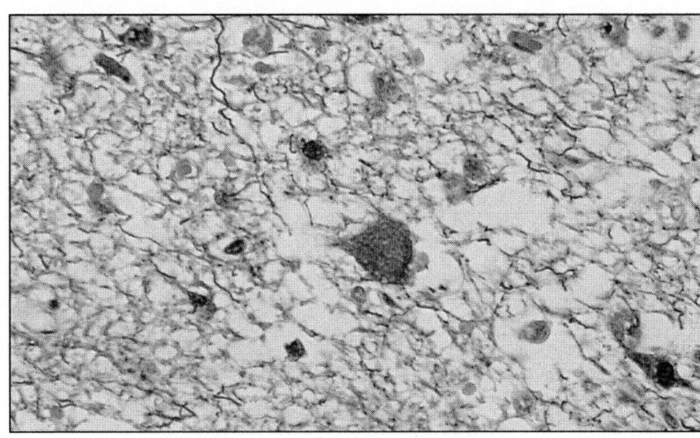

Fig. 3.205 As Fig. 3.204, but Palmgren silver stain. *(× 400.)*

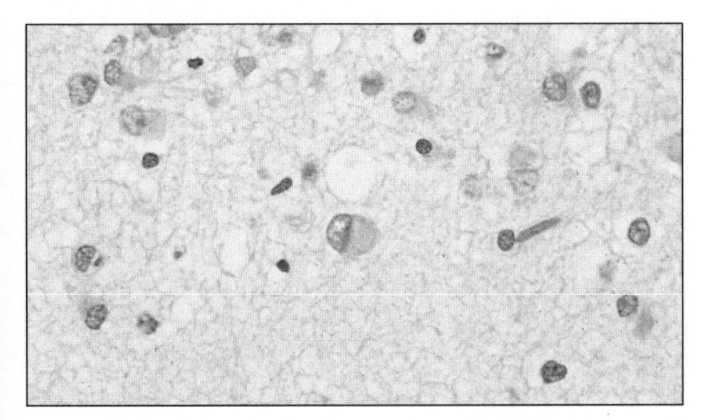

Fig. 3.206 Inclusion body in a pyramidal nerve cell of the temporal cortex (Pick body). *(Haematoxylin–eosin × 400.)*

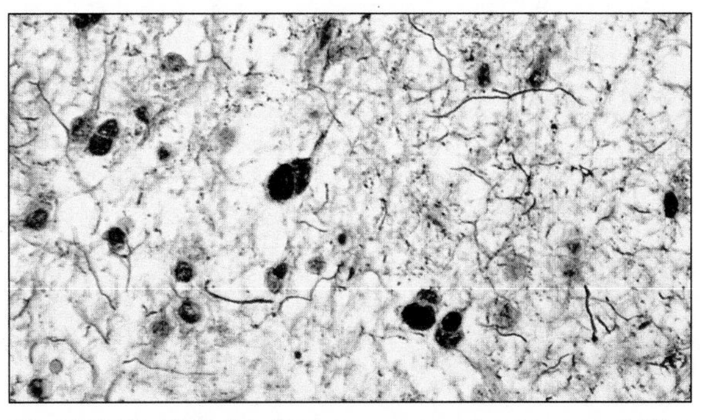

Fig. 3.207 Pick bodies are strongly argyrophilic. *(Palmgren silver stain × 400.)*

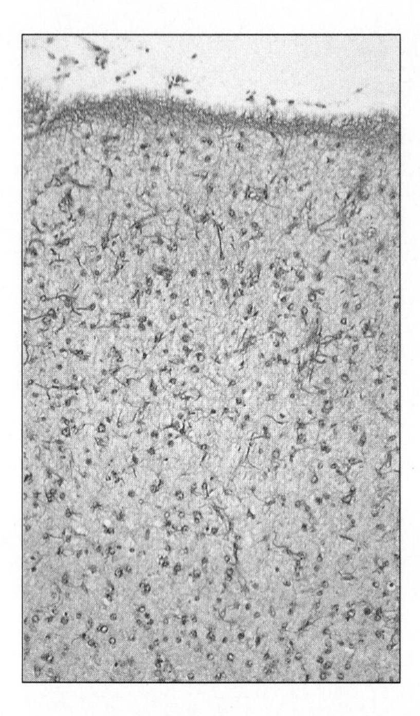

Fig. 3.208 (left) Astrocytosis in Pick-type histology. Note that all cortical laminae are severely affected. *(Phosphotungstic acid–haematoxylin × 100.)*

Fig. 3.209 (right) Severe cortical astrocytosis in fronto-temporal atrophy in the absence of Pick bodies and swollen neurones. *(Phosphotungstic acid–haematoxylin × 100.)*

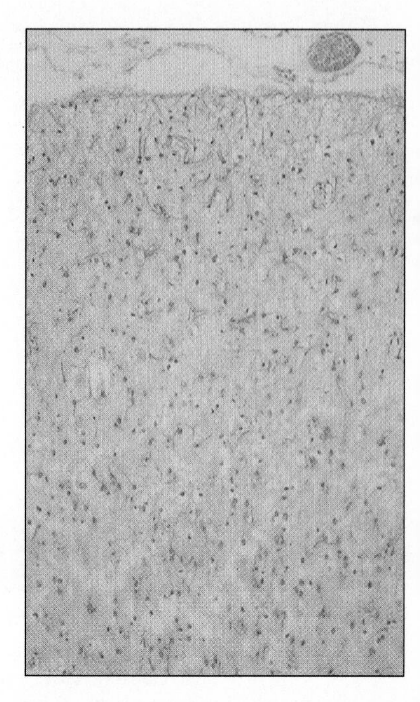

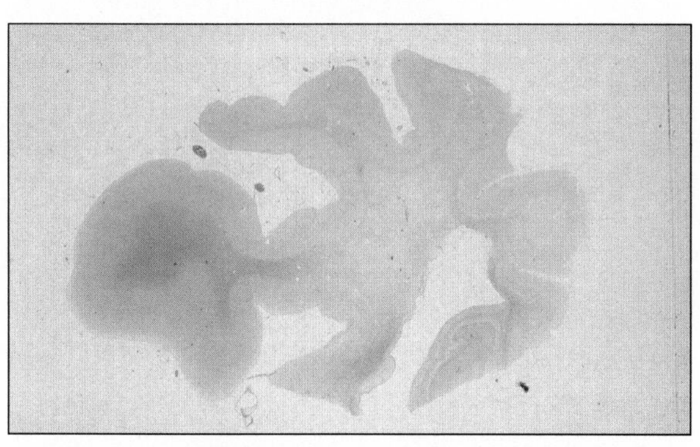

Fig. 3.210 Atrophy of the inferior and middle temporal gyri, with loss of myelin from white matter. Section of temporal lobe. The superior temporal gyrus is conspicuously spared. *(Haematoxylin–eosin × 0.5.)*

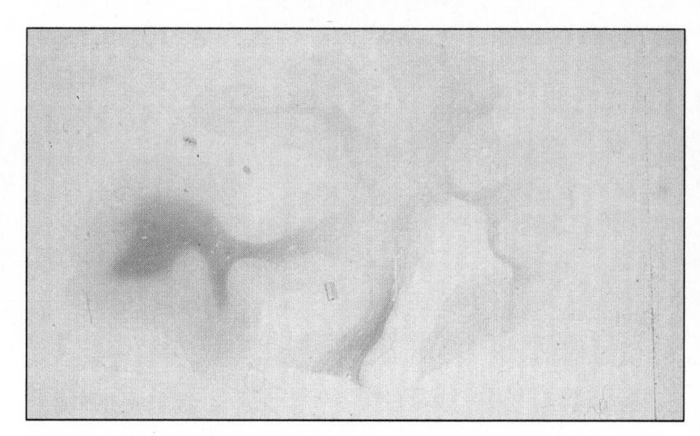

Fig. 3.211 As Fig. 3.210, but Luxol fast blue. *(× 0.5.)*

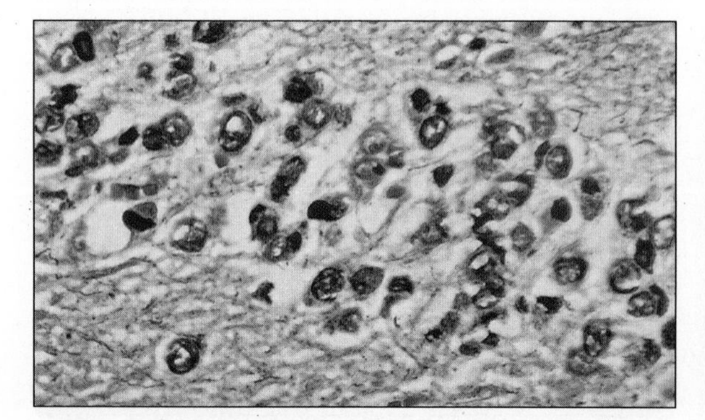

Fig. 3.212 Argyrophilic inclusions (Pick bodies) in granule cells of the dentate gyrus of the hippocampus. *(Palmgren silver stain × 400.)*

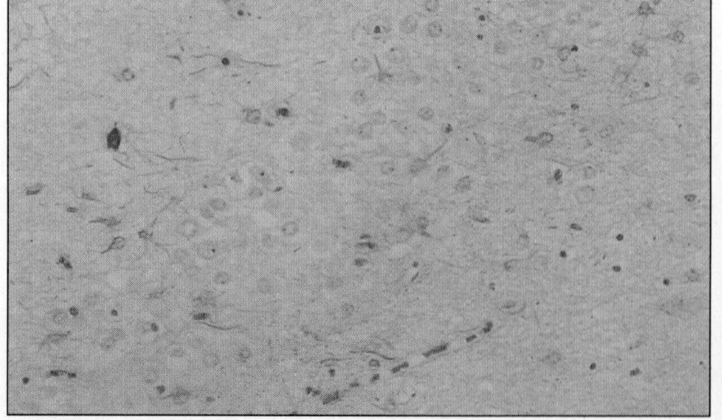

Fig. 3.213 Astrocytosis in the dentate gyrus of the hippocampus and the adjoining CA4/5 region of Ammon's horn. *(Phosphotungstic acid–haematoxylin × 100.)*

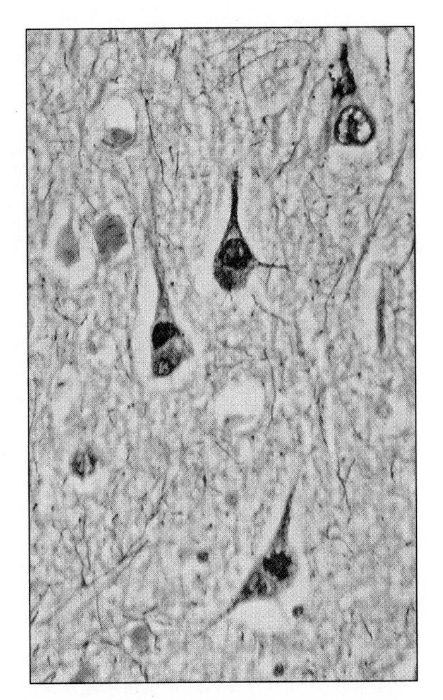

Other inclusions occur within the pyramidal cells of areas CA1 (**Fig. 3.214**) and subiculum, where an extensive cell loss is accompanied by an intense astrocytosis (**Fig. 3.215**). The basolateral nuclei of the amygdala are also severely affected. Although the basal ganglia are grossly atrophied, they do not generally display any histological change, although occasionally a mild astrocytosis is present. The major subcortical nuclei are largely unaffected, but the substantia nigra and locus caeruleus can sometimes be damaged. The cerebellum usually appears normal.

Both Pick cells (**Fig. 3.216**) and Pick bodies (**Figs 3.217–3.220**) are immunoreactive with antisera to tau (see **Figs 3.216–3.218**) and ubiquitin

Fig. 3.214 Pick bodies in pyramidal cells of area CA1 of the hippocampus. *(Palmgren silver stain × 400.)*

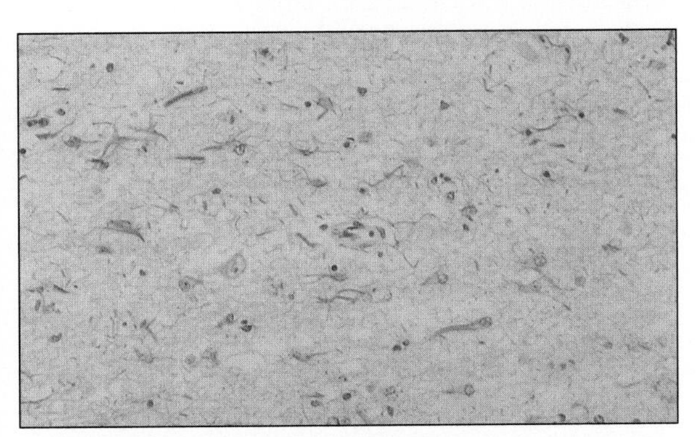

Fig. 3.215 Loss of nerve cells and severe astrocytosis in the subiculum of the hippocampus. *(Phosphotungstic acid–haematoxylin × 200.)*

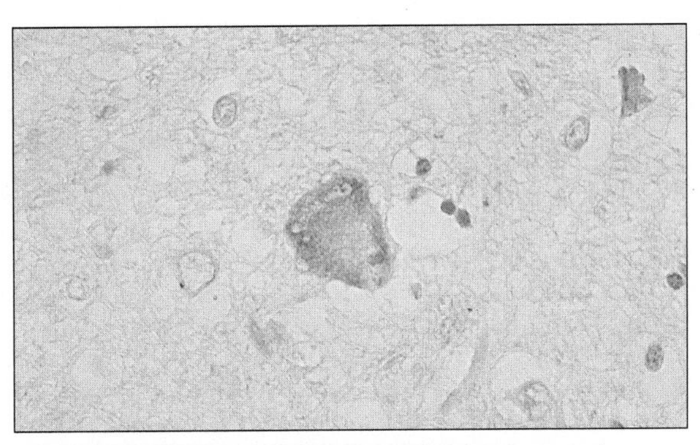

Fig. 3.216 Ballooned neurones in the temporal cortex showing tau immunoreactivity. *(Anti-tau × 400.)*

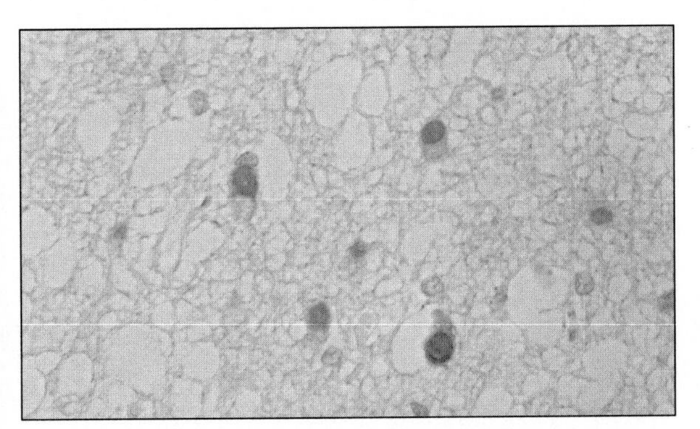

Fig. 3.217 Pick bodies in pyramidal cells of the frontal cortex showing tau immunoreactivity. *(Anti-tau × 400.)*

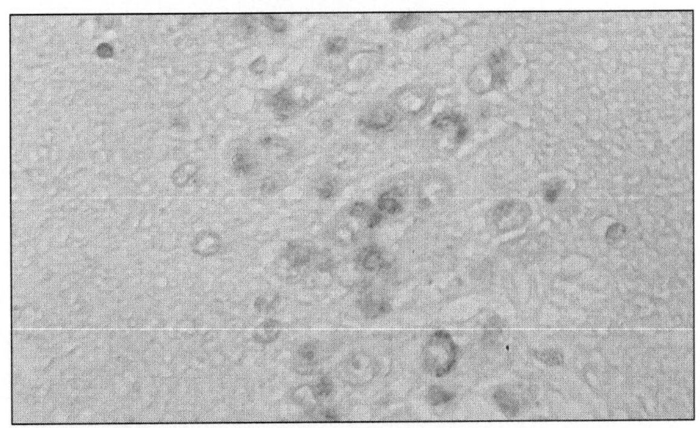

Fig. 3.218 Pick bodies in granule cells of the dentate gyrus of the hippocampus showing tau immunoreactivity. *(Anti-tau × 400.)*

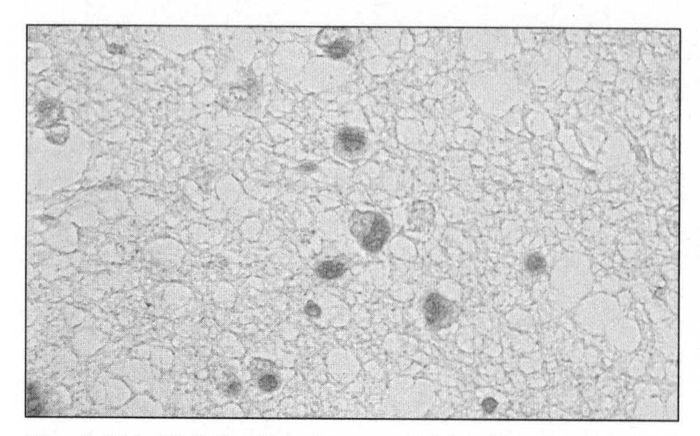

Fig. 3.219 Pick bodies in pyramidal cells of the frontal cortex showing ubiquitin immunoreactivity. *(Anti-ubiquitin × 400.)*

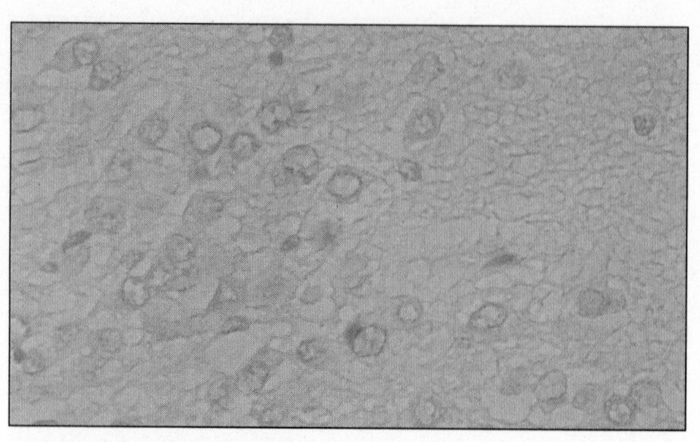

Fig. 3.220 Pick bodies in granule cells of the dentate gyrus of the hippocampus showing ubiquitin immunoreactivity. *(Anti-ubiquitin × 400.)*

(see **Figs 3.219** and **3.220**) proteins. The swollen cells are also strongly reactive with antibodies against αB crystallin (**Fig. 3.221**), but the inclusions do not react in this way. Ultrastructurally, Pick bodies comprise of intermingled crossing fibrils 12–18 nm in diameter with variable amounts of granular material.

The cytoplasmic source of Pick bodies remains unknown. They are thought to represent accumulated debris from the cytoskeleton of neurones, being formed either as a reaction to direct damage at their processes or as a consequence of transynaptic changes in connecting neurones.

In some patients brain weight is less reduced (**Fig.3.201** see page 73) and there is a more circumscribed atrophy affecting the temporal pole, the orbitofrontal cortex and the anterior insular cortex. Such patients have a gliotic type of degeneration, though Pick cells and Pick bodies may not occur. Fronto-temporal dementia showing a gliotic type of cortical degeneration, with or without the presence of Pick bodies and Pick cells, conforms histologically to what has in the past been recognised as **'Pick's disease'**.

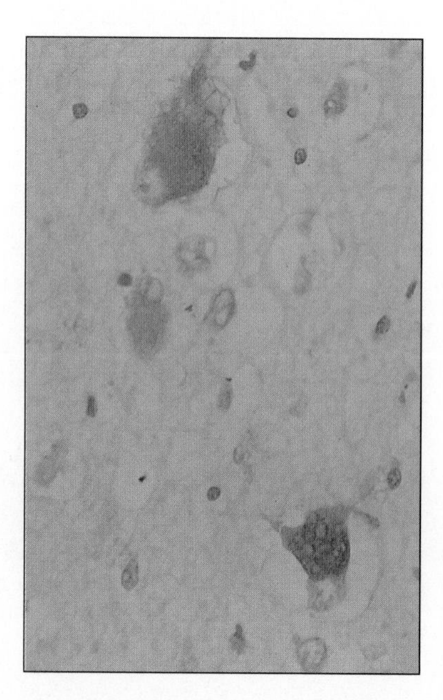

Fig. 3.221 Ballooned cells in the temporal cortex containing αB crystallin. *(Anti-αB crystallin × 400.)*

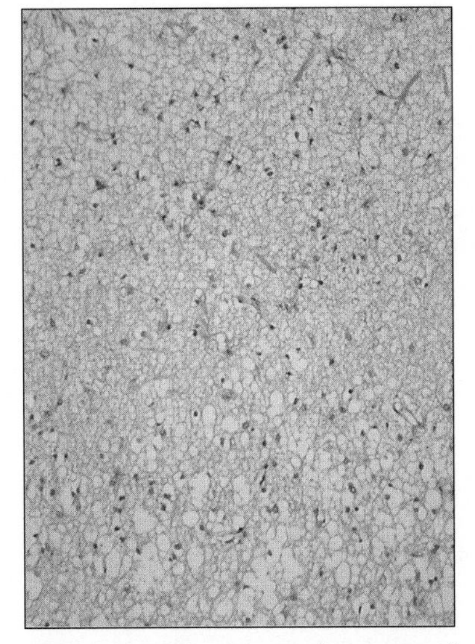

Fig. 3.222 Microvacuolar type of degeneration in the frontal cortex. There is a severe nerve cell loss with vacuolation of cortical lamina II. Astrocytosis is mild and confined to lamina I. *(Haematoxylin–eosin × 100.)*

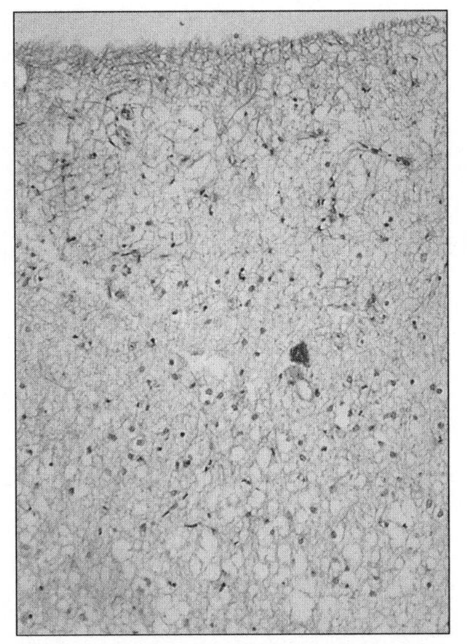

Fig. 3.223 As Fig. 3.222, but showing mild astrocytosis within lamina I only. *(Phosphotungstic acid–haematoxylin × 100.)*

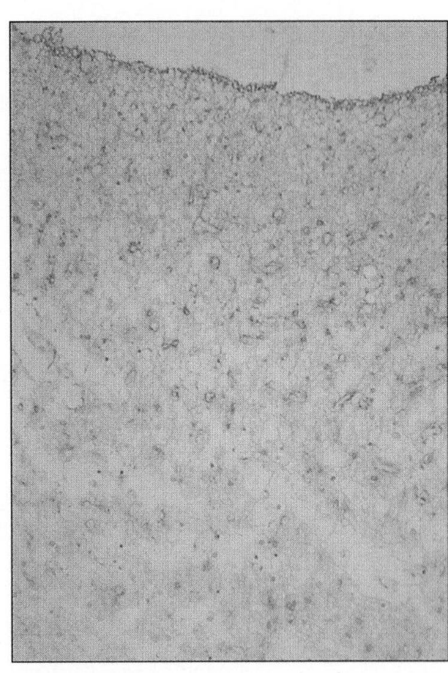

Fig. 3.224 As Fig. 3.221, but anti-GFAP. *(× 100.)*

Histopathological type characterised by microvacuolar degeneration of the cortex

Fronto-temporal dementia may also be associated with a quite different histological picture. In this second type, there are no Pick cells or Pick bodies in the cortex or hippocampus, even when sensitive immunohistochemical procedures for tau and ubiquitin are used. The histopathological features are characterised by a microvacuolar degeneration of the cortex, which is limited to layer II and the superficial parts of layer III (**Fig. 3.222**), and is caused by a loss of nerve cells from these layers (see **Fig. 3.222**). The pyramidal cells of layers V and VI are less affected, many of these still being present, though atrophied. Usually, there is only a little, or no, reactive astrocytosis (**Figs 3.223** and **3.224**); some mild subpial change is common and often a mild or moderate gliosis is also present at the junction of the grey and white matter (**Fig. 3.225**) near the U-fibres.

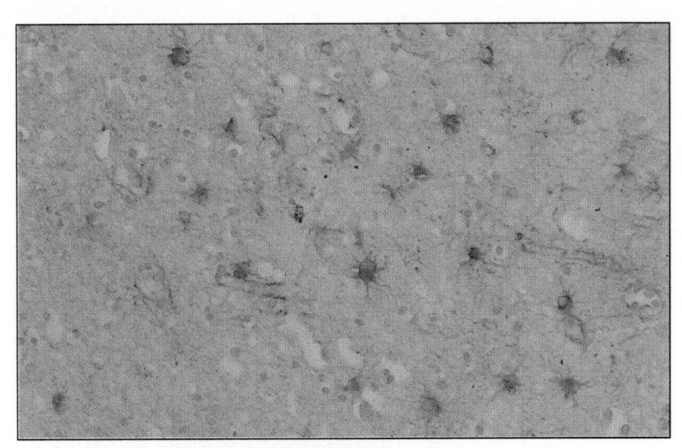

Fig. 3.225 Reactive astrocytosis at the junction between grey and white matter. *(Anti-GFAP × 200.)*

As in the Pick-type, the white matter is often grossly demyelinated (**Figs 3.226** and **3.227**) and shows a severe loss of axons, although without much, if any, reactive astrocytosis. Anti-ubiquitin immunostaining reveals a large amount of particulate material throughout the white matter (**Fig. 3.228**). The hippocampus, amygdala and basal ganglia show no major histopathological changes, though sometimes there is a mild astrocytosis. Again, the major subcortical nuclei in the mid-brain and brain stem are largely unaffected, although a mild loss of neurones from the substantia nigra and locus caeruleus can sometimes occur. The cerebellum is normal.

Within this clinical syndrome of fronto-temporal dementia there are pathological variants other than those so far described, particularly in association

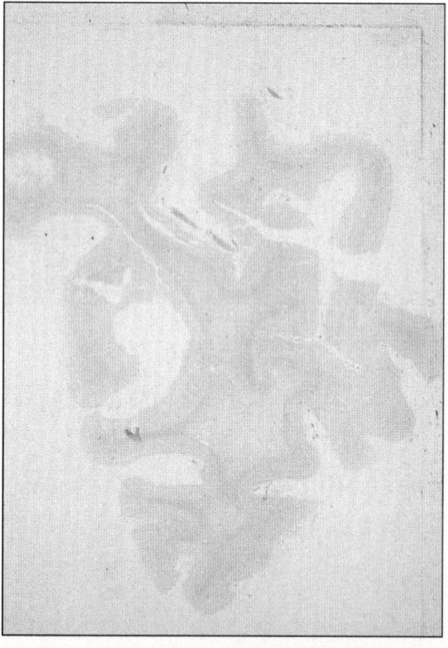

Fig. 3.226 Loss of myelin from deep white matter of the frontal cortex. There is some preservation of arcuate fibres. *(Haematoxylin–eosin × 0.5.)*

Fig. 3.227 As Fig. 3.226 but Luxol fast blue. *(× 0.5.)*

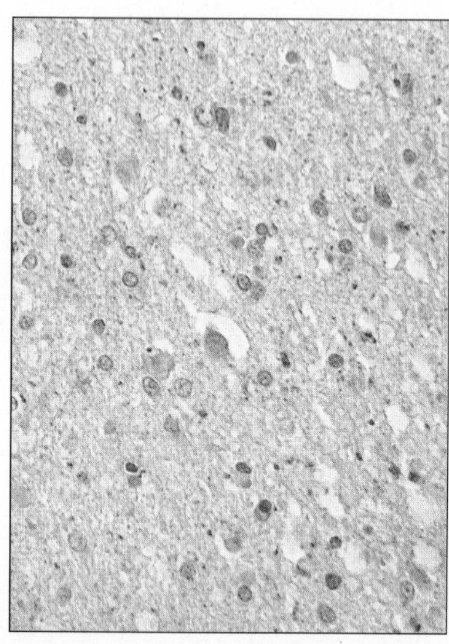

Fig. 3.228 Ubiquitinated particulate material. A large amount of ubiquitinated particulate material within the white matter of the frontal cortex. *(Anti-ubiquitin × 200.)*

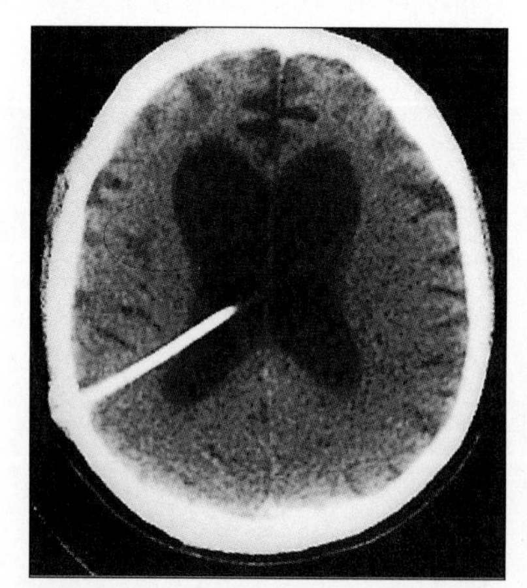

Fig. 3.229 Mild and diffuse atrophy within the frontal and temporal cortex, but considerable bilateral enlargement of the lateral ventricles. CT scan of a 50-year-old man. Note an A/V shunt has been inserted into the right ventricle.

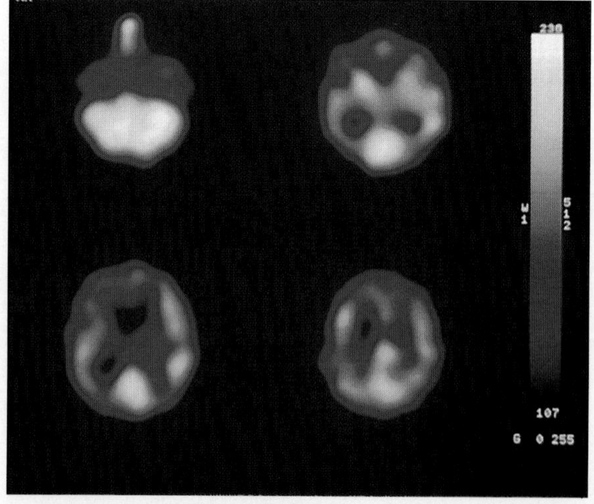

Fig. 3.230 Bilateral hypometabolism within the anterior cerebral hemispheres. SPET imaging of the brain of a 49-year-old man.

with those patients who demonstrate stereotypic behaviours. Such patients do not show preferential atrophy on CT scan (**Fig. 3.229**), and SPET imaging can be normal or show an anterior subcortical pattern to the hypometabolism (**Fig. 3.230**).

The brain is less reduced in weight (1100–1300 g) and externally shows a mild or moderate generalised atrophy, although in some instances a preferential temporal lobe involvement is seen. On slicing the brain coronally, a common and severe atrophy of the corpus striatum is evident in all cases, the caudate nucleus usually appearing concave in profile (**Figs 3.231** and **3.232**; see also **Fig. 3.236**).

Histologically, the striatum shows a severe, if not almost complete loss of nerve cells with a dense reactive astrocytosis (see **Figs 3.237** and **3.238**). In some patients there is a severe temporal lobe atrophy (**Fig. 3.231–3.234**) involving the medial and inferior temporal gyri (see **Figs 3.231–3.233**), the parahippocampal gyrus (see **Fig. 3.233**), the amygdala (see **Fig. 3.233**), but with sparing of the superior temporal gyrus (see **Fig.3.234**), the hippocampus (see **Fig. 3.234**), and the rest of the neocortex (see **Figs 3.231–3.235**).

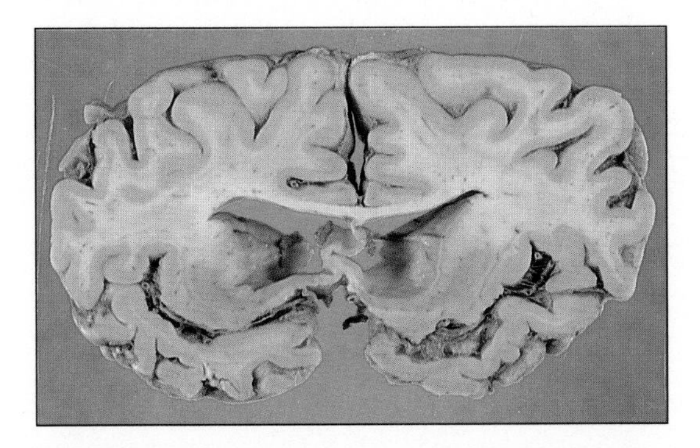

Fig. 3.231 Severe atrophy of the corpus striatum, dilatation of the lateral ventricles and atrophy of the temporal lobe. Coronal section of the brain of a 50-year-old man.

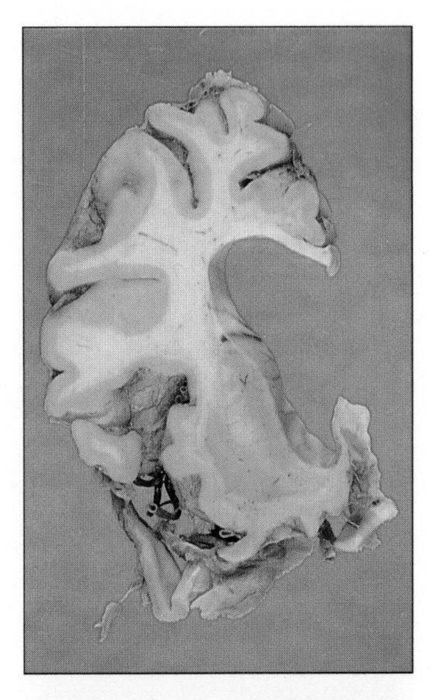

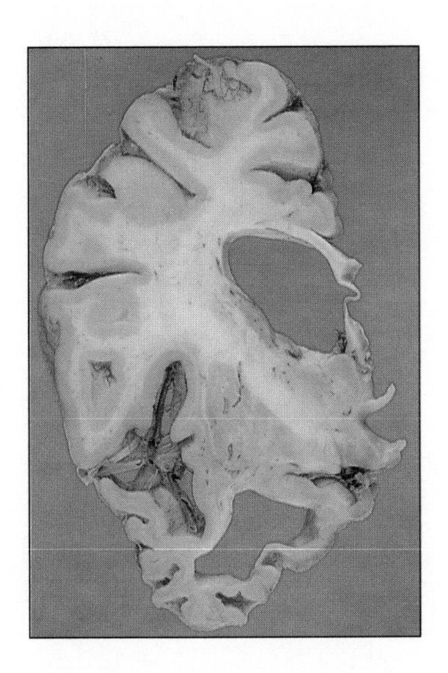

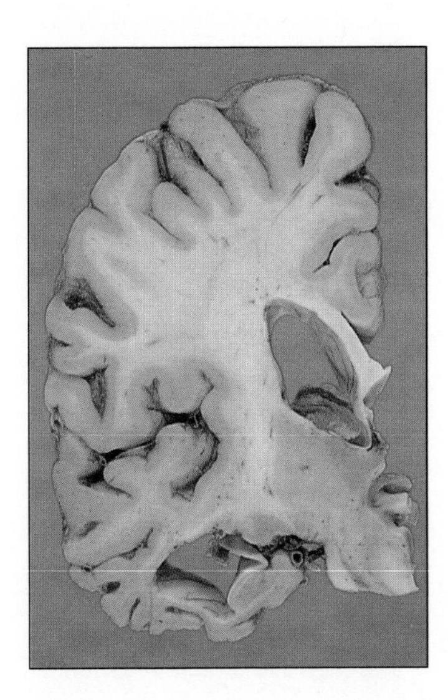

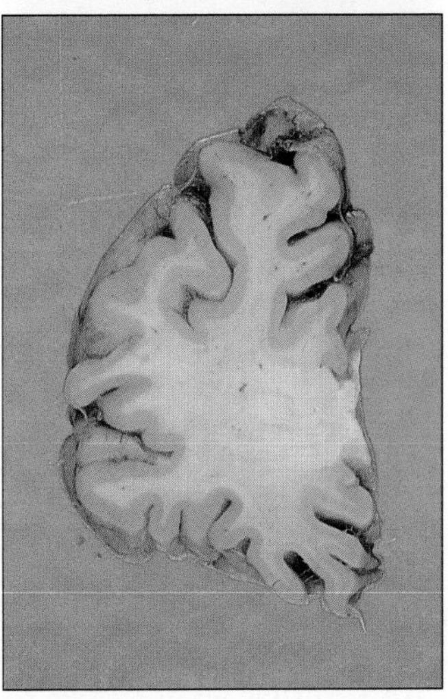

Figs 3.232–2.235 Severe atrophy of the corpus striatum and temporal lobe, and marked ventricular dilatations especially within the temporal horn. Coronal sections of the brain of a 73-year-old man. The parietal and frontal lobes show only little atrophy.

The cortical histology in these patients is a profound gliosis (see **Figs 3.239–3.241**), but without Pick cells or Pick bodies.

In other patients, there is frontal lobe involvement with sparing of the temporal lobes (**Fig. 3.236**), and here the changes comprise microvacuolar degeneration.

The precise nosology of these striato-cortical degenerations and their relationship to the more prototypical cases of fronto-temporal dementia remain uncertain. It is not clear whether they themselves form a 'distinct' group or whether their pathology and aetiology are heterogeneous.

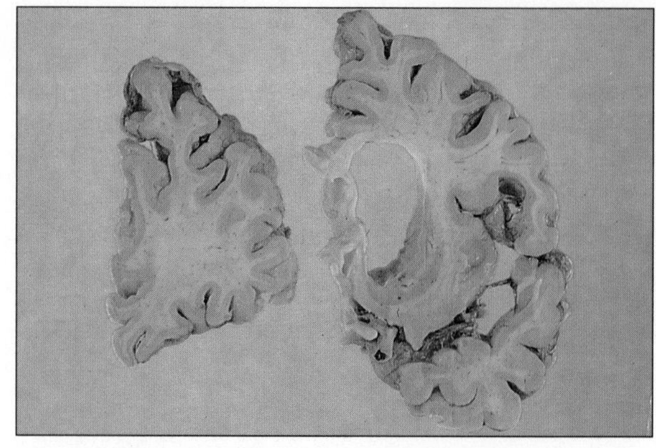

Fig. 3.236 Severe atrophy of the corpus striatum and moderate atrophy of the frontal lobes. Coronal sections of the brain of a 49-year-old man. The temporal lobe is conspicuously normal.

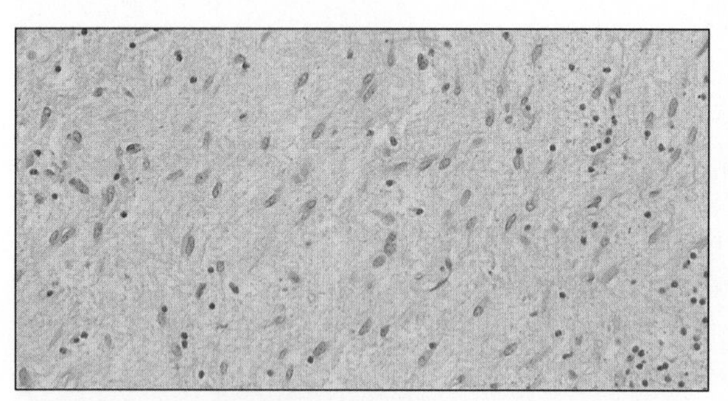

Fig. 3.237 Severe nerve cell loss and reactive astrocytosis in the corpus striatum. From the patient featured in **Fig. 3.236**. *(Haematoxylin–eosin × 200.)*

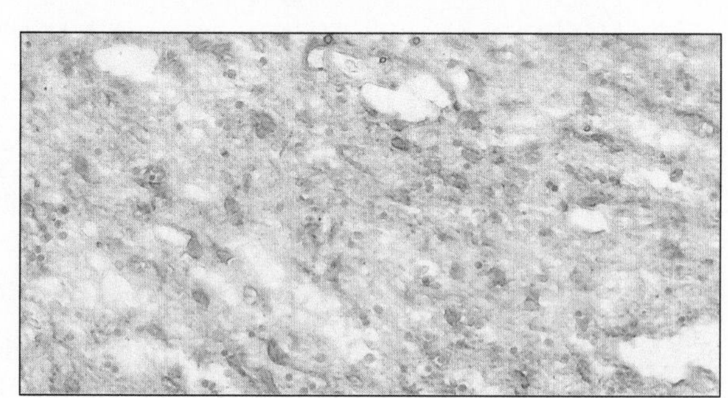

Fig. 3.238 As Fig. 3.237, but anti-GFAP. *(× 200.)*

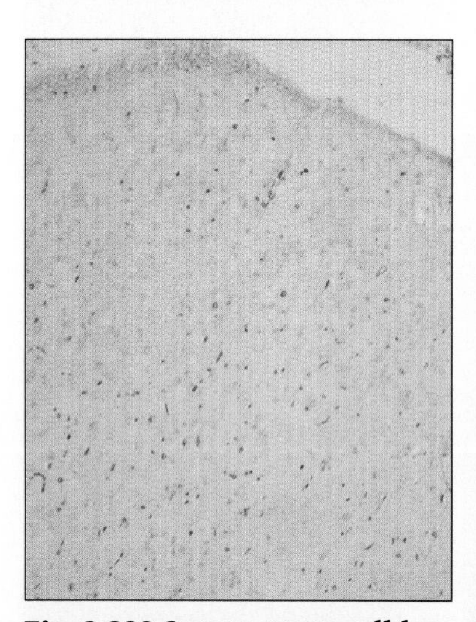

Fig. 3.239 Severe nerve cell loss and reactive astrocytosis in the temporal cortex. From the 73-year-old man featured in **Figs 3.232–3.235**. *(Haematoxylin–eosin × 100.)*

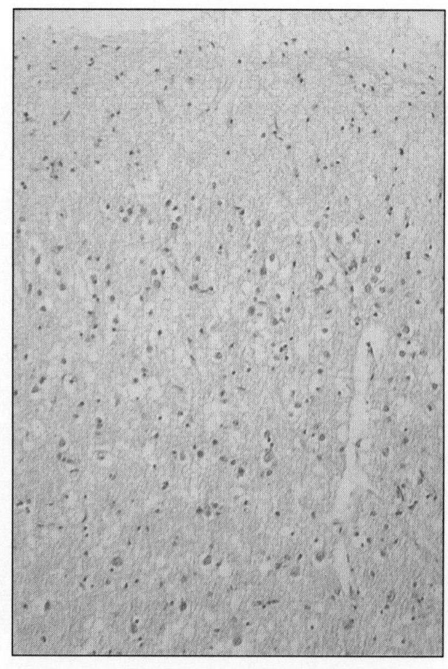

Fig. 3.240 As Fig. 3.239, but phosphotungstic acid–haematoxylin. *(× 100.)*

Fig. 3.241 As Fig. 3.239, but anti-GFAP. *(× 100.)*

Fronto-temporal dementia with motor neurone disease

Demographic features

An association between dementia and motor neurone disease was first noted in 1929 by Meyer, and has become increasingly recognised since, now being accepted as a distinct clinical and pathological entity falling under the 'umbrella' of those conditions that comprise the fronto-temporal dementias. Although uncommon, the disease appears to occur worldwide and displays similar demographic features.

Age of onset varies from 30–66 years, averaging about 55 years, and duration of the disease ranges from 1–6 years, averaging 2–3 years. Men appear to be affected slightly more often than women. Usually the disease is sporadic, but it can be familial.

Neurological signs
Dementia as presentation
Bulbar palsy and amyotrophy (late)
Investigations
Neurophysiology confirms MND
EEG: normal
SPET: frontal lobe abnormality

The demographic features of motor neurone disease with dementia closely parallel those of 'classic' motor neurone disease and there are many histopathological similarities between the two conditions.

Gross changes

The CT scan usually reveals bilateral atrophy within the frontal lobes, which as in fronto-temporal dementia alone (**Fig 3.192**) also show reduced metabolism under SPET imaging (**Fig. 3.242**). No abnormalities are seen elsewhere in the brain with either method.

At autopsy the brain shows only a slight reduction in weight, usually weighing 1150–1400 g. Macroscopically, there is a well-defined though usually mild atrophy affecting the frontal lobes and anterior-parietal cortex (**Figs 3.243** and **3.244**), with involvement of the temporal pole in some cases (see **Fig. 3.243**). All the other brain regions appear normal externally. Examination of the spinal cord reveals no macroscopic abnormalities

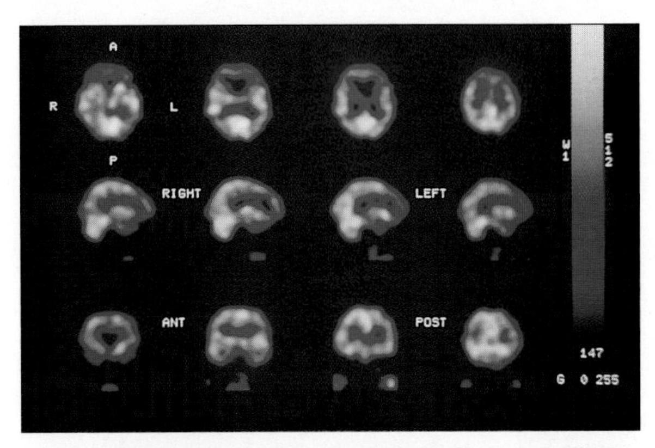

Fig. 3.242 Bilateral hypometabolism predominantly within the frontal lobes. SPET imaging of the brain of a 48-year-old man.

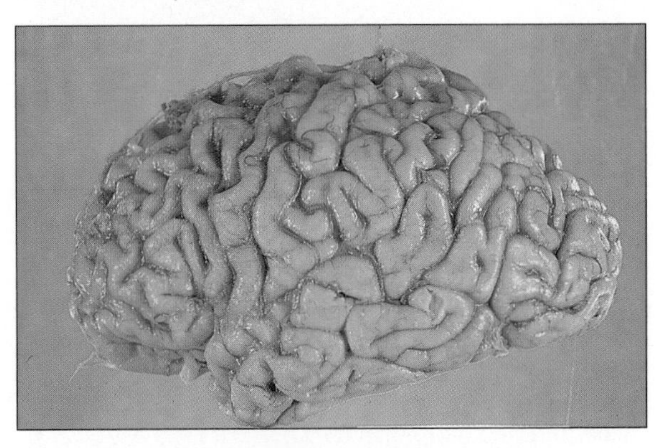

Fig. 3.243 Mild atrophy of the frontal lobes. Lateral view of the brain of a 76-year-old man.

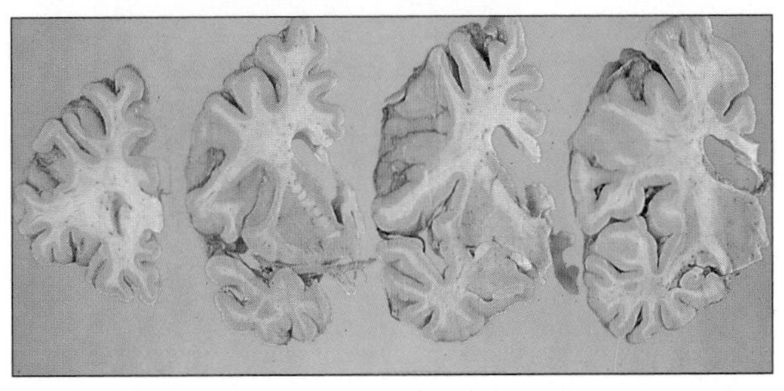

Fig. 3.244 Mild frontal and anterior parietal cortical atrophy and mild dilatation of the lateral ventricle. Coronal sections of the brain of the 76-year-old man featured in **Fig.3.243**. Note the preservation of the basal ganglia, temporal lobe structures and the posterior hemisphere.

Morphometric analysis (**Figs 3.245** and **3.246**) confirms this pattern of atrophy and shows that there is a greater loss of white than grey matter in most areas, leading to an elevation of the grey/white matter ratio. The basal ganglia are slightly reduced in size, particularly the caudate nucleus (see **Fig. 3.246**).

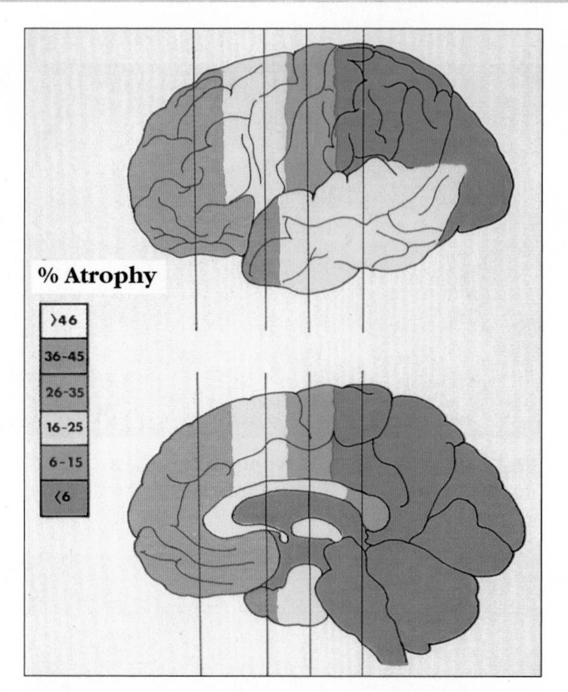

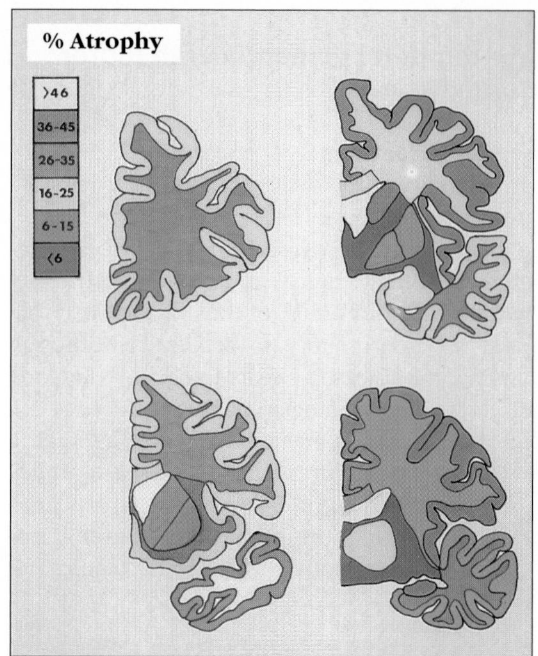

Figs 3.245 and 3.246 Morphometric analysis of regional brain atrophy. Note the preferential involvement of the frontal lobe and the anterior temporal cortex and thalamus. The white matter shows a greater atrophy than the corresponding grey matter.

Age of onset
Usually 40–65 years.

Sex incidence
Males affected more than females

Duration
Usually less than 5 years, sometimes less than 2 years

Gross features
Mild atrophy of frontal and anterior temporal lobes
Often depigmentation of the substantia nigra

Histopathology
- Affected areas of cortex show pyramidal nerve cell loss, microvacuolation of outer cortical laminae, mild astrocytosis
- Ubiquitinated, but not tau-containing, inclusions in hippocampus dentate gyrus cells and layer II neurones of frontal cortex
- Loss of neurones from substantia nigra. Severe astrocytosis
- Loss of anterior horn cells and motor cells of trigeminal and hypoglossus nuclei. Ubiquitinated inclusions in surviving cells
- Occasional cases associated with (Pick) inclusion bodies and astrocytosis in the cerebral cortex

Genetics
- Most cases appear to be sporadic
- Family history for about 15% of patients: genetic locus in these cases is unknown though point mutations in the superoxide dismutase gene on long arm of chromosome 21 are associated with 'classic' inherited motor neurone disease without dementia

Histopathological changes

Histologically, there is a loss of anterior horn cells from the spinal cord, this being more severe medially than laterally and affecting cervical levels (**Fig. 3.247**) more than lumbar regions (**Fig. 3.248**), where many cells are preserved. Surviving anterior horn cells often contain the ubiquitinated inclusion bodies (**Figs 3.249–3.253**) typically seen in people with classic (non-dementing) motor neurone disease. These inclusions appear as large rounded globular or 'solid' entities (see **Figs 3.249** and **3.253**) or, more commonly, are loosely 'woven' into skeins of material (see **Figs 3.250** and **3.252**).

Often cells are lost from the hypoglossus and trigeminal motor nuclei and some surviving cells contain the same kinds of inclusion as in the spinal cord. The Betz cells of the precentral gyrus are commonly shrunken, and can contain inclusions, but usually there is no cell loss. These neuronal inclusions are ubiquitin positive, but do not react with antisera to any cytoskeletal or other protein so far investigated. While some cells containing inclusions appear histologically normal, most show a loss of basophilia and a breakdown of the nuclear chromatin (see **Figs 3.251** and **3.252**), eventually appearing as 'ghost cells' (see **Fig. 3.252**). Following cell death and dissolution the ubiquitinated material is left behind in the extracellular space (see **Figs 3.252** and **3.253**).

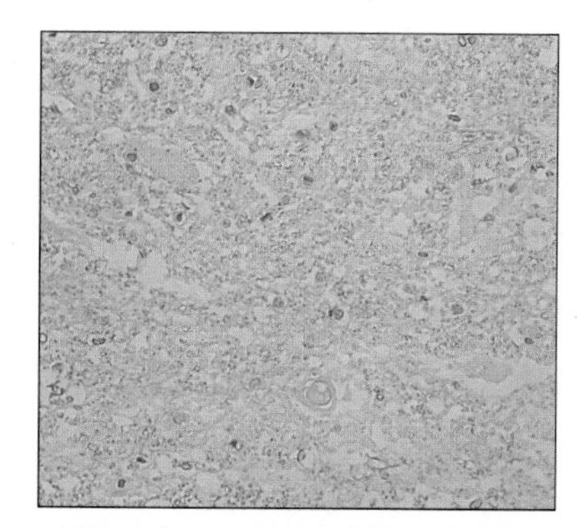

Fig. 3.247 Anterior horn of spinal cord at cervical level. There is an almost complete loss of motor neurones. *(Haematoxylin–eosin × 200.)*

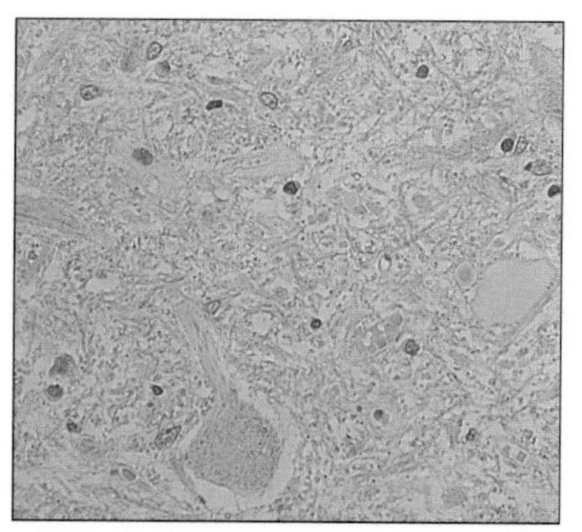

Fig. 3.248 Anterior horn of spinal cord at lumbar level. Motor neurones are better preserved, but there are large eosinophilic inclusions within the nerve processes. *(Haematoxylin-eosin x 200)*

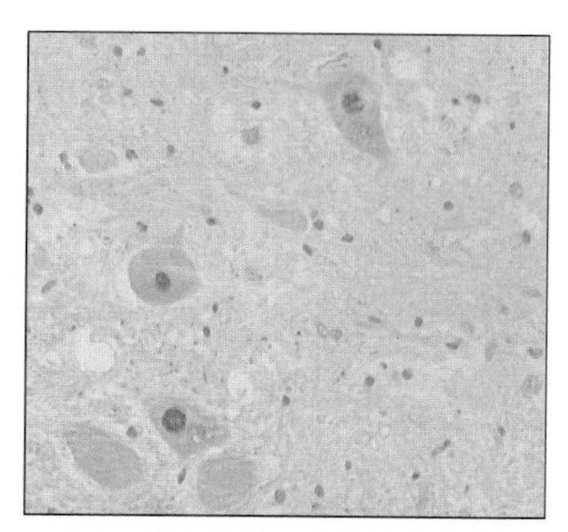

Fig. 3.249 Rouunded ubiquitinated inclusions in anterior horn cells of the spinal cord at cervical level. *(Anti-ubiquitin × 200.)*

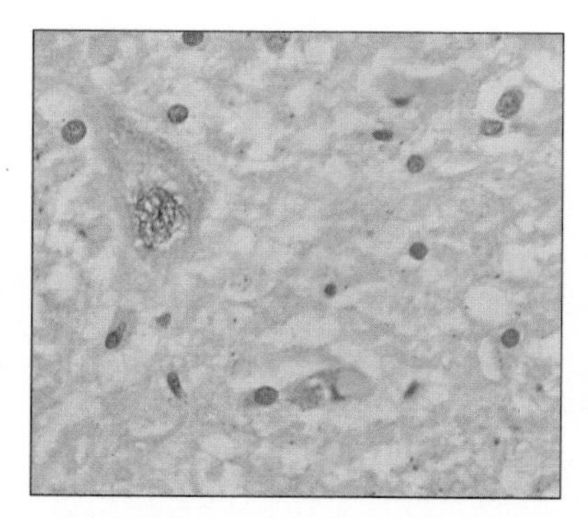

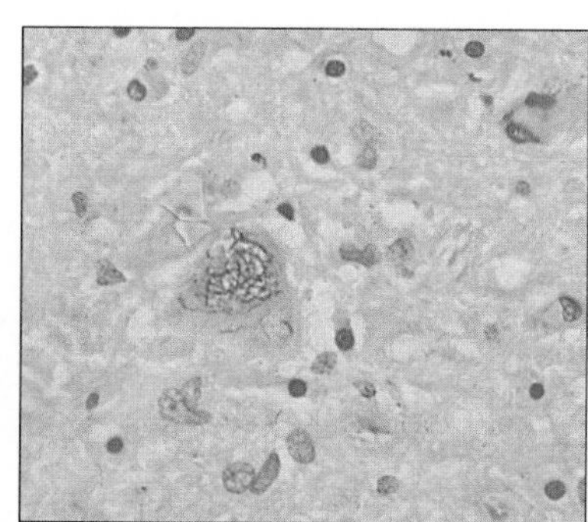

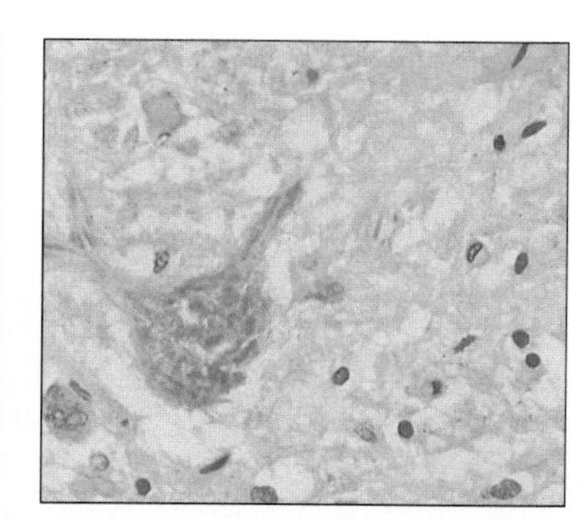

Figs 3.250–3.252 Skein-like inclusions in motor neurones of the trigeminal nucleus are ubiquitinated. Affected cells show a loss of Nissl substance and a nuclear disintegration, leaving behind 'ghost' cells. *(Anti-ubiquitin × 400.)*

Despite the loss of motor neurones, the long tracts within the spinal cord and brain stem remain well myelinated. Affected areas of frontal and temporal cortex show microvacuolar degeneration of the outer laminae (**Fig. 3.254**) similar to that seen in people with fronto-temporal dementia. There is a loss of layer III pyramidal cells (see **Figs 3.222–3.224**), while those of layers V and VI are shrunken rather than lost. Occasional surviving nerve cells, mostly in layers II and III, show ubiquitinated inclusions (**Fig. 3.255**) that do not react with other antisera and are not apparent on silver staining.

There is a mild astrocytosis within subpial regions, but a pronounced reaction is common at the grey/white matter interface (**Fig. 3.256**), and within the white matter itself (**Fig. 3.257**). Apart from a mild astrocytosis of the end-folium (**Figs 3.258** and **3.259**) and subiculum (**Fig. 3.260**), the hippocampus appears normal. On immunostaining,

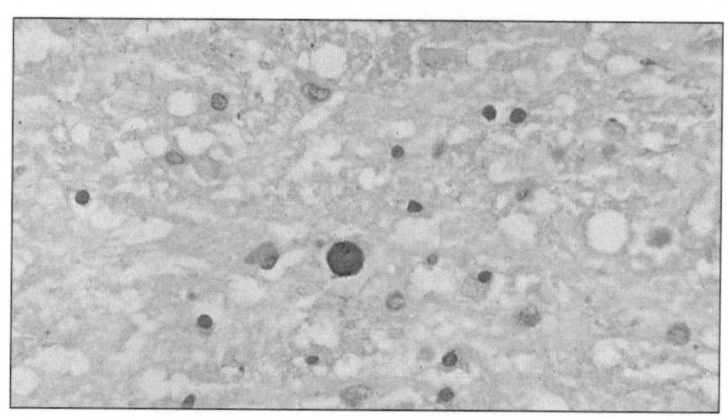

Fig. 3.253 Extraneuronal ubiquitinated inclusion in the neuropil of the trigeminal nucleus. *(Anti-ubiquitin × 400.)*

ubiquitinated inclusions are present in the granule cells of the dentate gyrus (**Fig. 3.261**).

The basal ganglia and cerebellum are histologically normal, as are the main subcortical nuclei, except for the substantia nigra which shows a substantial loss of nerve cells (**Fig. 3.262**) and a profound reactive astrocytosis (**Fig. 3.263**), but inclusions are absent. This latter change is not seen either in fronto-temporal dementia alone or in 'typical' motor neurone disease.

A few deposits of β/A4 protein (as diffuse plaques) in the cerebral cortex and occasionally neurofibrillary tangles, chiefly within the hippocampus, can be seen in some of the more elderly patients.

Clinical dementia in these patients presumably relates to disruption and disconnection of cortical processing caused by damage in the outer laminae of the cortex to nerve cells and fibres that make up cortico-cortical pathways. The pathological substrate underlying this damage appears to involve the presence of ubiquitinated inclusions within affected cells. Although the presence of similar material within cortical and motor neurones implies a pathogenetic mechanism common to all such affected cells, the nature of this neurodegenerative process remains unknown.

While a microvacuolar-type degeneration of the cortex seems to be normal, sometimes fronto-temporal dementia with motor neurone disease appears to relate to a histology comprised of nerve cell swelling and profound astrocytosis (changes reminiscent of a 'Pick' type of pathology, (see page 74).

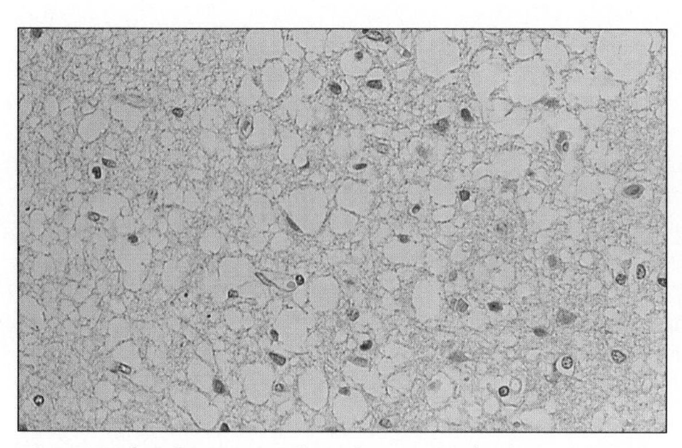

Fig. 3.254 Microvacuolar change in lamina II of the frontal cortex. *(Haematoxylin–eosin × 200.)*

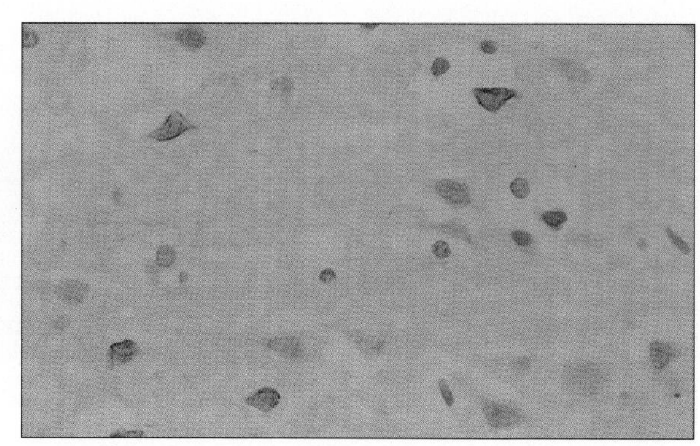

Fig. 3.255 Neurones of layer II of the frontal cortex contain ubiquitinated inclusions. *(Anti-ubiquitin × 200.)*

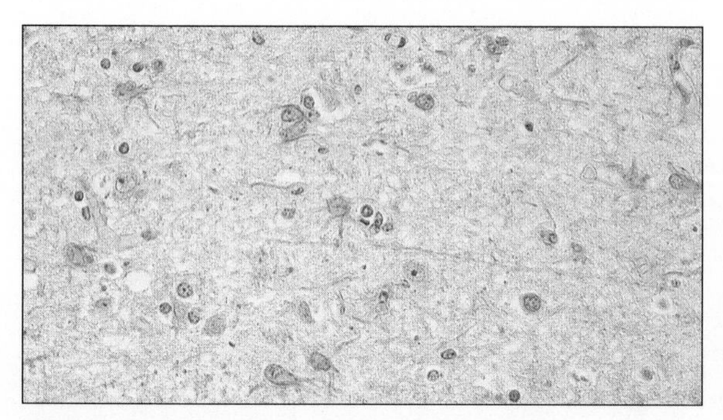

Fig. 3.256 Reactive astrocytosis at the junction of the grey and white matter of the frontal cortex. *(Phosphotungstic acid–haematoxylin × 200.)*

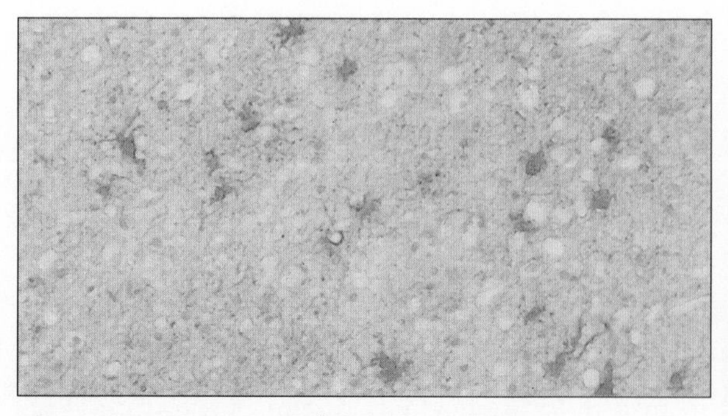

Fig. 3.257 As Fig. 3.256, but anti-GFAP.

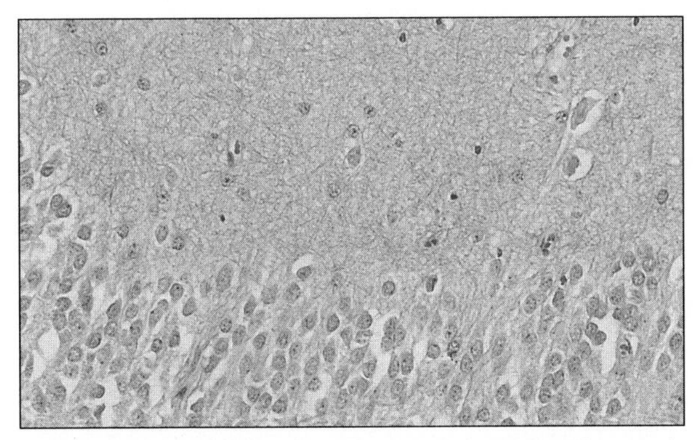

Fig. 3.258 Reactive astrocytosis within the endfolium of the hippocampus. *(Phosphotungstic acid–haematoxylin × 200.)*

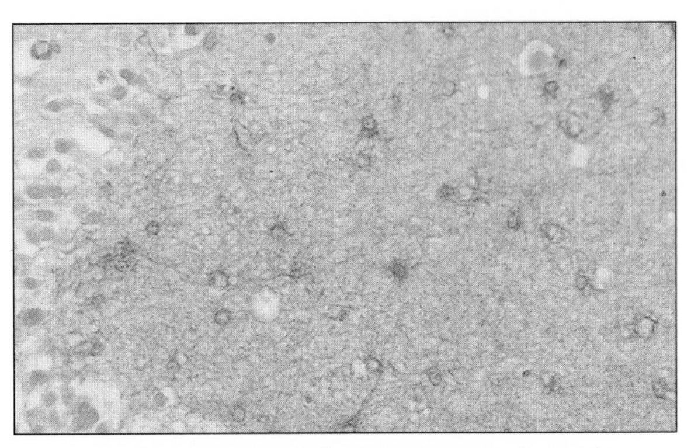

Fig. 3.259 As Fig. 3.258, but anti-GFAP. *(× 200.)*

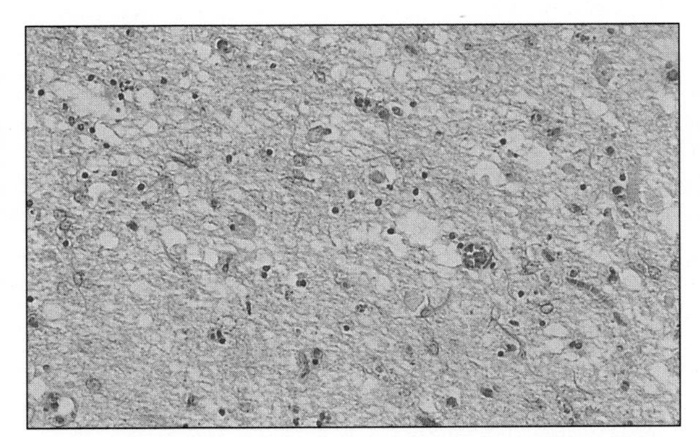

Fig. 3.260 Reactive astrocytosis in the subiculum of the hippocampus. *(Phosphotungstic acid–haematoxylin × 200.)*

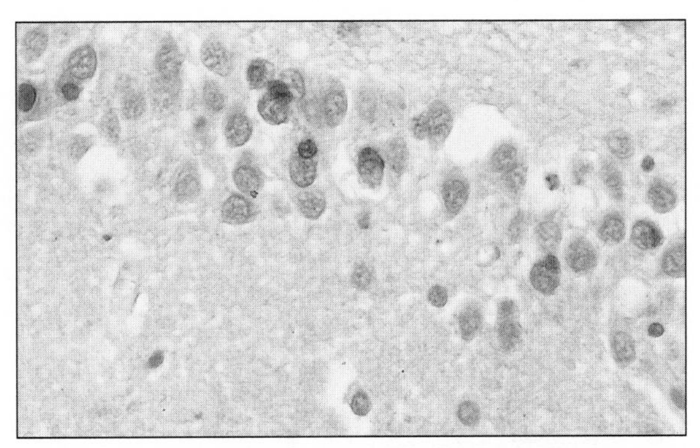

Fig. 3.261 Ubiquitinated inclusions within granule cells of the dentate gyrus of the hippocampus. *(Anti-ubiquitin × 400.)*

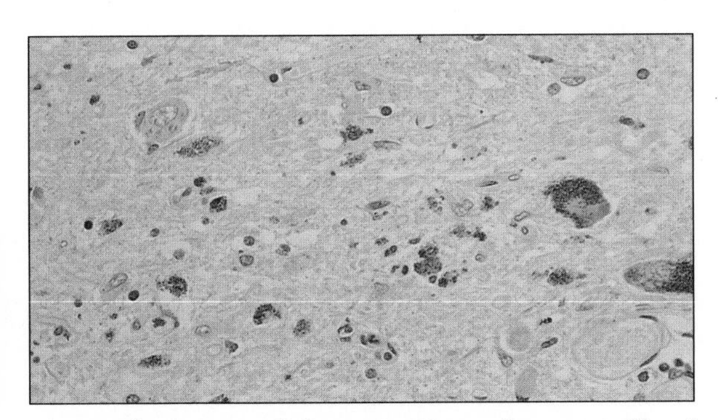

Fig. 3.262 Loss and degeneration of nerve cells of the substantia nigra. *(Haematoxylin–eosin × 200.)3*

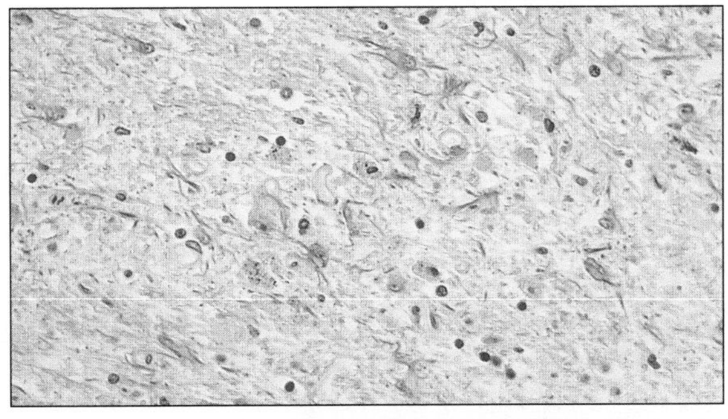

Fig. 3.263 Reactive astrocytosis within the substantia nigra. *(Phosphotungstic acid–haematoxylin × 200.)*

Progressive aphasia

The clinical entity of progressive aphasia comprises two distinct profiles: profile A and profile B.

Profile A: non-fluent aphasia

Profile A, the more common form of progressive aphasia, is characterised by a non-fluent aphasia with anomia, impaired repetition, and phonemic errors. Comprehension is generally preserved. Behavioural changes, similar to those of fronto-temporal dementia, occur usually late in the disease, but sometimes start soon after the linguistic difficulties. Neurological signs are commonly absent in the early stages, but extrapyramidal signs appear later.

Pathological features

A CT scan (**Fig. 3.264**) will show a cortical atrophy affecting mainly the left side, while SPET imaging (**Fig. 3.265**) reveals a reduced uptake of tracer preferentially in the left hemisphere. At autopsy, the brain shows a markedly asymmetrical atrophy (**Figs 3.266–3.274**), which is slight and generalised on the right but gross on the left. The left anterior temporal cortex can show 'knife-edge' atrophy (see **Figs 3.267** and **3.269**).

NON-FLUENT

Neurological signs
Agrammatic
Impaired repetition
Impaired word-finding
Literal and verbal paraphasias
Reading paralexias
Writing telegrammatic
Mild comprehensive disorder

Investigations
SPET: left hemisphere, frontal and temporal abnormality

FLUENT

Neurological signs
Severe comprehension disorder
Severe naming disorder
Verbal (semantic) paraphasias
Preserved repetition and series speech
Preserved reading aloud
Preserved writing to dictation

Investigations
SPET: bilateral frontal and temporal abnormality

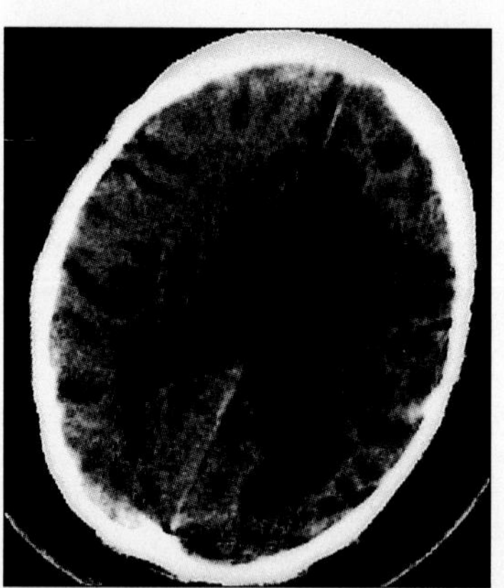

Fig. 3.264 Severe asymmetrical atrophy of the left cerebral hemisphere with lesser involvement of the right hemisphere. CT scan of the brain of a 71-year-old man. The lateral ventricles are grossly and asymmetrically enlarged.

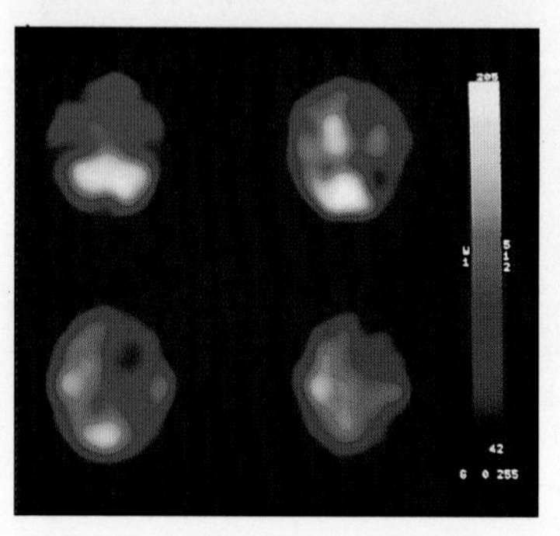

Fig. 3.265 Asymmetrical hypometabolism in favour of the left cerebral hemisphere. SPET imaging of the brain of the 71-year-old man featured in **Fig. 3.262**. Note that the cerebellum shows normal metabolism.

Age of onset
Usually 40–65 years

Sex incidence
Males and females equally affected

Duration
Long, often over 10 years.

Gross features
- Asymmetrical atrophy of left hemisphere, particularly involving frontal and temporal regions

Or
- Bilateral atrophy of temporal lobes

Histopathology
- Affected areas of cortex show loss of pyramidal cells, microvacuolation of outer cortical laminae, mild astrocytosis. No inclusion bodies or swollen neurones
- Occasionally (Pick) inclusion bodies and severe astrocytosis

Genetics
- About 50% of patients appear to inherit the disorder in an autosomal dominant manner, but the genetic locus is unknown

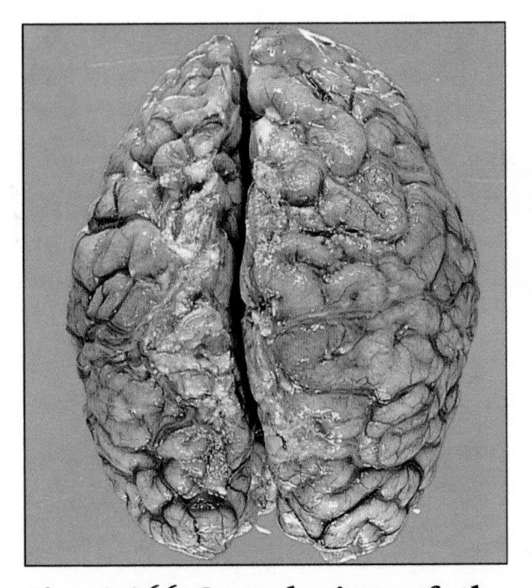

Fig. 3.266 Dorsal view of the brain of the 71-year-old man featured in Figs 3.264 and 3.265. This shows an asymmetrical atrophy of the left hemisphere.

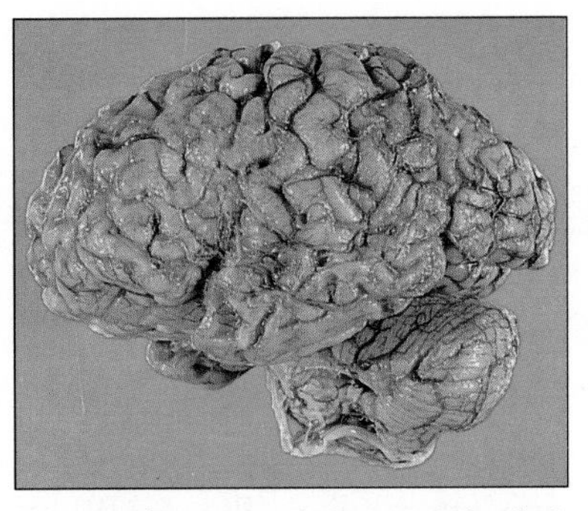

Fig. 3.267 Lateral view of the left hemisphere of the 71-year-old man featured in Figs 3.264– 3.266. This shows the severe atrophy of the frontal and temporal lobes.

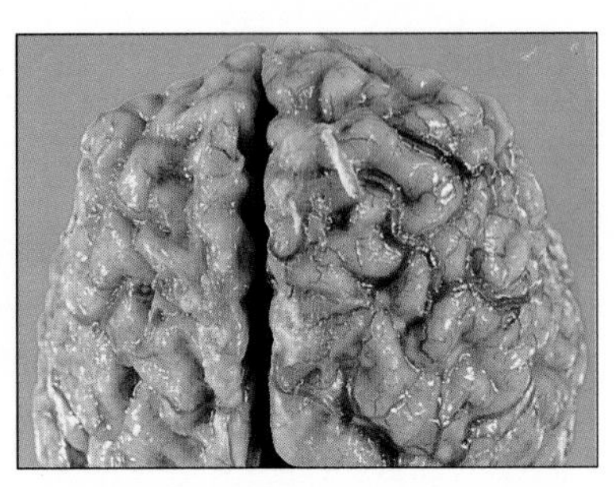

Fig. 3.268 Anterior view of the brain of the 71-year-old man featured in Figs 3.264–3.267. This shows the preferential atrophy of the left frontal lobe.

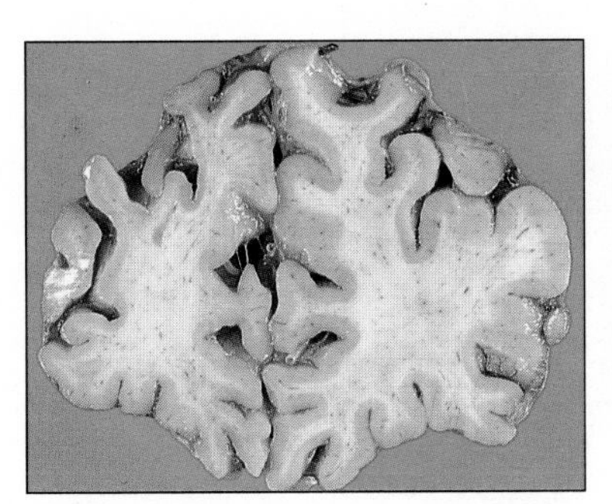

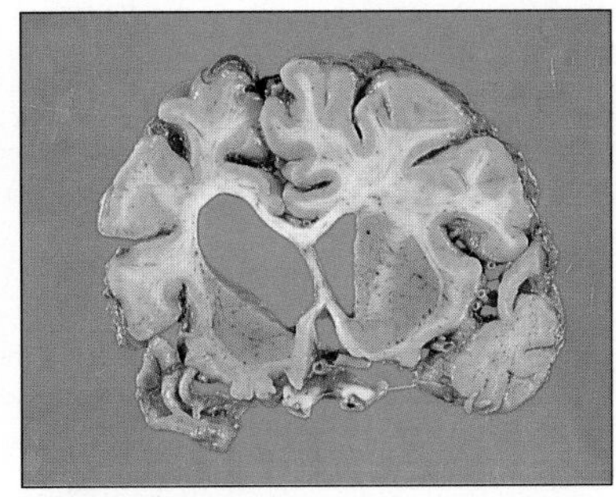

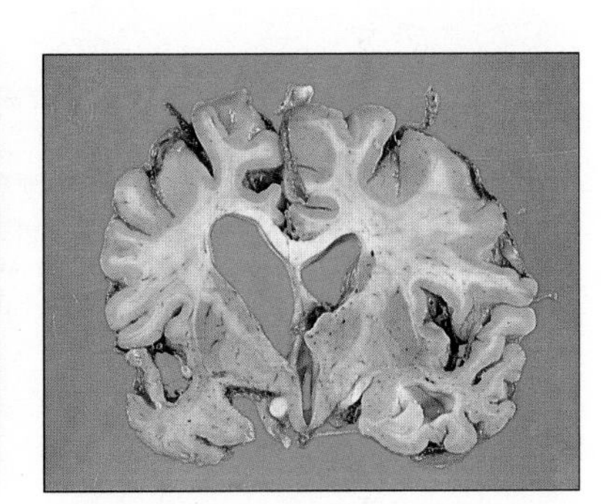

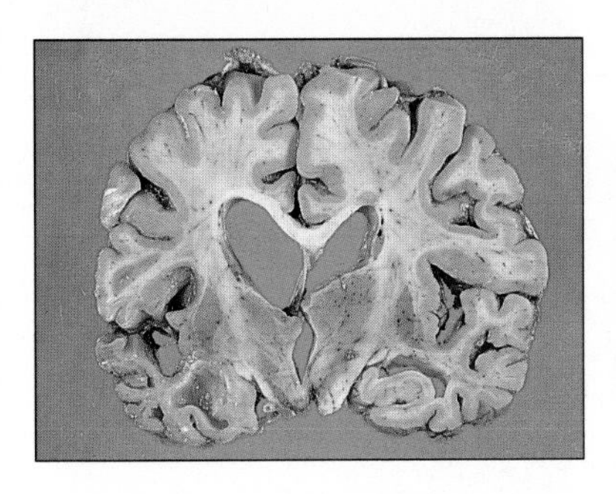

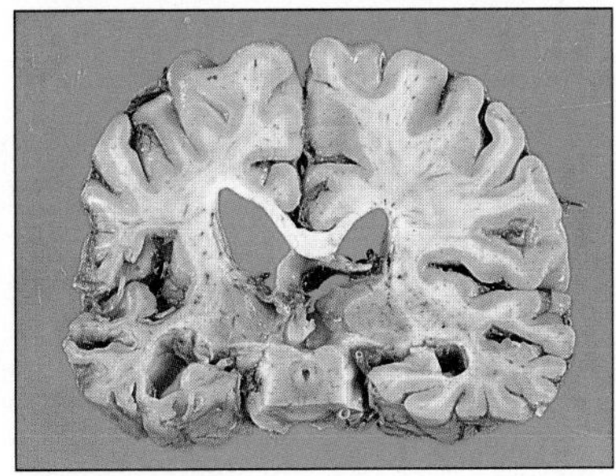

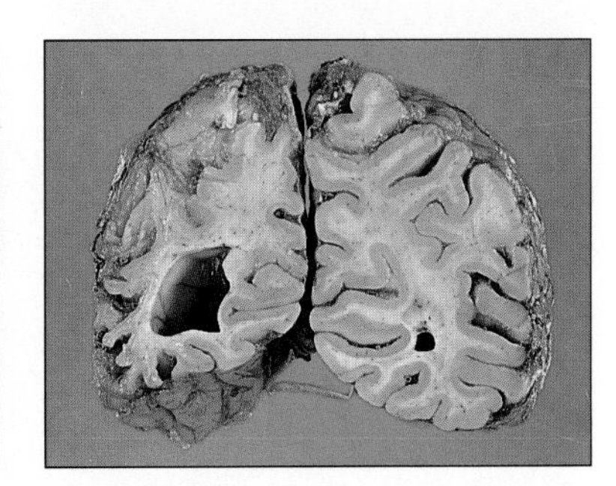

Fig. 3.269–3.274 Coronal sections of the brain of the 71-year-old man featured in Figs 3.264–3.268. These show asymmetrical atrophy of the left hemisphere involving particularly the frontal and temporal lobes. The corpus striatum and thalamus are also affected on the left side.

The brain atrophy also involves the hippocampus, amygdala, caudate, putamen, globus pallidus and thalamus on the left side alone (see **Figs 3.270–3.272**).

Morphometry (**Fig. 3.275**) confirms the atrophy, and reveals that the right hemisphere is also involved, but to a much lesser degree.

Histopathological changes

Histopathologically, frontal, fronto-parietal and anterior temporal cortices on the left side show an almost complete loss of large pyramidal cells from layers III and IV (**Fig. 3.276**). There is a widespread microvacuolar change due to neuronal fallout, particularly in layers II and III, though this change is best seen in lesser affected regions (**Fig. 3.277**) because in severely affected areas tissue necrosis and collapse can obliterate the vacuolation (see **Fig. 3.276**). Reactive astrocytosis is mild (**Fig. 3.278**), even in severely affected tissue. There are no Pick or Lewy-type inclusion bodies or inflated cells. A mild or moderate deposition of β/A4 amyloid protein is often present in less affected regions (**Fig. 3.279**), especially in the more elderly patients, but there is little if any such protein in severely affected regions (**Fig. 3.280**).

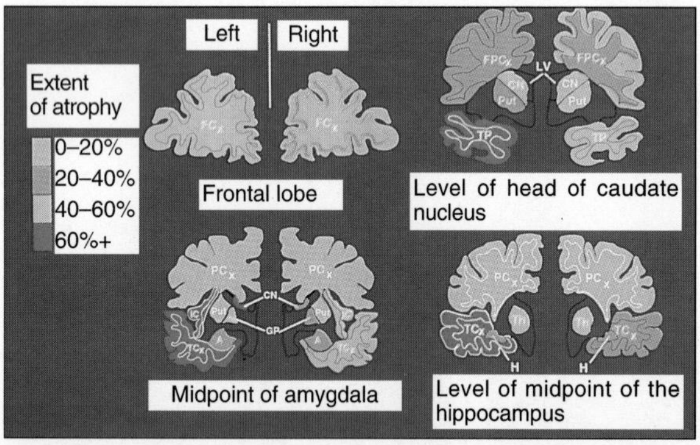

Left
Right
Extent of atrophy
0–20%
20–40%
40–60%
60%+
Frontal lobe
Level of head of caudate nucleus
Midpoint of amygdala
Level of midpoint of the hippocampus

Fig. 3.275 Morphometric analysis of regional brain atrophy in the 71-year-old man featured in Figs 3.264–3.274. The frontal and temporal lobes of the left hemisphere and the thalamus are severely atrophied, and there is also a mild to moderate atrophy of the right hemisphere.

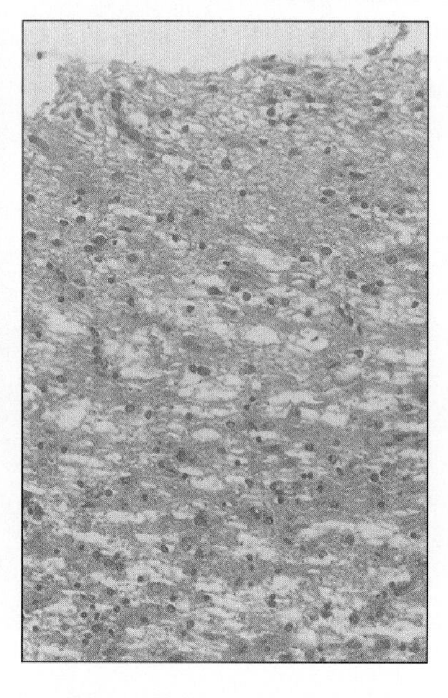

Fig. 3.276 Loss of pyramidal nerve cells from the frontal cortex with 'collapse' of the remaining cortex. (*Haematoxylin-eosin × 100*)

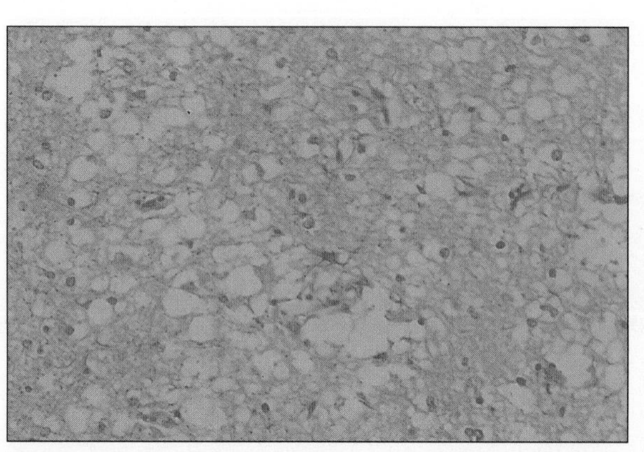

Fig. 3.277 Less affected regions of the parietal cortex show a microvacuolar change in lamina II. (*Haematoxylin–eosin × 200.*)

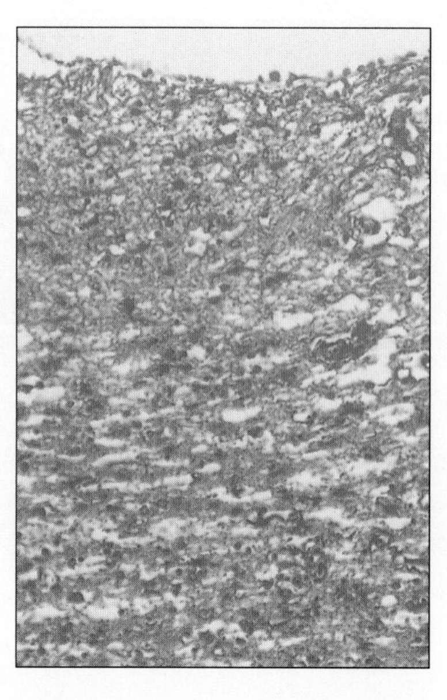

Fig. 3.278 Mild reactive astrocytosis in the frontal cortex. (*Phosphotungstic acid–haematoxylin × 100.*)

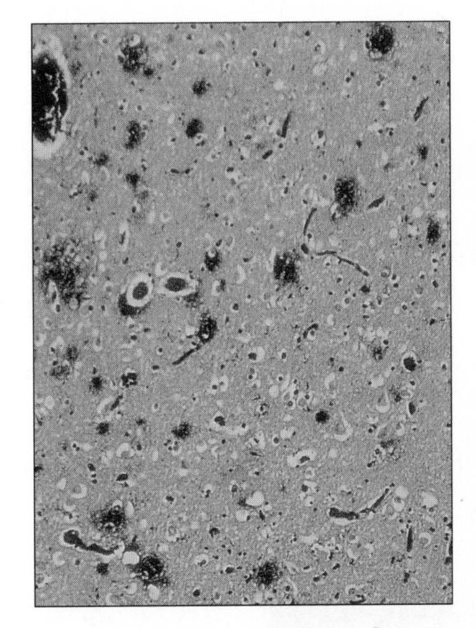

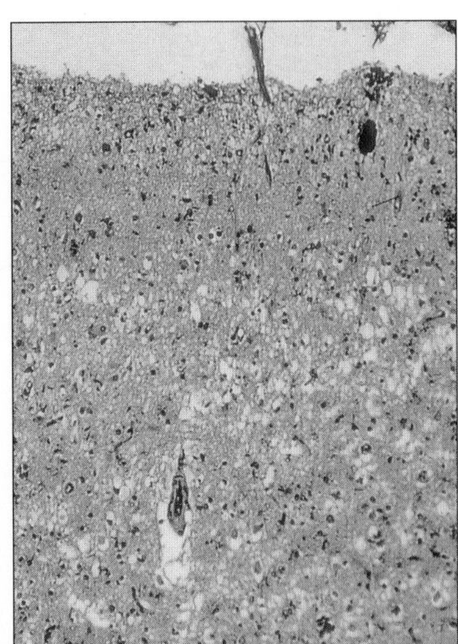

Fig. 3.279 (left) Less affected regions of the parietal cortex containing a few diffuse deposits of β/A4 protein. *(Methenamine silver stain × 100.)*

Fig. 3.280 (right) Severely affected regions of the temporal cortex. These do not contain diffuse amyloid plaques. *(Methenamine silver stain × 100.)*

Although the right hemisphere may appear grossly unaffected, the histology shows similar changes to those on the left side in equivalent areas, but to a much lesser extent.

Basal ganglia, although atrophic, are histologically normal, as are the substantia nigra, brain stem, and cerebellum.

Family studies

Progressive aphasia has a strong familial trait: about 50% of patients have relatives with the disease. In one family, the brother of a patient with profile A presented with identical linguistic breakdown, but shortly afterwards developed the behavioural changes of fronto-temporal dementia. His brain showed asymmetrical atrophy predominantly of the temporal lobes, but in this instance it was more marked on the right side (**Figs 3.281–3.285**). An asymmetrical involvement of the basal ganglia was noted, again with right-sided predominance (see **Figs 3.283–3.285**).

Morphometry (**Fig. 3.286**) clearly showed the right-sided emphasis within the temporal lobes, but also demonstrated the relatively symmetrical involvement of the frontal lobes. The histological changes were identical to those of his brother, as described on page 92.

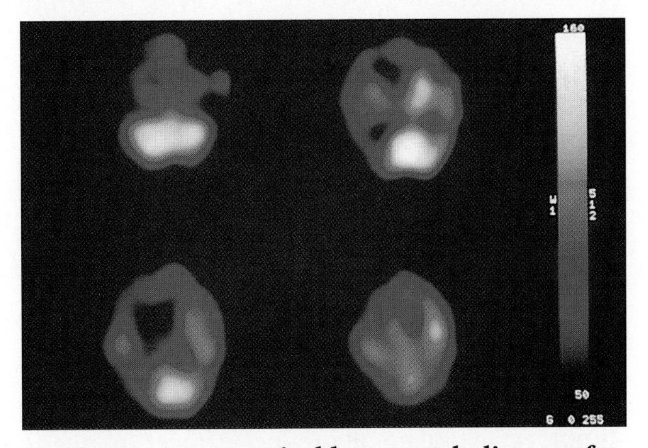

Fig. 3.281 Asymmetrical hypometabolism preferentially affecting the right cerebral hemisphere. SPET imaging of the brain of a 70-year-old man (brother of the 71-year-old man featured in **Figs 3.262–3.273**). There is, however, bilateral frontal involvement. Again, the cerebellum shows normal metabolism.

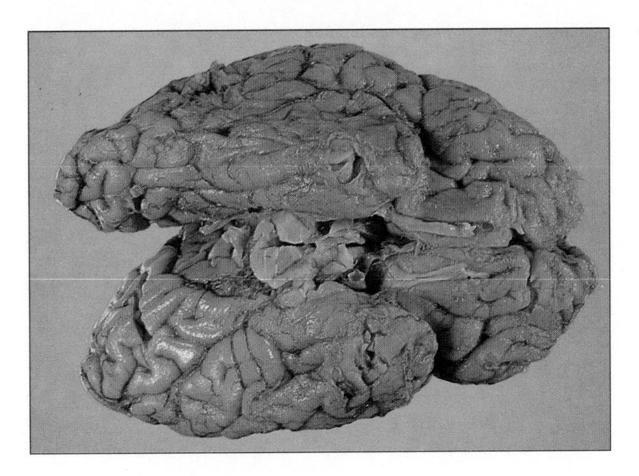

Fig. 3.282 Ventral view of the brain of the 70-year-old man featured in Fig. 3.281. This shows asymmetrical atrophy, preferentially involving the right hemisphere.

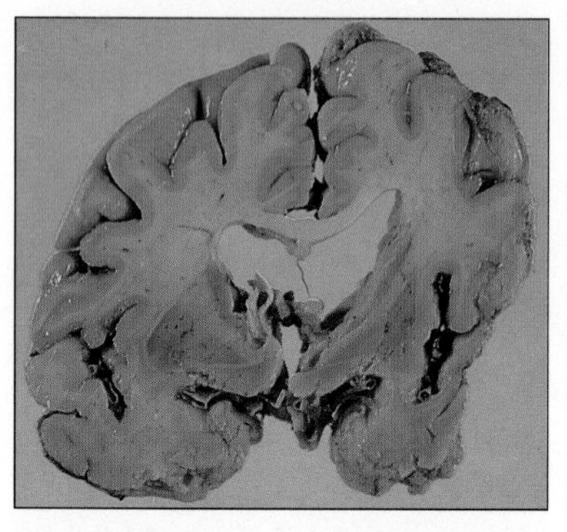

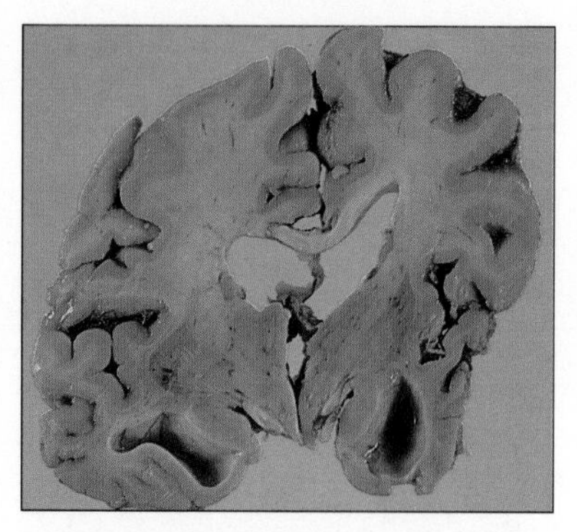

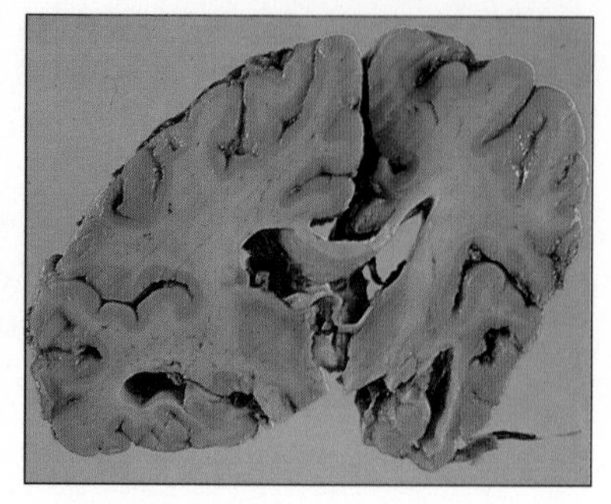

Figs 3.283–3.285 Coronal sections of the brain of the 70-year-old man featured in Figs 3.281 and **3.282** These show asymmetrical atrophy of the right hemisphere. Atrophy is severe in the temporal lobe, corpus striatum and thalamus.

Profile B: fluent aphasia and associative agnosia

Profile B is characterised by a fluent aphasia with preserved repetition and verbal paraphasias. There are profound problems with comprehension, though reading aloud and writing to dictation are preserved. Some patients go on to develop a visual associative agnosia (semantic dementia). Behavioural changes like those of fronto-temporal dementia sometimes occur in the late stages of disease. There are no significant neurological signs.

Pathological features

A CT scan (**Fig. 3.287**) will show a bilateral fronto-temporal atrophy and SPET imaging (**Fig. 3.288**) reveal bilaterally reduced tracer uptake in the anterior hemisphere.

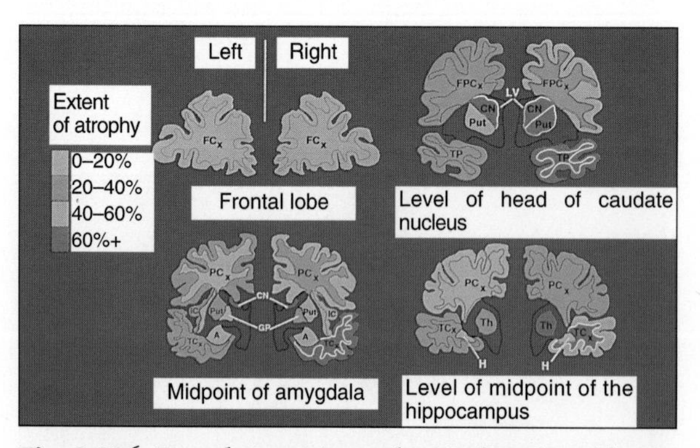

Fig. 3.286 Morphometric analysis of regional brain atrophy in the 70-year-old man featured in Figs 3.281–3.285. The frontal and temporal lobes of the right hemisphere are severely atrophied, as is the corpus striatum and thalamus. The left hemisphere also shows a mild to moderate atrophy, particularly within the frontal and temporal regions.

At autopsy, the brain appears grossly normal. There is slight ventricular enlargement and mild asymmetrical atrophy of the temporal lobes.

Histological changes affect chiefly the middle and inferior temporal gyri, with relative preservation of the superior temporal gyrus and occipital and frontal cortex. The histopathological changes are identical to those of patients with profile A.

The microvacuolar type of histology usually prevails in progressive aphasia irrespective of clinical profile, but rarely patients show different tissue changes (i.e. gliosis with typical Pick-type inclusions and swollen neurones, see page 74).

Clinico-pathological correlations

The distinct clinical syndromes of fronto-temporal dementia, fronto-temporal dementia with motor neurone disease, and progressive aphasia occurring in patients with atrophy of the frontal and temporal lobes appear to reflect a varying topographical distribution of a pathology. This seems to be common to them all rather than each being dictated by a distinct and separate type of histological change.

- When the frontal lobes are predominantly involved bilaterally and symmetrically, the patient develops the behavioural changes that characterise the clinical syndrome of fronto-temporal dementia.
- When the left dominant cerebral hemisphere is predominantly affected, the patient develops the syndrome of non-fluent progressive aphasia (profile A).

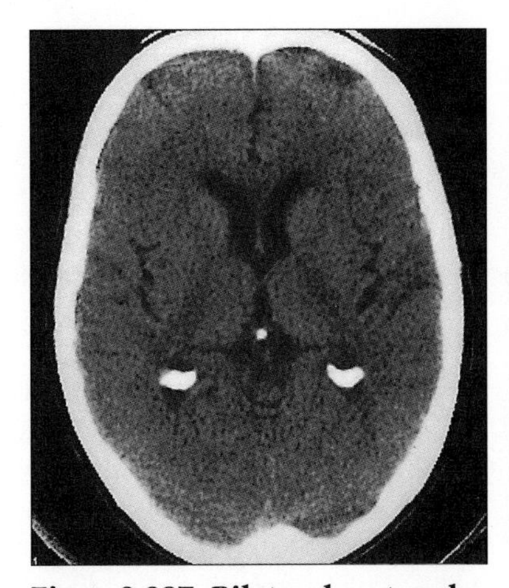

Fig. 3.287 Bilateral atrophy within perisylvian regions and mild ventricular enlargement. CT scan of the brain of a 63-year-old woman.

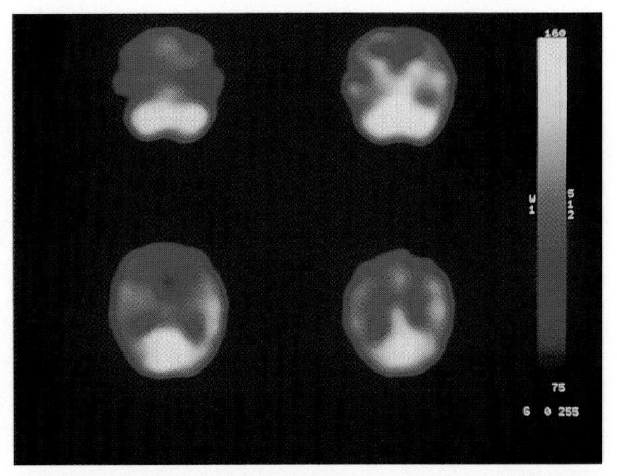

Fig. 3.288 Hypometabolism within frontal and temporal lobes, slightly favouring the right side. SPET imaging of the brain of the 63-year-old woman featured in **Fig. 3.287.**

- Bilateral involvement of the temporal lobes, with relative sparing of the frontal lobes, leads to a progressive fluent aphasia (profile B) with associative visual agnosia.
- Spread of pathology from the temporal to the frontal lobes is associated with the onset of a progressive aphasia followed by the behavioural disorder of fronto-temporal dementia as in the two brothers described.
- Motor neurone disease is mainly associated with fronto-temporal dementia, but an association with progressive aphasia has occasionally been observed.

Clinico-histological correlations

A distinction has been made histologically between those cases that assume a microvacuolar appearance to the degeneration and those that have a gliotic change, with or without Pick cells and Pick bodies.

The clinical syndrome of fronto-temporal dementia appears to be associated with either histology, in roughly similar proportions, both with a broadly similar familial incidence. There is nothing to distinguish the two histologies in terms of the severity of the brain atrophy, or in respect of the way in which that atrophy is distributed throughout the brain. The macroscopic appearance of the tissue is similar in both histological situations. Consequently, as might be expected, no distinctions can be made in terms of the clinical presentation or neuropsychological profiles of patients with either histology. The cardinal question therefore is whether the different histologies are of aetiological significance (i.e. do they represent different disease entities that share a common topographic localisation of pathological change within the brain), or are they different phenotypes of a single disease that can manifest with a spectrum of pathological change.

In the past, Pick's disease has been used, often 'loosely', to describe fronto-temporal atrophy, whether or not the pathognomic Pick cells or Pick bodies were actually present. When used in this way *all* fronto-temporal dementia could be called Pick's disease. In addition, if it is accepted that a microvacuolar degeneration of the cortex is one of the pathological phenocopies of Pick's disease, then the clinical syndromes of fronto-temporal dementia with motor neurone disease and progressive aphasia would also fall under this umbrella. However, if Pick's disease is to be more strictly defined by the histological change of astrocytic gliosis and the presence of neuronal inclusions that are immunoreactive to tau and ubiquitin,then it accounts for only a minority of cases of fronto-temporal atrophy.

Gustafson, Brun and Risberg have described a series of cases in Sweden closely parallelling the authors' own case material. They use the term 'frontal lobe degeneration (FLD)' to describe a clinical syndrome in which underlying atrophy of the frontal and temporal lobes is associated with a microvacuolar degeneration of the outer cortex and an *absence* of gliosis, swollen cells, and inclusions. They also draw a distinction between this syndrome and the clinical syndrome of fronto-temporal dementia associated with a fronto-temporal atrophy characterised by astrocytosis and cellular inclusions, which they refer to as Pick's disease. In addition, as if to emphasise that the clinical syndrome cannot be used to implicate the underlying pathology, Gustafson comments that there are 'only small and non-systematic clinical differences between frontal lobe degeneration and Pick's cases.

Constantinidis and colleagues from Switzerland have reviewed their own series of patients and describe a clinical syndrome of fronto-temporal dementia that includes three categories under the histological description of Pick's disease:

- Gliosis.
- Gliosis with swollen neurones.
- Gliosis with neuronal swellings and argyrophilic inclusions.

There were apparently no patients with microvacuolation but without gliosis.

Knopman in the USA has described patients with fronto-temporal dementia displaying a microvacuolar degeneration of the superficial cortex with minimal gliosis. This condition was designated as 'dementia lacking distinctive histological features'. Some of these patients also had amyotrophy with appropriate pathological changes in the spinal cord and hypoglossal nucleus, and would therefore correspond to our group of patients with fronto-temporal dementia and motor neurone disease.

It is clear that fronto-temporal dementia, due to a pathology other than that typified by gliosis and neuronal inclusions, is not a new disorder and has been reported on other occasions. Often ,however, the condition has probably been 'submerged' under the title of 'Pick's disease'. Whether this is justifiable or not remains unclear in the absence of a distinctive biochemical or pathological marker that 'segregates' or clearly differentiates these histological variants, or brings them together under a unified molecular pathological abnormality.

The processes that induce tissue vacuolation and gliosis remain to be explained. It is possible that in some instances, as is the case with tangles in Alzheimer's disease, the neuronal inclusions and swollen cells may eventually vanish from the tissue along with the neurones, giving an appearance of gliosis without inclusions. Whether microvacuolation and gliosis are interchangeable aspects of a similar process is not known.

Spongiform encephalopathies display phenotypic variation in pathological presentation (see page 145) despite being driven by particular mutations within the prion gene or resulting from a possible 'mismetabolism' of the product of that gene. It is possible that a similar situation is involved in fronto-temporal dementias.

It appears, therefore, that the distinctive clinical syndromes that encompass fronto-temporal dementia are dictated by topography and that the syndromes do not, in themselves, predict the underlying histology. This appears to comprise a spectrum of pathological alterations, rather than clear and well demarcated entities. Familial cases exist for each syndrome and for each histological type.

If descriptive distinctions are to be made between the clinical syndromes, the anatomical distributions of atrophy and the histological changes, then Pick's disease can be viewed as a separate histology that can cause fronto-temporal atrophy in each of the syndromes of fronto-temporal dementia, fronto-temporal dementia with motor neurone disease, and progressive aphasia. The other histology (that of microvacuolar change) can likewise direct these very same clinical syndromes.

The processes driving these different, though possibly interrelated or interchangeable histologies, remain obscure and require delineation. Given the high familial incidence associated with each syndrome, however, it is likely that a genetic cause will account for a large majority of cases (perhaps all of them), which could then be explained on a molecular biological basis.

THE GENETICS OF LOBAR ATROPHY

In about 50% of patients with lobar atrophy, a clear family history of a similar disorder is present. This is true for fronto-temporal dementia, fronto-temporal dementia with motor neurone disease and progressive aphasia with both microvacuolar and Pick-type histologies being implicated. However, proper family studies are rare with only a few full pedigrees having been reported. Our own cohort of patients has yielded several pedigrees, one concerning a family with fronto-temporal dementia, dates back to 1695 and postmortem examination on one deceased member has revealed a microvacuolar degeneration. In another pedigree, one patient has a similarly affected sister and a degeneration due to Pick-type histology. In yet another pedigree a patient with the microvacuolar type of degeneration had 4 other affected siblings. Familial progressive aphasia has been described by us in two brothers (see page 91).

The gene(s) responsible for producing the pathological changes of lobar atrophy is consequently unknown; insufficiently extensive pedigrees with lack of enough samples from affected and unaffected members has so far precluded linkage analysis. Nonetheless, we have been able to investigate sufficient cases of disease in each clinical (fronto-temporal dementia, fronto-temporal dementia with motor neurone disease, progressive aphasia) and histological (micro-vacuolar and Pick-type) category using a candidate gene approach in order to test whether particular genetic loci already implicated in other forms of neurodegenerative disease (and mostly leading to dementia) are involved. In this way we have been able to exclude the likelihood that any of the clinical or histological variants of lobar atrophy are associated with mutations in the prion gene (as in the spongiform encephalopathies, see page 160). There is an absence of proteinase resistant prion protein on immunohistochemistry or immuno-blotting. Likewise, mutations in codon 717 of the APP gene (as in familial Alzheimer's disease, see page 59), mutations in the superoxide dismutase gene (as in familial motor neurone disease), or excessive CAG repeats in the IT15 gene (as in Huntington's disease, see page 103) do not occur. The disorders are not associated with any unusual allelic variations in the Apolipoprotein E gene (as in late onset familial Alzheimer's disease, see page 59).

At present it is not clear whether this kind of 'shot in the dark' candidate gene approach will, in the absence of a specific molecular marker associated with lobar atrophy, lead to the prospect of an early identification of the genetic locus(i), although because a loss of glutamatergic pyramidal cells is fundamental to the pathology a search of glutamate markers (e.g. subgroups of glutamate receptor) might be informative. Alternatively, and perhaps more likely, it may prove necessary to carry out a systematic search of the genome in sufficiently extensive pedigrees to produce the required linkage data.

Alcoholic encephalopathy

Sometimes, the neuropsychological changes associated with chronic alcoholism stem directly from the effect of thiamine deficiency resulting from an impoverished diet. Affected individuals display an impairment of memory and concentration, ataxia, nystagmus with extraocular palsies, and peripheral neuropathies.

The main lesions lie in the mammillary bodies and in regions around the III and IV ventricles and the aqueduct. Macroscopically, petechial haemorrhages may be apparent, usually in the mammillary bodies (**Fig. 3.289**), but also elsewhere in the mid-brain and brain stem. Microscopically, there is capillary dilatation and haemorrhage. Demyelination may occur, but neuronal loss is not apparent; older lesions, however, indicate loss of neurones with gliosis. A patchy loss of Purkinje cells, particularly from the vermis, is common, with some reaction by the Bergmann glia of the Purkinje cell layer. These changes represent the *acute* lesions of *Wernicke's encephalopathy* and progress into the *chronic* changes of *Korsakoff's psychosis* when there is continued exposure to alcohol.

In *Korsakoff's psychosis* the mammillary bodies are shrunken (**Fig. 3.290**), showing severe neuronal loss and reactive astrocytosis (**Fig. 3.291**). Neuronal loss and gliosis may also be apparent within the wall of the medial thalamus. Atrophy of frontal and parietal lobes may occur in some patients with meningeal thickening and ventricular dilatation. Histologically, neurones may be lost from the III layer (along with some astrocytic proliferation) and from the nucleus of Meynert and locus caeruleus.

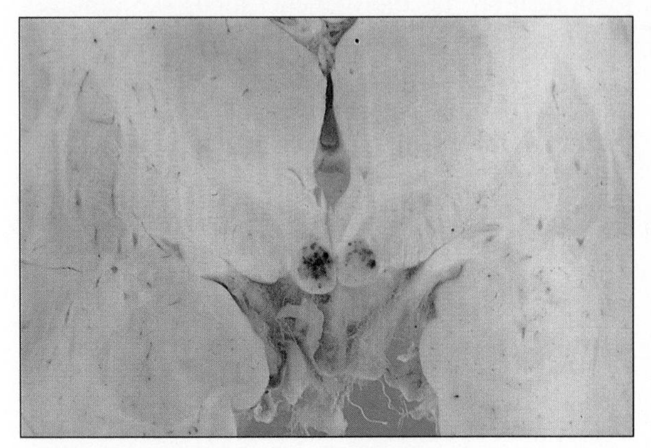

Fig. 3.289 Wernicke's encephalopathy. Acute haemorrhagic changes in the mammillary bodies occur in Wernicke's encephalopathy.

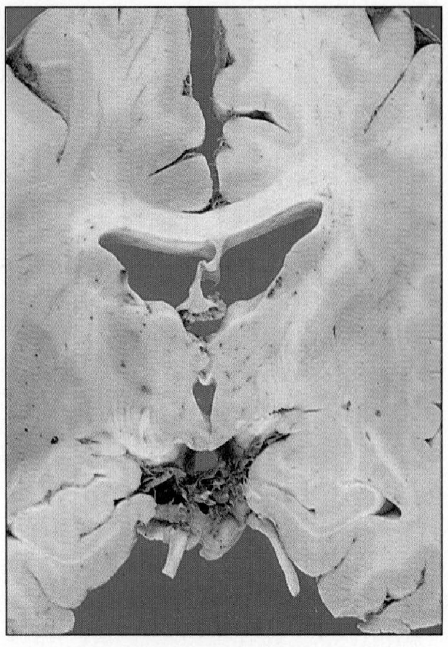

Fig. 3.290 Korsakoff's psychosis. Chronic atrophy of the mammillary bodies is a major feature in Korsakoff's psychosis.

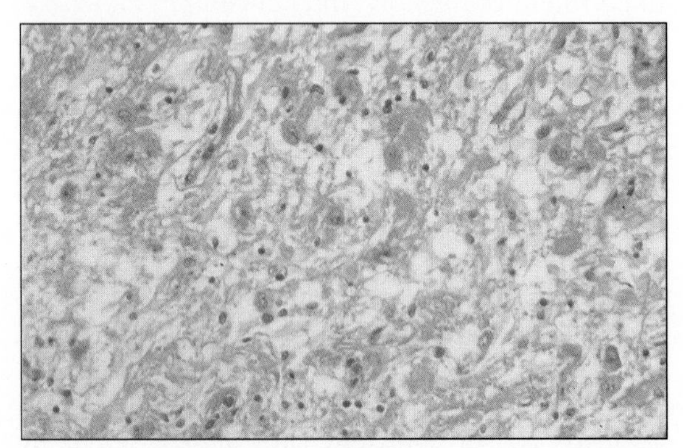

Fig. 3.291 Korsakoff's psychosis. Loss of nerve cells and astrocytosis in the mammillary bodies in Korsakoff's psychosis. *(Haematoxylin–eosin × 200.)*

4. Subcortical encephalopathies

Certain disorders, such as progressive supranuclear palsy, Huntington's disease and Parkinson's disease affect chiefly subcortical structures within the basal ganglia or brain stem, or both, leaving the cerebral cortex largely, but not always wholly, undamaged. Impaired function of these non-cortical brain regions affects the cerebral cortex by slowing reactions and failing to regulate responses in an orderly fashion. Neuropsychological deficits are usually subordinate to the profound neurological problems that occur.

PROGRESSIVE SUPRANUCLEAR PALSY

Demographic features

In 1964, Steele, Richardson, and Olszewski reported nine male patients with a syndrome of progressive paralysis of vertical eye movement, dysarthria, and muscular rigidity, especially involving the neck muscles. Many other similar patients have since been identified and all display a dementia considered to be prototypical of subcortical dementia, especially in the later stages of the disease.

From reported cases, twice as many men are are affected as women. Age of onset is variable, ranging from 40–70 years, while the duration of the illness can be prolonged. Familial cases have only rarely been identified.

Neurological symptoms and signs (early)
Supranuclear gaze
Pseudobulbar palsy
Nuchal rigidity
Disturbed posture
Ataxia
Psychological symptoms (late)
Mental slowness
Inefficient memory
Investigations
SPET: frontal lobe abnormality

Pathological features

The brain shows no distinctive features on CT scan (**Fig. 4.1**), though sometimes there may be mild cerebral atrophy and ventricular enlargement. SPET imaging (**Fig. 4.2**) usually reveals bilateral subcortical hypometabolism in the frontal lobes with preservation of the cortical margin.

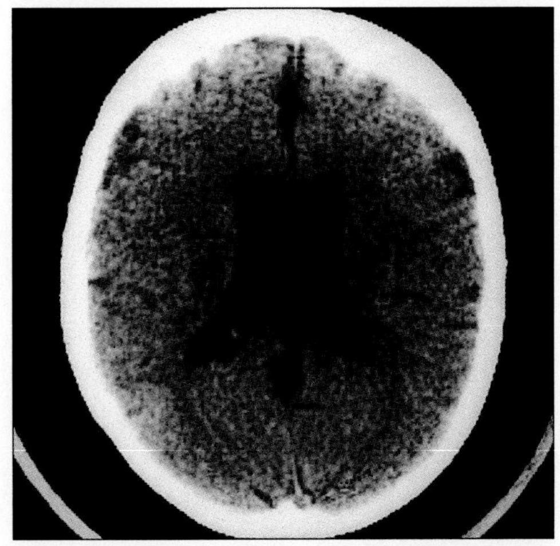

Fig. 4.1 Mild and diffuse cortical atrophy with moderate enlargement of the lateral ventricles and widening of the interhemispheric fissure. CT scan of the brain of a 56-year-old woman.

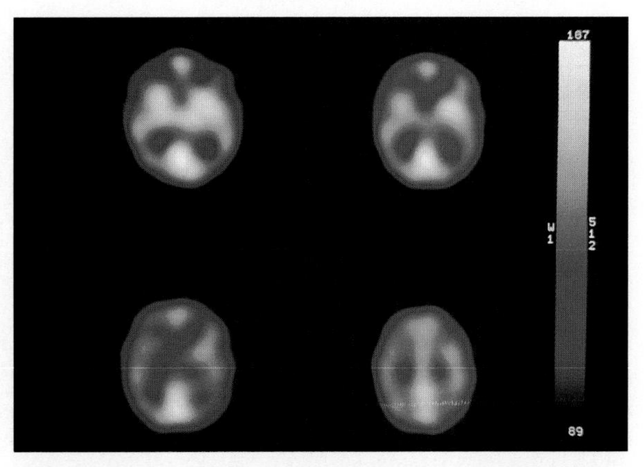

Fig. 4.2 Bilaterally reduced brain metabolism in the frontal lobes. SPET imaging in a 60-year-old woman.

At autopsy, brain weight may be slightly reduced or is normal; gross alterations in brain size do not occur. There may be some mild atrophy in the frontal and anterior temporal regions. On coronal section there are no consistent abnormalities in the cerebral cortex (**Fig. 4.3**), but gross depigmentation of the substantia nigra and locus caeruleus is apparent in the brain stem regions. Morphometry (**Fig. 4.4**) shows that cortical grey matter is on the whole preserved, but there is atrophy of the white matter and a reduction in the size of subcortical regions such as the globus pallidus and thalamus.

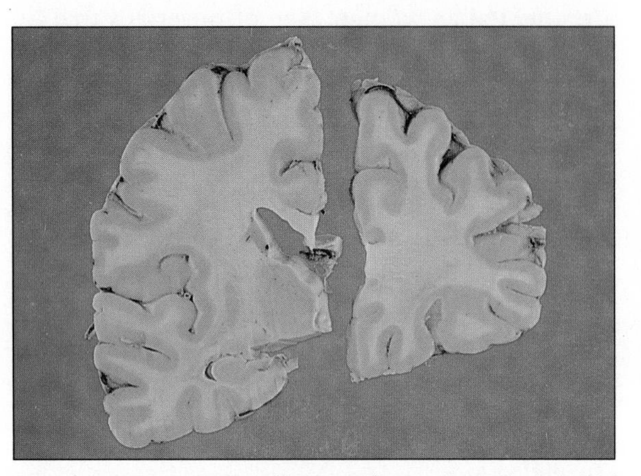

Fig. 4.3 No specific abnormality. Coronal slices of brain of the 66-year-old woman.

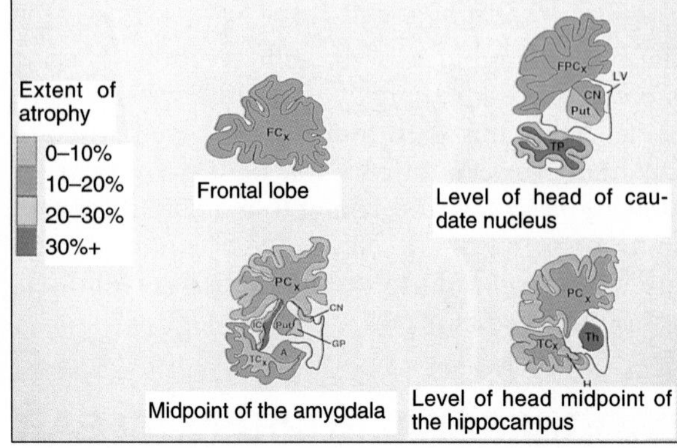

Fig. 4.4 Mild though preferential atrophy of the cerebral cortical white matter with greater involvement of the temporal lobe. Morphometric analysis of regional brain atrophy. Atrophy is greater in the globus pallidus and thalamus than other subcortical regions.

Age of onset
40–65 years.

Sex incidence
Slightly more common in males

Duration
Variable, usually 5–10 years.

Gross features
Mild cerebral atrophy, usually of the frontal lobes
Depigmentation of the substantia nigra

Histopathology
- Loss of nerve cells from the substantia nigra, with tangles
- Other regions such as locus caeruleus, nucleus basalis of Meynert, pontine nuclei, dentate nucleus also affected
- Tangles are tau, but not ubiquitin positive
- Dentate nucleus often shows severe astrocytosis
- Sometimes there are tangles in the hippocampus, entorhinal cortex (especially), and neocortex (occasionally)

Genetics
- Usually appears to occur spontaneously
- Occasional familial cases, but the genetic basis of these is unknown

Histological changes

Histologically, the most characteristic change involves a neurofibrillary degeneration and loss of neurones in certain brain stem, mid-brain, and basal ganglia regions. Of these, the substantia nigra is most consistently and severely affected (**Fig. 4.5**), but similar though lesser changes occur in the locus caeruleus (see **Fig. 4.12**), nucleus basalis of Meynert, dorsal raphe and pontine (**Fig. 4.6**; see also **Fig. 4.14**) and olivary nuclei. Often there is also involvement of the globus

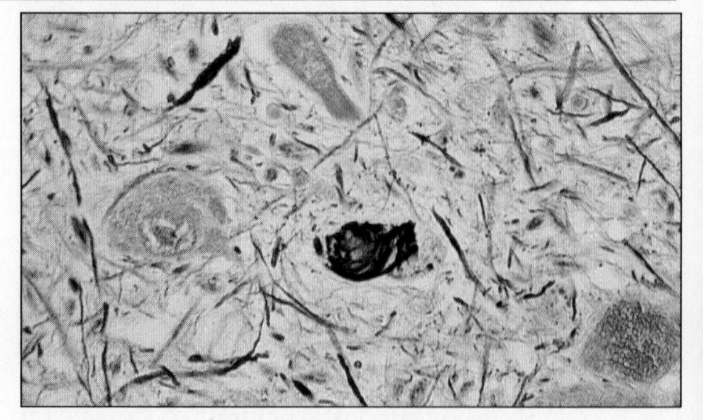

Fig. 4.5 Neurofibrillary tangle in a nerve cell of the substantia nigra. *(Palmgren silver stain × 400.)*

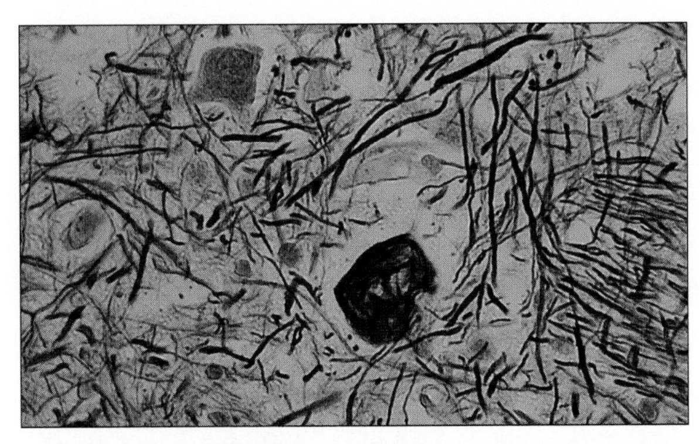

Fig. 4.6 Neurofibrillary tangles in nerve cells of the pontine nuclei. *(Palmgren silver stain × 400.)*

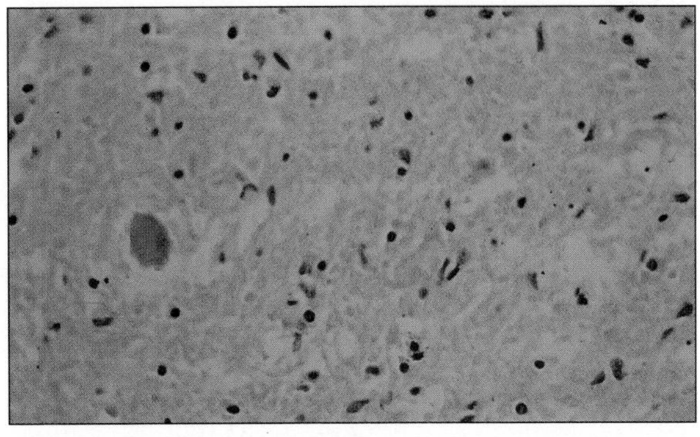

Fig. 4.7 Loss of nerve cells from the dentate nucleus of the cerebellum. *(Haematoxylin–eosin × 200.)*

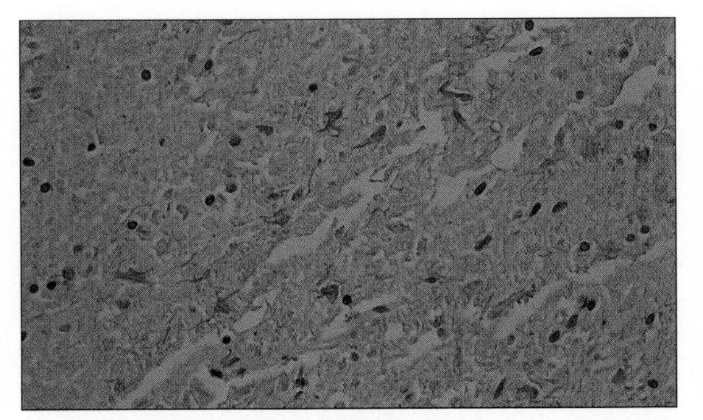

Fig. 4.8 Reactive astrocytosis in the dentate nucleus of the cerebellum. *(Phosphotungstic-acid–haematoxylin × 200.)*

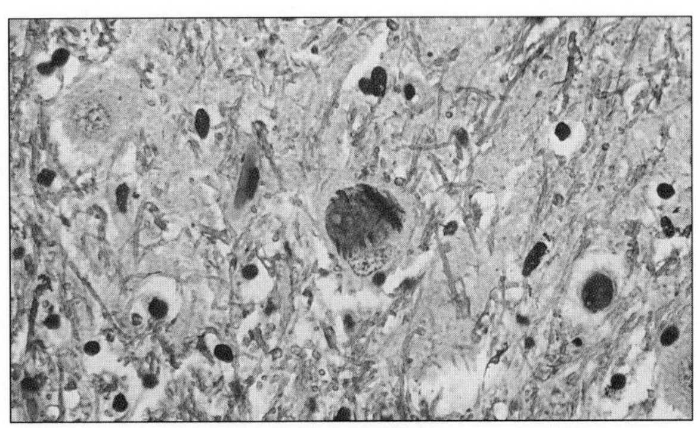

Fig. 4.9 Neurofibrillary tangle in a nerve cell of the dentate nucleus. *(Palmgren silver stain × 400.)*

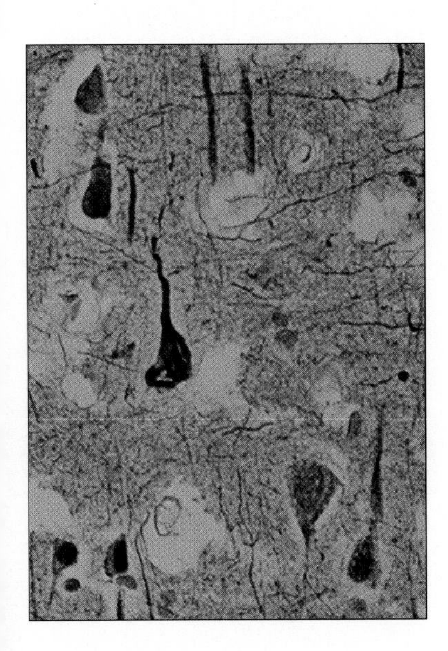

Fig. 4.10 (left) Neurofibrillary tangle in a pyramidal nerve cell of the temporal cortex. *(Palmgren silver stain × 400.)*

Fig. 4.11 (right) Many neurofibrillary tangles in the stellate neurones of layer II of the entorhinal cortex. *(Palmgren silver stain × 200.)*

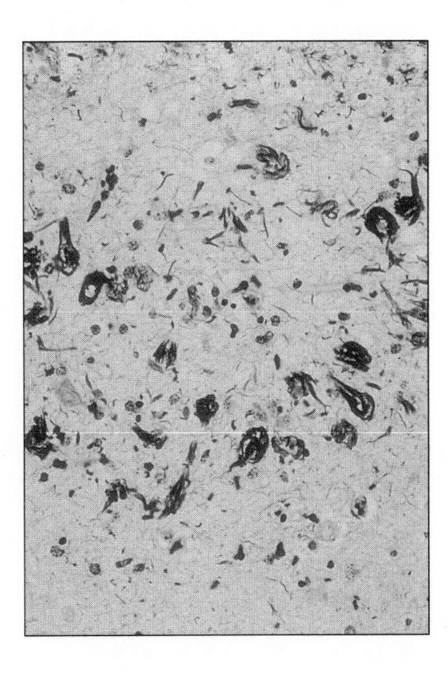

pallidus, thalamus, subthalamic nucleus, red nucleus and dentate nucleus; in the latter region nerve cell loss and intense gliosis are common (**Figs 4.7** and **4.8**), although neurofibrillary degeneration (**Fig. 4.9**; see also **Figs 4.13** and **4.17–4.18**) is less frequent.

The cerebral cortex and hippocampus are inconsistently involved, with isolated pyramidal cells in the frontal (**Fig. 4.10**, see also **Fig. 4.16**) and temporal, and even motor cortex, showing neurofibrillary tangles. Often, although it is the stellate cells in layer II of the entorhinal cortex (**Fig. 4.11**) that are mainly affected (see **Fig.4.22**), as are many neurones in the subiculum and CA1 region of Ammon's horn.

The neurofibrillary tangles of progressive supranuclear palsy are composed mainly of 'straight' filaments of 15 nm diameter, but variable quantities of 10 nm paired helical filaments (PHFs) of the type seen in Alzheimer's disease are sometimes present. Like the tangles of Alzheimer's disease, those of progressive supranuclear palsy are immunoreactive with antisera to tau protein (**Figs 4.12–4.18**). In contrast to Alzheimer's disease, those in subcortical regions do not react with anti-ubiquitin antibodies, though cortical tangles usually do. Neuropil threads that are also tau but not ubiquitin immunoreactive are widely present in cortical regions, especially in the entorhinal cortex (**Figs 4.11** and **4.22**)

White matter tracts in the brain stem contain a large amount of 'granular' ubiquitinated material (**Fig. 4.20**), this is probably being axons. Nonetheless, as in Alzheimer's disease it is likely that neurofibrillary degeneration provides the mechanism underlying neuronal loss in progressive supranuclear palsy: ghost tangles (**Figs 4.18, 4.21** and **4.22**) and cells with tangle, but without other organelles (see **Fig. 4.17**) are common. How this change is aetiologically produced is not known.

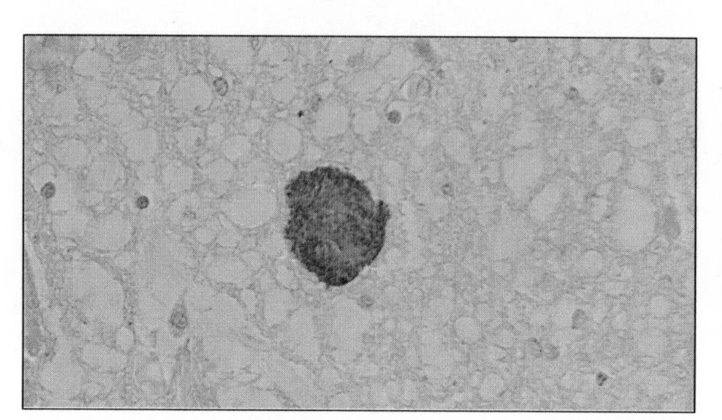

Fig. 4.12 Neurofibrillary tangles in the locus caeruleus, containing tau proteins. *(Anti-tau × 400.)*

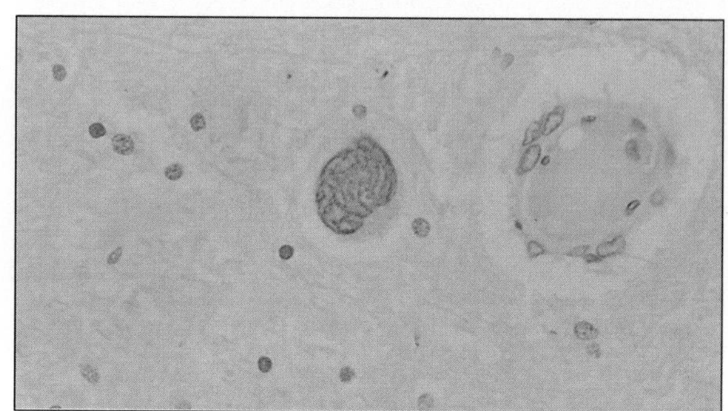

Fig. 4.13 Neurofibrillary tangles in the dentate nucleus, also containing tau protein. *(Anti-tau × 400.)*

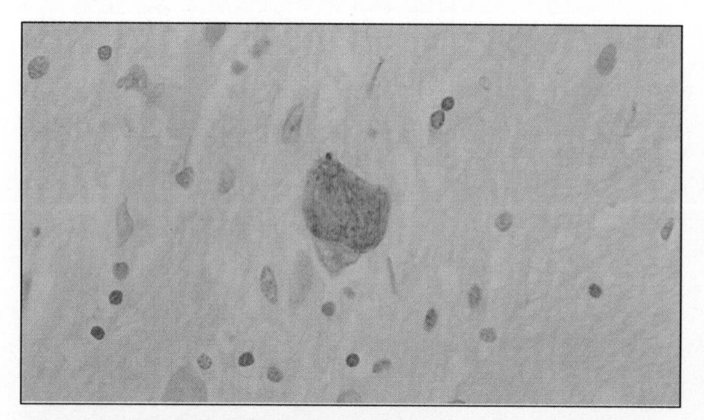

Fig. 4.14 Neurofibrillary tangles in the pontine nuclei, again containing tau protein. *(Anti-tau × 400.)*

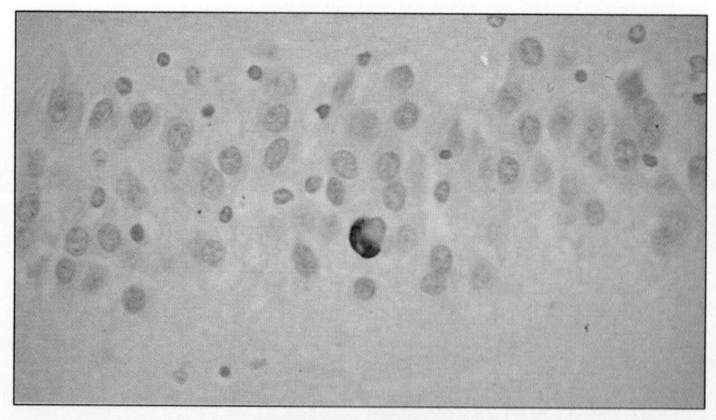

Fig. 4.15 Neurofibrillary tangle in a granule cell of the dentate gyrus of the hippocampus. *(Anti-tau × 400.)*

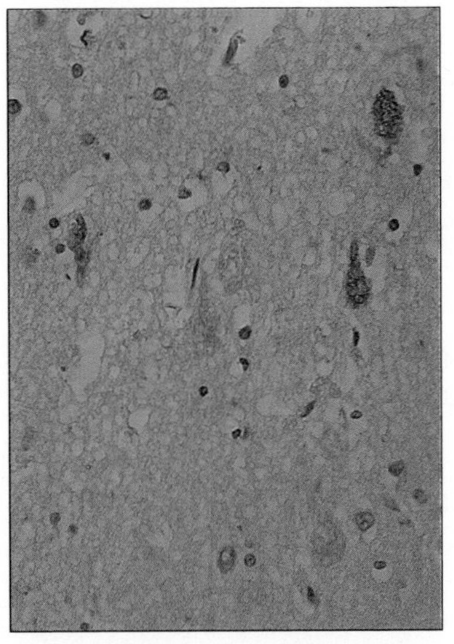

Fig. 4.16 This pyramidal cell in the temporal cortex is tau-reactive. *(Anti-tau × 400.)*

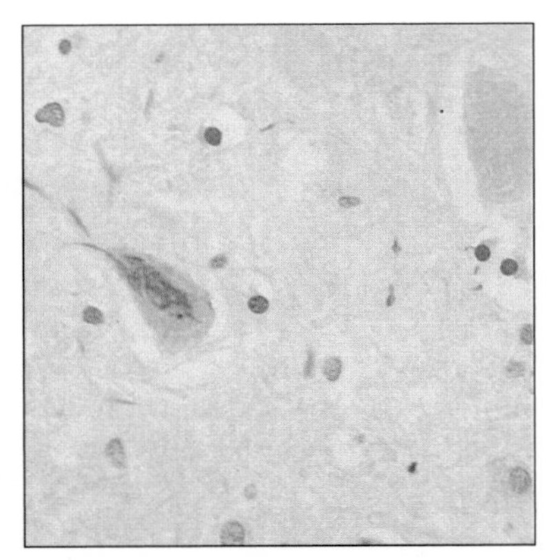

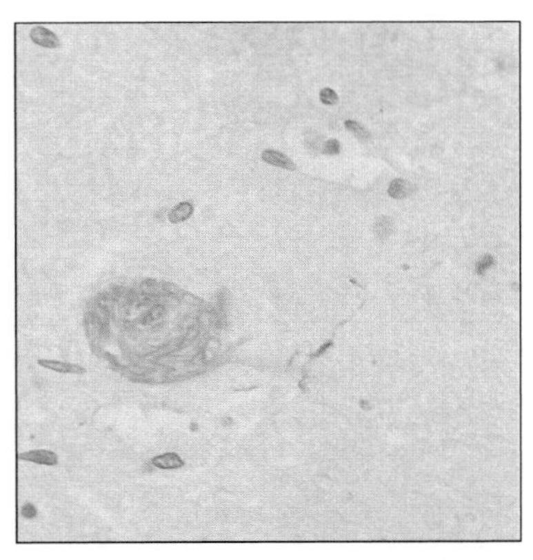

Figs 4.17 and **4.18 'Ghost' cells** in the dentate nucleus show only the remains of neurofibrillary tangle, but no Nissl substance or nucleus. *(Anti-tau × 400.)*

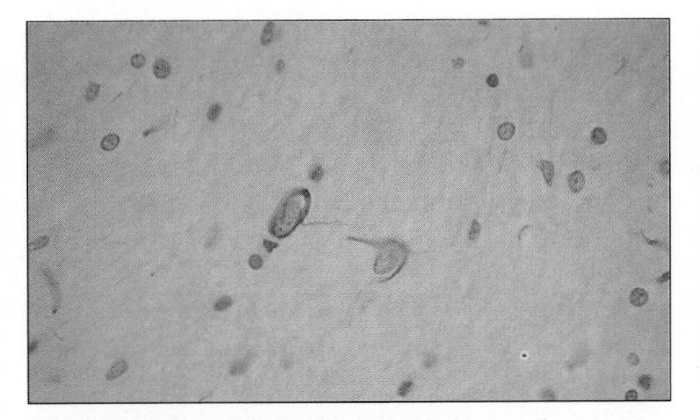

Fig. 4.19 Astrocytes in the internal capsule containing tau protein. *(Anti-tau × 200.)*

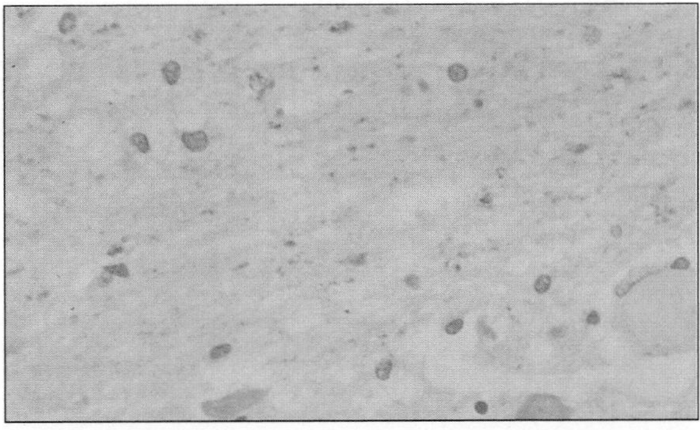

Fig. 4.20 Ubiquitin immunoreactive particulate material. There is a large amount of ubiquitin immunoreactive particulate material in the corticospinal tract. *(Anti-ubiquitin × 200.)*

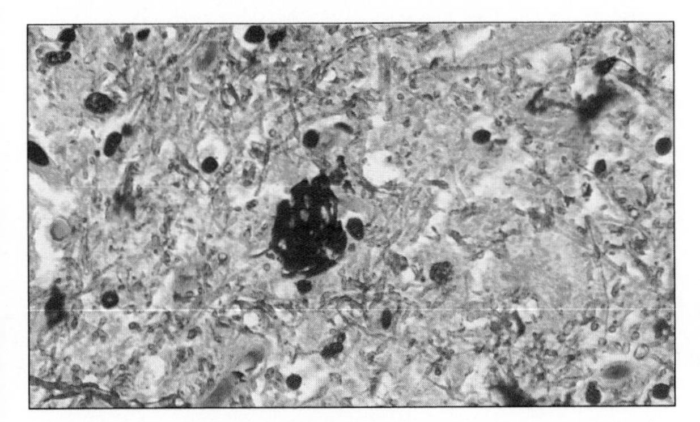

Fig. 4.21 An extracellular tangle in the dentate nucleus. *(Palmgren silver stain × 400.)*

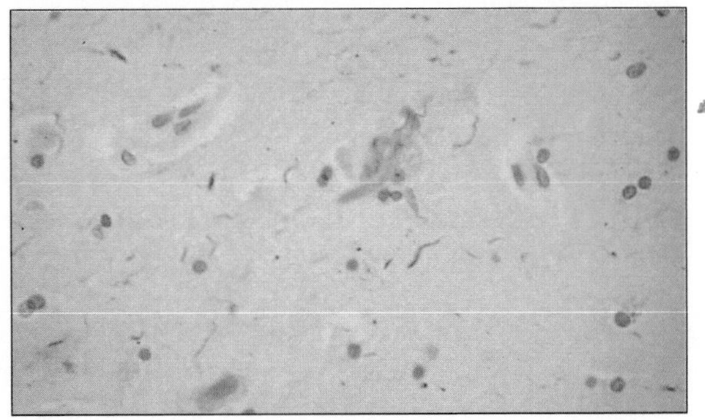

Fig. 4.22 An extracellular tangle and neuropil threads in the entorhinal cortex. *(Palmgren silver stain × 400.)*

Astrocytes, sometimes binucleate, containing tau proteins have been identified in the striatum, thalamus and frontal cortex (**Fig. 4.19**). Such astrocytes are rarely present in other neurodegenerative disorders; tau protein is not usually present in normal, or typical reactive, astrocytes. Furthermore, tau positive oligodendrocytes are widely present in white matter tracts, these differing from astrocytes by the possession of anti-ubiquitin immunoreactivity. The significance of these glial cell alterations is unknown.

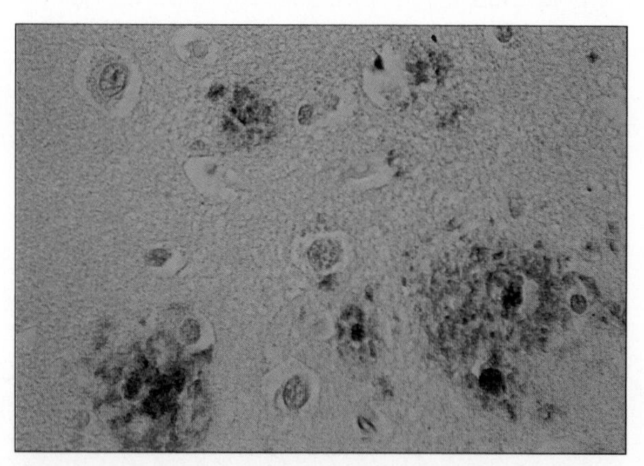

Fig. 4.23 Diffuse deposits of β/A4 protein in the temporal cortex. *(Anti-β/A4 × 200.)*

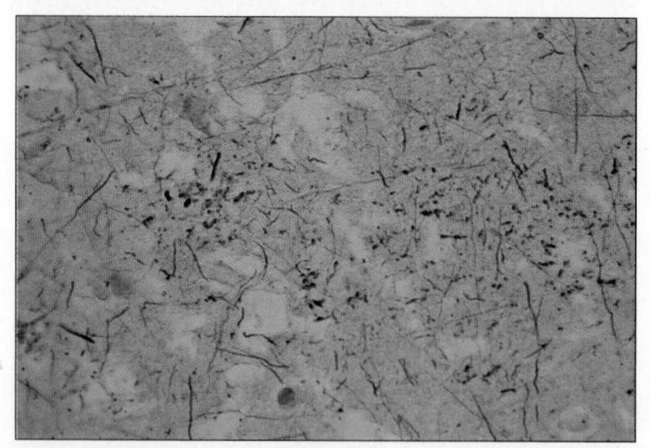

Fig. 4.24 Such diffuse plaques do not contain neurites. *(Palmgren silver stain × 200.)*

A few to many diffuse deposits of β/A4 protein are widely present in the cerebral cortex in some of the more elderly patients (**Figs 4.23** and **4.24**). These deposits, like those seen in normal ageing, are not associated with a neuritic change, but it is not certain whether their quantity is entirely appropriate to, or excessive for, the age of the patient.

Clinico-pathological characteristics of progressive supranuclear palsy

Patients have a subcortical dementia and on tests sensitive to frontal lobe dysfunction perform poorly. As there appear to be no significant pathological changes in the frontal lobes it is presumed that the clinical changes (and the SPET images) reflect a functional deafferentation of the frontal lobes due to disease in other brain regions projecting to the frontal cortex. In this context, specific pathway alterations between the thalamus and basal ganglia and the frontal lobes would play an important role, as would contributions from the diffusely projecting cortical afferents from the nucleus basalis, locus caeruleus and dorsal raphe. Collectively, loss of these afferent fibres could account for the reduction in quantity of white matter. The destruction of the entorhinal cortex and hippocampus may also contribute to the cognitive impairment.

Nothing is known about the aetiology of progressive supranuclear palsy, nor is it clear how the neurofibrillary changes of the disorder are caused. Whether the disease has aetiological relationships with idiopathic Parkinson's disease (with which it shares loss of neurones from the substantia nigra) or Alzheimer's disease (with which it shares tangle formation and occasionally a particularly heavy deposition of amyloid β/A4 protein) is uncertain.

HUNTINGTON'S DISEASE

Demographic features

Huntington's disease occurs in all races with a frequency in Europe and North America of about 4–7 cases/100,000 population, while the prevalence in Japan is about 10% of this. Worldwide local areas of high incidence can occur where population movement is restricted. Males and females are equally affected, with age of onset at any time but usually 25–45 years of age. The duration of the illness averages about 15 years.

Autosomal dominant inheritance
Presenile onset

Neurological symptoms and signs
Choreiform movements
Rigidity
Corticospinal signs
Ataxia
Subcortical dementia
Juvenile rigid form

Investigations
Neuroimaging: caudate nucleus atrophy

Genetic aspects

The disease is inherited in an autosomally dominant fashion with full penetrance; sporadic cases and "new mutations" are rare. The disease is due to a single gene defect located on the short arm of chromosome 4 close to the marker S10 (also known as the G8 locus). The precise genetic locus (termed IT 15) for the disease has now been identified and this may cause the disease in the great majority, if not all, patients.

The mutation is an expanded and unstable triplet repeat (CAG) located at the 5' end of the gene. This sequence varies in both normals and Huntington's disease patients and while normals (unaffecteds) have between 9 and 37 such repeats (98% of normal chromosomes have less than 28 repeats and are meiotically stable), Huntington's patients have between 38 and 121 (unstable) repeat units. Within the Huntington's disease population there appears to be a strong inverse relationship between age at onset and repeat size though environmental effects, genetic modifiers or other stochastic events also influence the time of onset.

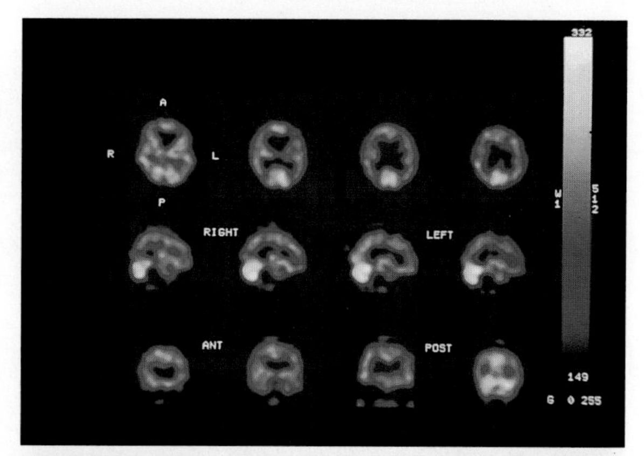

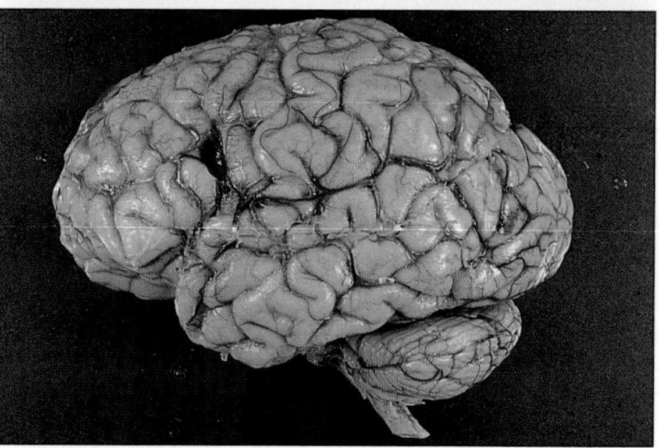

Fig. 4.25 (above left) Huntington's disease. This CT scan of the brain of a 50-year-old man with Huntington's disease is normal.

Fig. 4.26 (above right) Hypometabolism within the subcortical grey structures. SPET imaging of the brain of a 35-year-old man.

Fig. 4.27 (right) Mild generalised atrophy. Lateral view of the brain of a 70-year-old woman.

The disease can be transmitted through either paternal or maternal genes, paternal transmission producing slightly larger sized repeat units than maternal. Moreover, repeat size in affected children can vary from that in the affected parent being either larger (usually) or smaller with paternal transmission producing more variability.

A number of what were once thought of as 'sporadic' cases of disease or 'new mutations' have now been assigned to the (relatively) rare situation where one parental allele, usually paternal, is an unstable 30-37 repeat unit size. These latter individuals are clinically unaffected though if expansions into the Huntington's disease range take place in their children they (the offspring) then succumb to disease. These 'intermediate alleles' may be considered as a 'premutation' which do not themselves cause disease but can, with appropriate expansion, do so in later generations. These apparently sporadic cases can then in turn transmit

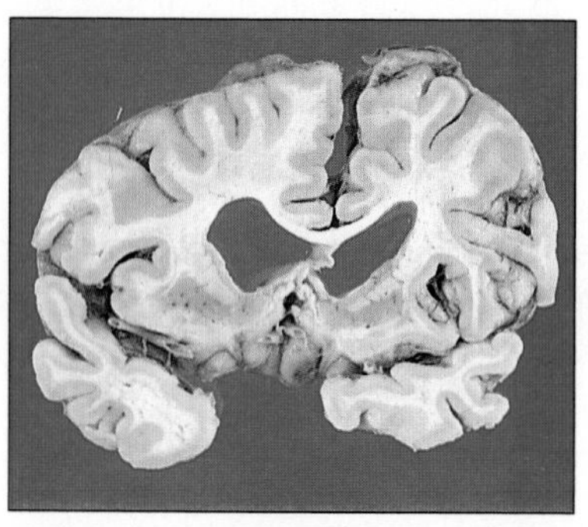

Fig. 4.28 Gross atrophy of the corpus striatum with marked ventricular dilatation. Coronal section of brain of the 70-year-old woman featured in **Fig.4.27**.

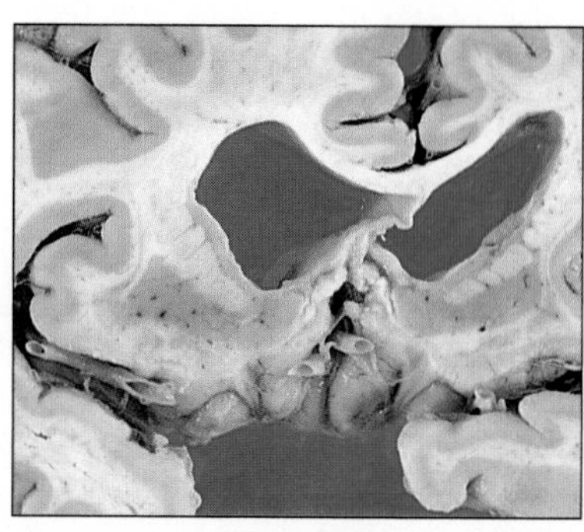

Fig. 4.29 As Fig. 4.28, but with a higher power view of the corpus striatum.

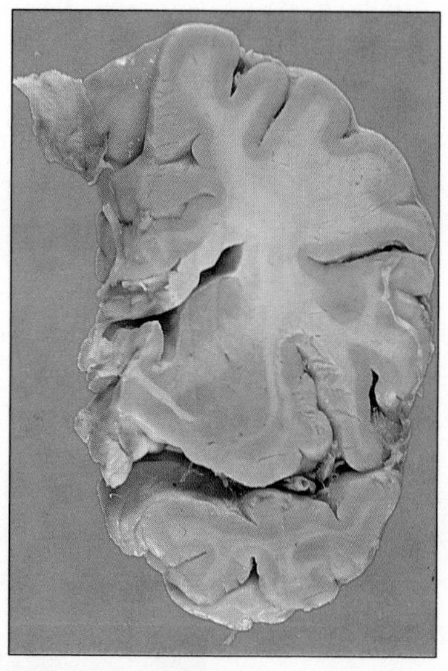

Fig. 4.30 Minimal change in the corpus striatum. Coronal section of the brain of a 73-year-old woman.

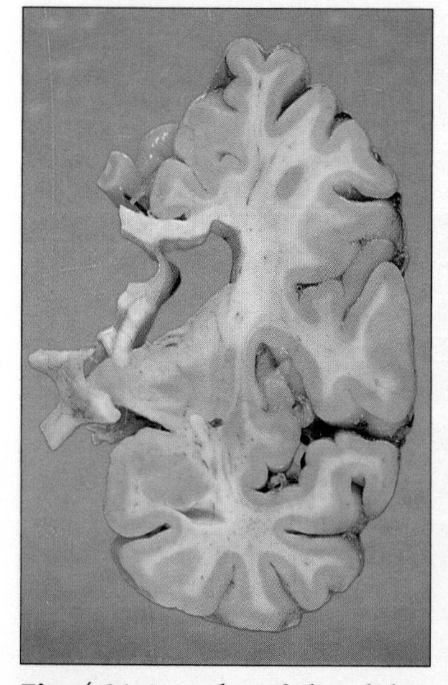

Fig. 4.31 Atrophy of the globus pallidus. Coronal section of the brain of a 64-year-old woman.

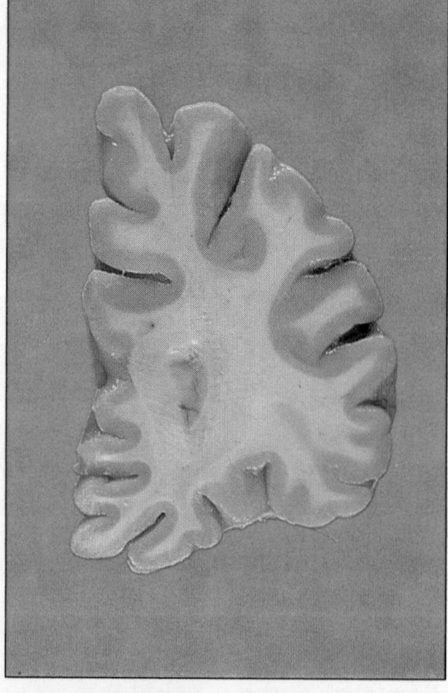

Fig. 4.32 Mild atrophy of the frontal lobes. Coronal section of the brain of the 64-year-old woman featured in **Fig. 4.31**.

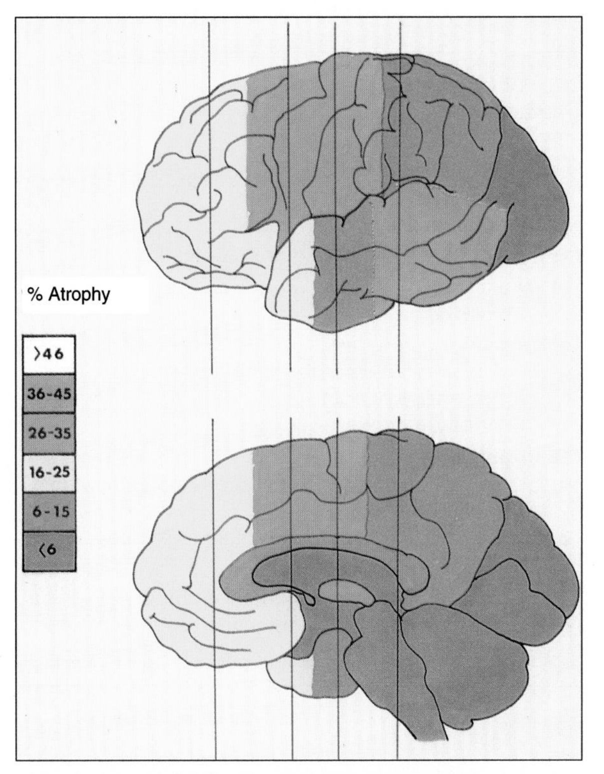

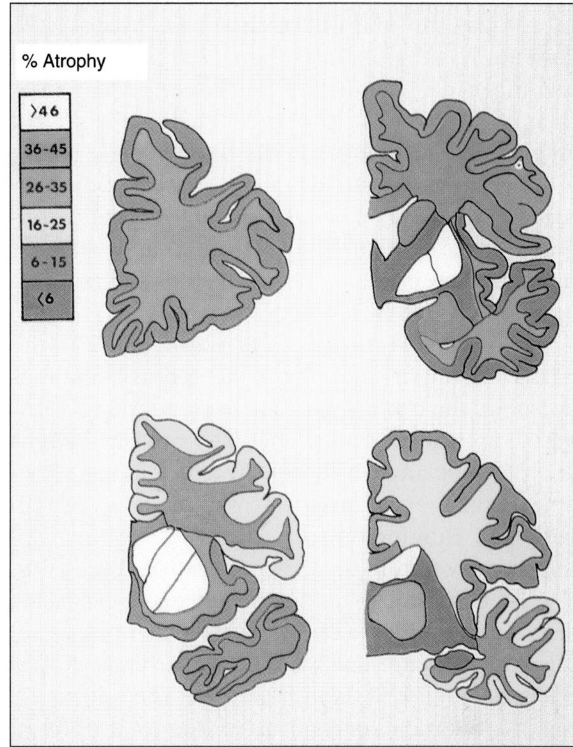

Figs 4.33 and 4.34 Morphometric analysis of regional brain atrophy showing involvement of the corpus striatum and thalamus. There is also atrophy of the anterior parietal cortex, frontal and temporal lobes, with more white matter being lost than grey matter.

the disease to their own offspring in the usual way by maintaining, or even further enlarging, the gene expansion 'acquired' from their parent. Again, expansion of intermediate alleles is greater and occurs most frequently when the possessor is male. Truly sporadic instances of disease are thus rare. Nonetheless, clinically diagnosed cases of apparently sporadic disease do occur where the genotype of both the affected individual and parents are within the normal range of repeat units. Such cases either represent a misdiagnosis or are clinical phenocopies of idiopathic chorea, not associated with gene expansion, in which the underlying cause is obscure.

The product of the genetic locus for Huntington's disease remains to be identified though it relates to a 10 kilobase transcript producing a protein of predicted molecular weight of 348KDa. The function of such a protein is unknown. Nonetheless, the gene is normally expressed strongly by neurones in neural tissues but is also expressed at low levels in non-neural tissues. Interestingly within the CNS expression seems most intense in the hippocampus and cerebellum; the basal ganglia show only low expression.

A differential expression, or an over- or under-expression, of the gene in areas of the brain preferentially involved in the Huntington's disease process does not seem to occur. Hence the manner whereby the presence or the size of the genetic disorder produces the pathological changes, and the regional specificity, of the disease is still unknown.

Pathological features

Gross changes

In established Huntington's disease a CT scan can show bilateral atrophy of the corpus striatum with a variable degree of cortical atrophy, and obvious ventricular enlargement, especially anteriorly. In other instances, especially in early stages of the disease, the CT images can apparently be normal (**Fig.4.25**). SPET imaging (**Fig. 4.26**) shows bilaterally decreased blood flow and glucose utilisation in the subcortex, sometimes with hypometabolic changes in the cerebral cortex, particularly in frontal regions.

At autopsy the brain is often smaller than usual, commonly weighing less than 1100 g. The leptomeninges are frequently thickened and rather opaque. External inspection reveals insignificant atherosclerotic changes in the basal vessels. There is a mild to moderate, rather generalised, cortical atrophy (**Fig. 4.27**), although sometimes some preferential involvement of the frontal and anterior parietal lobes is seen. The brain stem and cerebellum appear normal.

When sliced coronally (**Figs 4.28** and **4.29**), the characteristic gross atrophy of the corpus striatum is apparent, the caudate nucleus often adopting a flattened or even concave profile. The caudate nucleus and putamen are usually equally affected, but sometimes a preferential involvement of either is seen. In early Huntington's disease, however, the corpus striatum may appear normal (**Fig. 4.30**). The lateral ventricles are grossly enlarged, especially anteriorly (see **Figs 4.28** and **4.29**). Other basal ganglia structures are involved, particularly the globus pallidus (**Fig. 4.31**) and thalamus. The substantia nigra is often darker than usual due to atrophy of the pars reticulata. The atrophy of these basal structures cannot account for the reduction in brain weight and usually there is some cortical atrophy in the frontal (**Fig. 4.32**), fronto-parietal, and anterior temporal regions.

Morphometric estimations of cross-sectional area confirm the atrophy of the basal ganglia, with the caudate nucleus, putamen and globus pallidus to be all being reduced in size by 50%, with less atrophy of the thalamus (**Figs 4.33** and **4.34**). The frontal and anterior parietal and temporal lobes are also atrophied (see **Fig. 4.34**), with a greater loss of white matter than grey matter (see **Fig. 4.34**). This increases the ratio in the amount of grey to white matter.

Histological features

The characteristic histopathological changes in the corpus striatum involve a loss of the medium spiny neurones (**Fig. 4.35**) containing GABA/substance P and GABA/enkephalin, projecting to the globus pallidus and pars reticulata of substantia nigra. The small spiny interneurones that contain neuropeptide Y/somatostatin/NADPH diaphorase are spared, as are the larger aspiny cholinergic interneurones. Nerve cells are also lost from the globus pallidus, ventrolateral thalamus, and subthalamic nucleus.

Age of onset
Any age
Juvenile onset is rare
Usually30–50 years of age

Sex incidence
Males and females affected equally

Duration
Prolonged, up to 20 years

Gross features
- Atrophy of corpus striatum
- Ventricular enlargement
- Cerebral atrophy (fronto-parietal) in patients who have a long duration of disease

Histopathology
- Loss of small neurones from corpus striatum with astrocytic proliferation
- Cerebral cortex shows no distinctive changes

Genetics
- Autosomally dominant inheritance: the genetic locus is on chromosome 4, but the gene product has not yet been identified

In severe disease there is vacuolation of the neuropil of the caudate nucleus, particularly in medial parts (see **Fig. 4.38**), due to neuronal fallout. In addition, because of the compacting down of surviving tissue, reactive astrocytes become more apparent (**Fig. 4.36**) and immunostaining with antibodies against GFAP reveals a dense meshwork of cells and fibres (**Figs 4.37** and **4.38**), giving the appearance of a proliferative astrocytosis. Similar histopathological changes occur in the putamen (**Figs 4.39** and **4.40**), but often to a lesser extent than in the caudate nucleus. However, cell counting has shown that while the *density* of astrocytes increases, due to compacting of residual tissue, the *absolute number* of cells does not increase; indeed, there may be some loss. The 'gliosis' of Huntington's disease is therefore artefactual: there is no increase in number, although pre-existing astrocytes do become 'reactive', enlarging their processes and producing more fibrillar protein. Similarly, the 'gliosis' in the globus pallidus is due to compacting of remaining tissue.

The 'subcortical nuclei' of the substantia nigra, locus caeruleus, nucleus basalis of Meynert, and raphe are normal.

Despite being atrophied, affected regions of cortex do not show any consistent histological abnormality. Claims of nerve cell loss, on the basis of visual inspection alone, have been vigorously asserted and denied. Recently, cell counting has shown a variable loss of pyramidal cells from layers III, V and VI of the frontal cortex and from area CA1 of the hippocampus. However, no reactive astrocytosis is seen in either region. Surviving nerve cells show no consistent abnormalities. Despite a gross loss of white matter, the remaining tissue is well myelinated with no change in axon density.

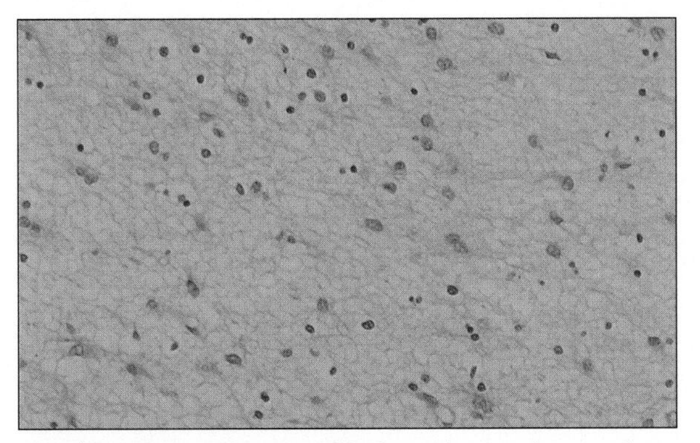

Fig. 4.35 Loss of nerve cells from the caudate nucleus. *(Haematoxylin–eosin × 200.)*

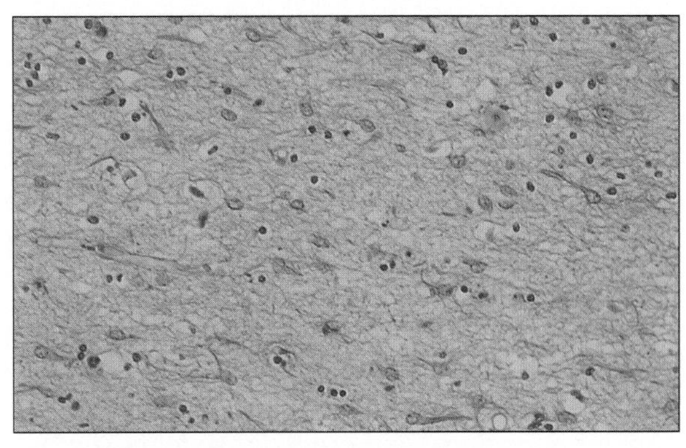

Fig. 4.36 Severe reactive astrocytosis in the caudate nucleus. *(Phosphotungstic acid–haematoxylin × 200.)*

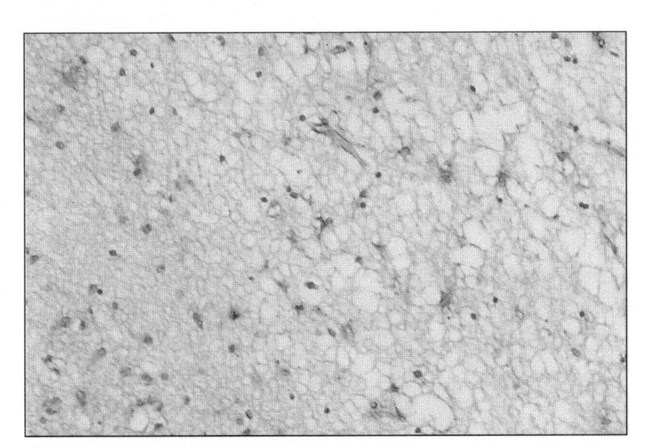

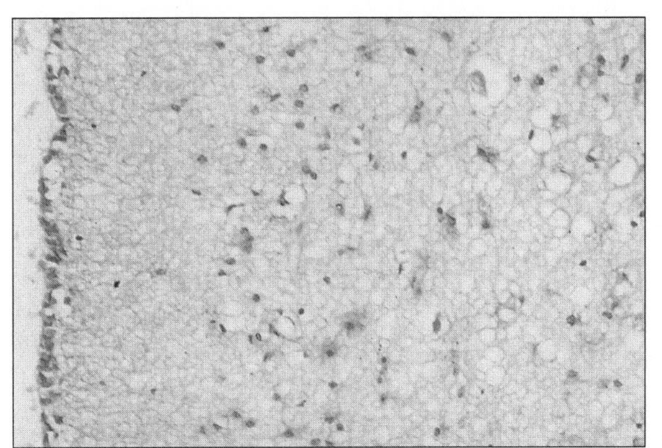

Figs 4.37 and 4.38 Reactive astrocytosis in the caudate nucleus. Note the vacuolation of the tissue (**Fig. 4.37**). *(Anti-GFAP × 200.)*

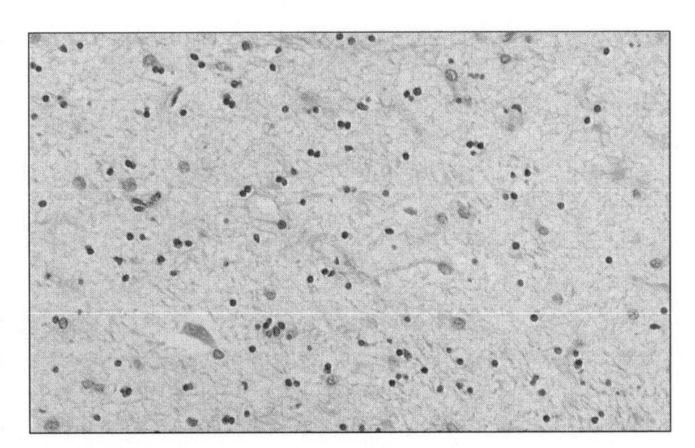

Fig. 4.39 Loss of nerve cells from the putamen. *(Haematoxylin–eosin × 200.)*

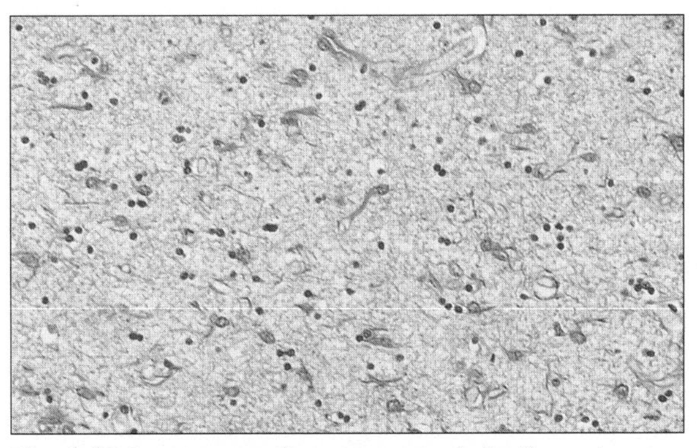

Fig. 4.40 Severe reactive astrocytosis in the putamen. *(Phosphotungstic acid–haematoxylin × 200.)*

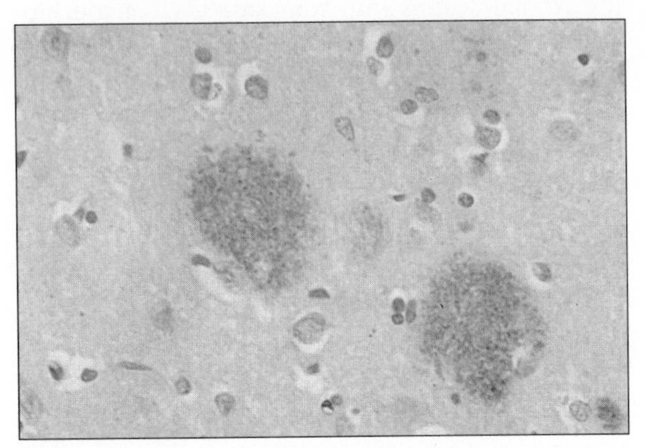

Fig. 4.41 Diffuse amyloid deposits in the frontal cortex. *(Anti-β/A4 × 200.)*

Some elderly people may have variable amounts of amyloid β/A4 protein in the cortex (**Fig. 4.41**) and hippocampus, although these deposits are nearly always diffuse and without any neuritic changes. Similarly, there may be occasional neurofibrillary tangles in the cortex, hippocampus and amygdala. Such changes are indicative of the patient's age and do not represent a concurrent Alzheimer's disease, although rarely the numbers of plaques and tangles have been sufficient to warrant this diagnosis.

Clinico-pathological correlations

Atrophic changes in the caudate/putamen, globus pallidus and subthalamic nucleus combine to cause the characteristic choreoathetoid movement disorder. Loss of striatal efferents cause a disinhibition of the lateral globus pallidus, which in turn results in a decreased activity of the subthalamic nucleus. The loss of input from the subthalamic nucleus into the medial globus pallidus and the reticulata of the substantia nigra (which also loses its direct projection from the striatum) lead to disinhibition of thalamic projections to the motor cortex. This results in the motor disturbances of the disorder.

As might be expected, the extent of caudate atrophy correlates with the degree of movement disorder, but it is not clear whether loss of striatal connections to the frontal cortex is responsible for the cognitive impairment. Functional imaging studies show a frontal hypometabolism that correlates with the degree of dementia, but these do not differentiate between a basic loss of pyramidal cells intrinsic to the cortex and a functional deafferentation from non-cortical regions. The 'clinical syndrome' of Huntington's disease may result from a combination of both pathologies with a loss of striatal afferents causing the 'slowing' of action and mood changes, the cortical pathology relating to behavioural alterations. To what extent the degree of pathological change (that is the severity of the pathology and regional distribution) are dependent upon the size of the genetic mutation is unclear, nor is it known whether clincal phenotype is under genetic control.

Pathogenesis

The cause of the nerve cell loss and how this relates to the genetics of the disease is not understood. In contrast to the pathologies of Alzheimer's disease, Pick's disease, Parkinson's disease, and Lewy body disease, no 'cytoskeletal' alterations have been detected in Huntington's disease. It is clear that the regional distribution of the Huntington's disease gene message is not correlated with the pathology; the hippocampus and cerebellum are essentially normal histologically, even in end-stage disease. Nor does it seem to be the case that differential expression, affecting principally the corpus striatum, takes place; overall gene expression levels and the regional pattern of gene expression seem similar in Huntington's disease and controls.

The cause of the pattern of pathology may lie in some aspect of the neurobiology of the particular sub-sets of striatal neurones that degenerate that makes them especially vulnerable to the changes in expression of the mutant gene; vulnerable cells might express the gene more strongly than others or may in turn be more dependent upon the (normal) product of that gene or more sensitive to the abnormal product.

The vulnerable neurones in the striatum in Huntington's disease are glutamate-receptive. Animal models, based on the postulate that an excess of excitatory amino acids (or other derivatives) could cause degeneration through their affect on the glutamate (NMDA) receptor leading to excess calcium influx, have been put forward. However, as yet there is no evidence that such amino acid excesses exist in humans; indeed, reductions in cortical glutamate, in line with pyramidal nerve cell loss, have been detected. Nonetheless, it is possible that the genetic changes affecting striatal neurones may render them especially sensitive to damage even in the context of a normal level of excitatory amino acid neurotransmission.

PARKINSON'S DISEASE

A subcortical type of dementia occurs in about 15–40% of patients with idiopathic Parkinson's disease, usually appearing late in the course of the illness and well after the onset of the motor symptoms. Like that in progressive supranuclear palsy and Huntington's disease, it is characterised by a slowing of mental processes with deficiences in attention and motivation; memory disturbance is mild. Speech is poor and slowly articulated, and apathy and depression are common. This pattern contrasts with the cortically based disorders of Alzheimer's disease and fronto-temporal dementia, although sometimes in Parkinson's disease memory and cognitive defects are severe and appear to be derived from 'cortical disease'.

Pathological features

As defined histopathologically, Parkinson's disease represents a loss of the catecholaminergic neurones of the mid brain and brain stem, particularly those of the substantia nigra (**Figs 4.42** and **4.43**) and locus caeruleus (**Figs 4.44** and **4.45**). There is often gross depigmentation of these regions due to neuronal fallout. However, a large amount of residual pigment can be freely present in the neuropil or in macrophages (**Fig. 4.46**).

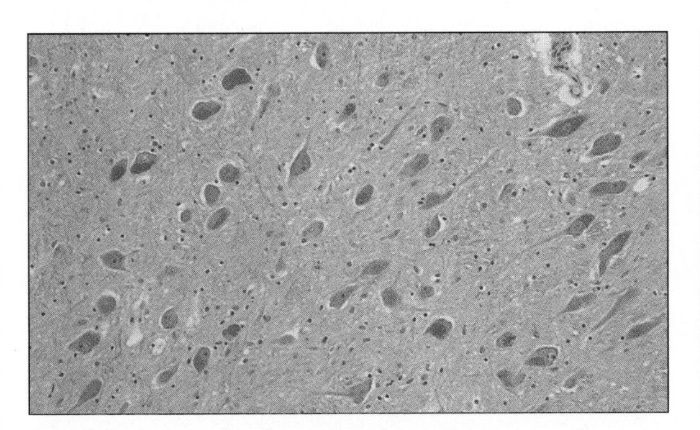

Fig. 4.42 Normal substantia nigra. *(Haematoxylin–eosin × 100.)*

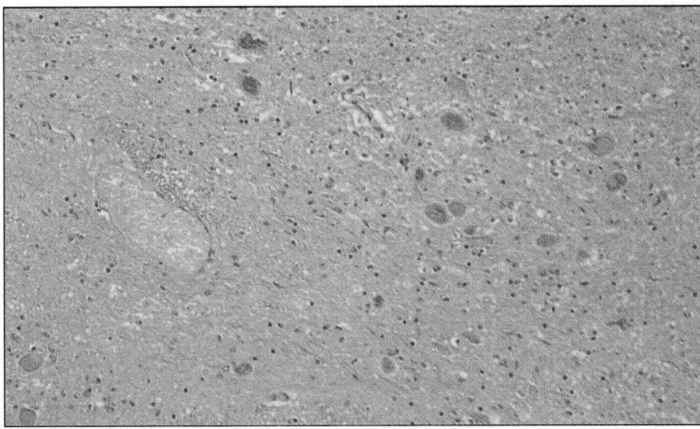

Fig. 4.43 Substantia nigra in Parkinson's disease. There is a severe loss of pigmented nerve cells. *(Haematoxylin–eosin × 100.)*

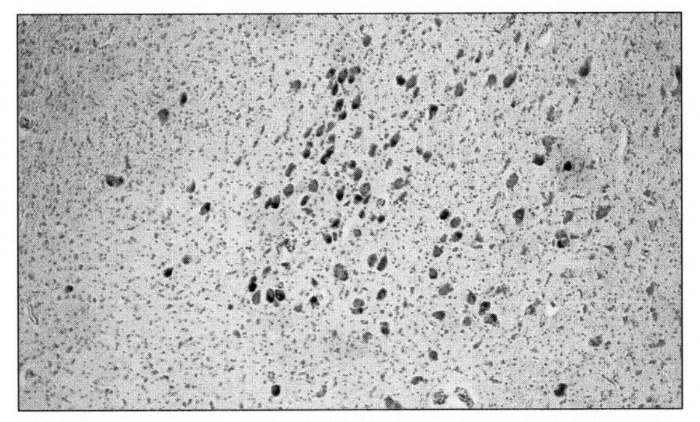

Fig. 4.44 Normal locus caeruleus. *(Nissl stain × 100.)*

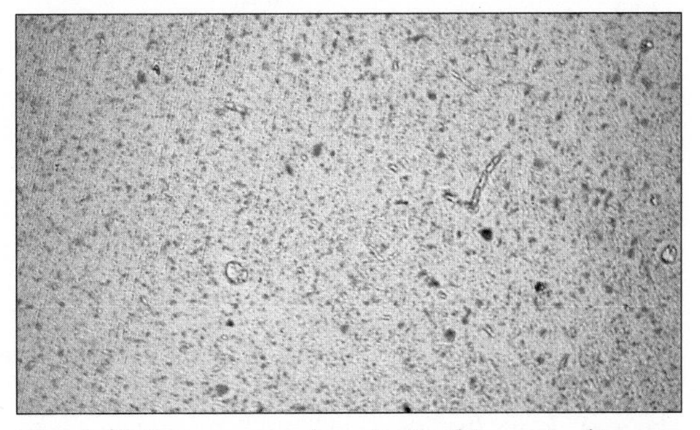

Fig. 4.45 Locus caeruleus in Parkinson's disease. There is a severe loss of nerve cells. *(Nissl stain × 100.)*

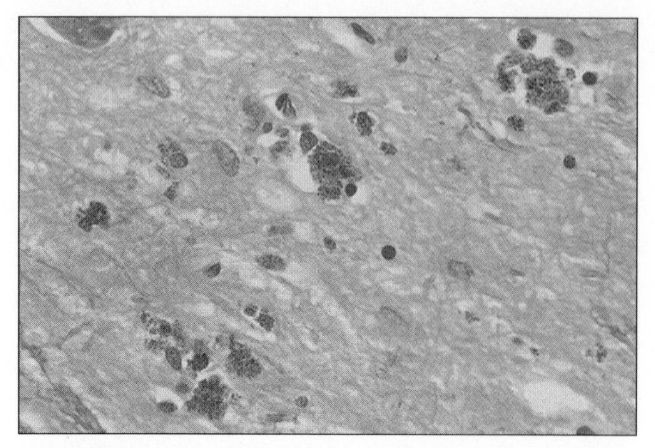

Fig. 4.46 Extraneuronal deposits of neuromelanin pigment in the neuropil or within macrophages. *(Haematoxylin–eosin × 200.)*

Some of the surviving neurones display the characteristic cytological change of the disease, the Lewy inclusion body (**Figs 4.47–4.49**). Lewy bodies are eosinophilic structures, sometimes with a denser core, giving a concentric laminated appearance and measuring more than 15μm in diameter. They are immunoreactive to antibodies against ubiquitin (**Fig. 4.50**), neurofilament protein, tubulin and high molecular weight microtubule-associated proteins (MAP1 and 2), but *not* to those against tau protein. Pale bodies (**Fig. 4.51**) in nigral cells may be morphological forerunners of the Lewy body.

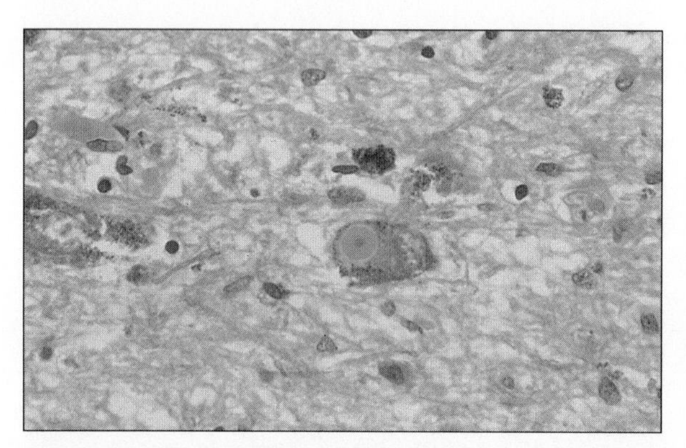

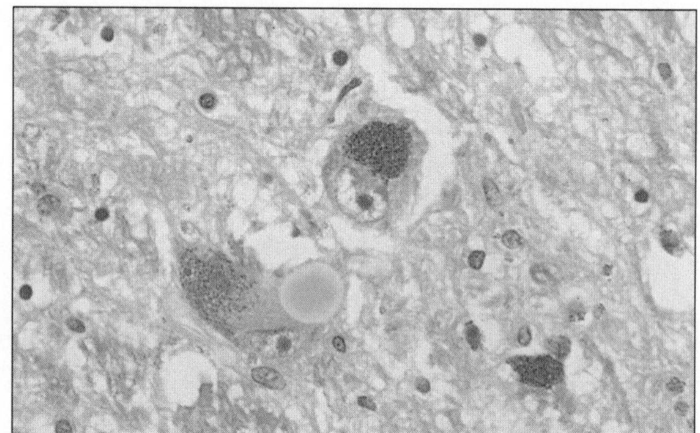

Fig. 4.47 and 4.48 Lewy body within a surviving neurone of the substantia nigra. Note the concentric laminated appearance, with a deeper staining central core. *(Haematoxylin–eosin × 200.)*

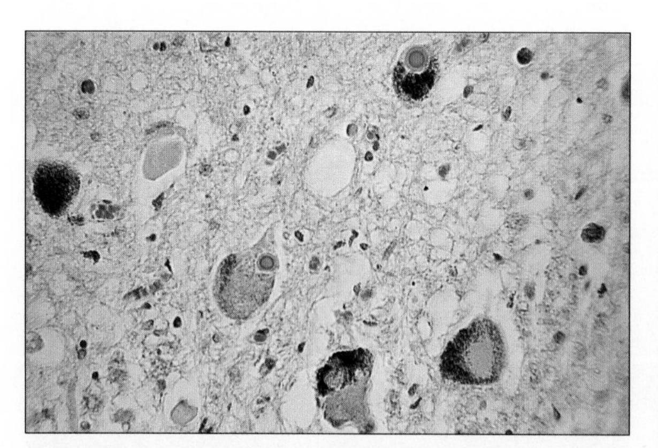

Fig. 4.49 Lewy bodies within surviving nerve cells of the locus caeruleus. *(Phloxine-tartazine × 200.)*

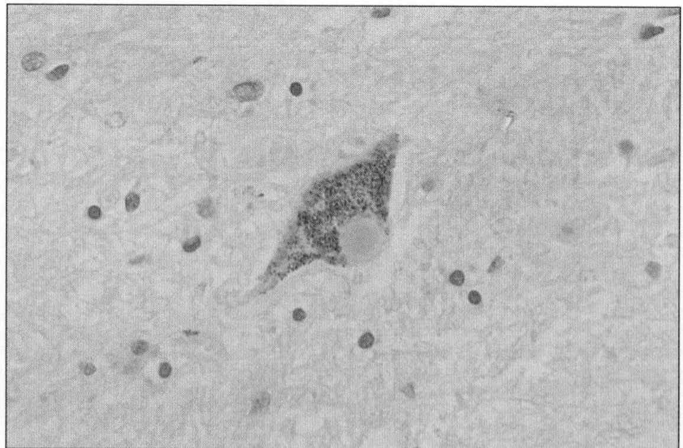

Fig. 4.50 Lewy bodies in neurones of the substantia nigra containing ubiquitin. *(Anti-ubiquitin × 400.)*

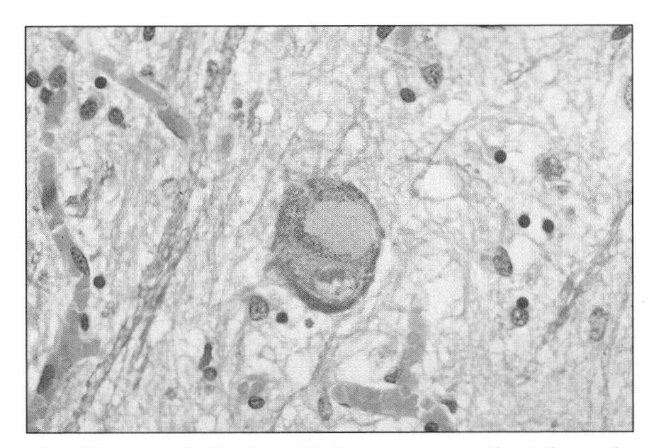

Fig. 451 A pale body within a nerve cell of the substantia nigra. *(Haematoxylin–eosin × 400.)*

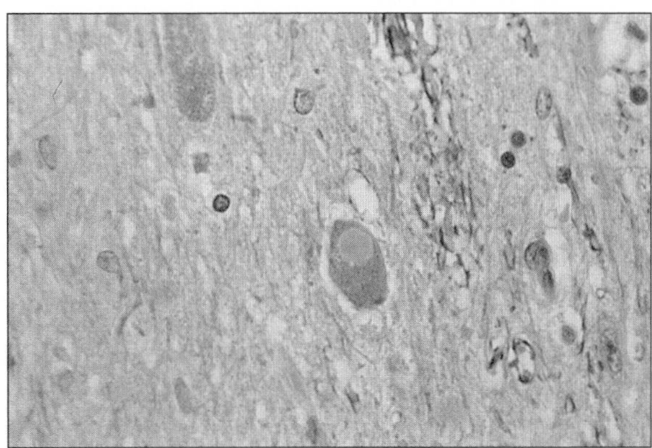

Fig. 4.52 A Lewy body in a nerve cell in the dorsal raphe nucleus. *(Haematoxylin–eosin × 400.)*

Ultrastructurally, Lewy bodies are comprised of randomly arranged (neuro) filaments of 11 nm diameter mixed with mitochondria, lipofuscin and smooth endoplasmic reticulum.

Lewy bodies can be widely found in non-pigmented neurones of the mid brain and brain stem, particularly those of the raphe nuclei (**Fig. 4.52**) and nucleus basalis of Meynert, but are typically absent from cortical regions.

The extent of pathology in the nigra does not seem to differ between demented and non-demented patients. Demented patients with Parkinson's disease show no distinguishing features on CT scanning, although a mild cortical atrophy and ventricular dilatation may be evident in some instances. On SPET imaging a mild hypometabolism within the posterior hemisphere may occur (**Fig.4.53**)

At autopsy the brain may be mildly to moderately diffusely atrophic with some ventricular dilatation. Depigmentation of the substantia nigra and locus caeruleus are the only macroscopic features of note.

Many, and particularly the more elderly, patients with Parkinson's disease and dementia have a few neuritic plaques and neurofibrillary tangles in the neocortex but more tangles can occur in the entorhinal cortex and hippocampus (**Fig. 4.54**).

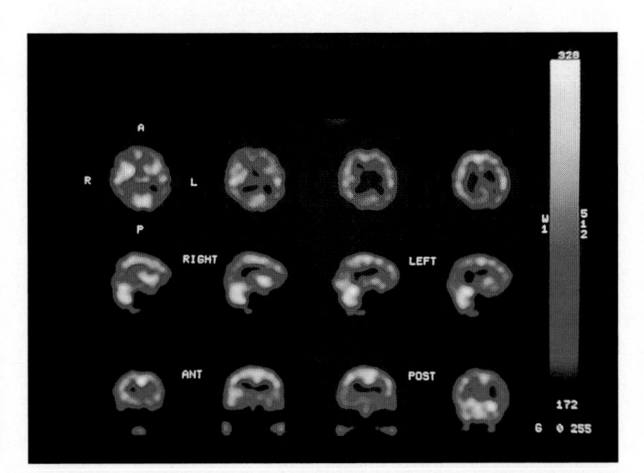

Fig. 4.53 Mild hypometabolism in posterior hemisphere regions. SPET imaging of the brain of a 65-year-old woman.

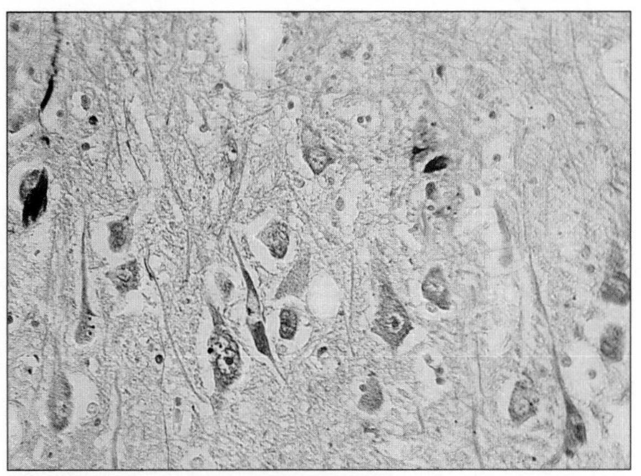

Fig. 4.54 Nerve cells in the pyramidal layer of the hippocampus show neurofibrillary tangle formation and granulovacuolar degeneration. *(Bielschowsky silver stain × 200.)*

An extensive deposition of β/A4 amyloid, mostly in the form of diffuse plaques, may also be found in the neocortex, but not elsewhere (**Figs 4.55** and **4.56**). In general, however, such changes are no more than would perhaps be expected for the age of the patient and do not in themselves represent a coincidental Alzheimer's disease. Occasionally, though, especially in the hippocampus and entorhinal cortex (**Fig. 4.57**), these Alzheimer-type changes can be excessive, being of a magnitude normally associated with Alzheimer's disease. Conversely, many patients with Alzheimer's disease have occasional Lewy bodies in the substantia nigra (**Fig. 4.58;** see also **Figs. 153–154**, p. 55), but usually without gross nigral cell loss. This change is again likely to be age-related. In truly combined cases of Alzheimer's disease and Parkinson's disease there is an extensive cell loss from the nigra with Lewy body formation.

Other patients with Parkinsonism and dementia have extensive Lewy body formation in the neocortex with or without plaques and tangles. These probably represent the condition of cortical Lewy body disease.

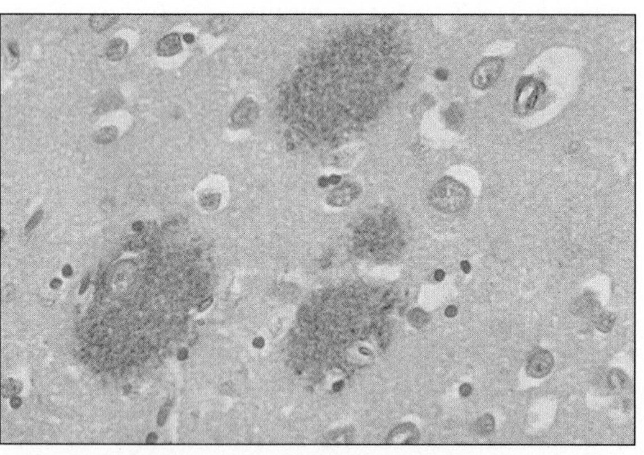

Fig. 4.55 Diffuse deposits of amyloid β/A4 protein in the temporal cortex. *(Anti-β/A4 × 200.)*

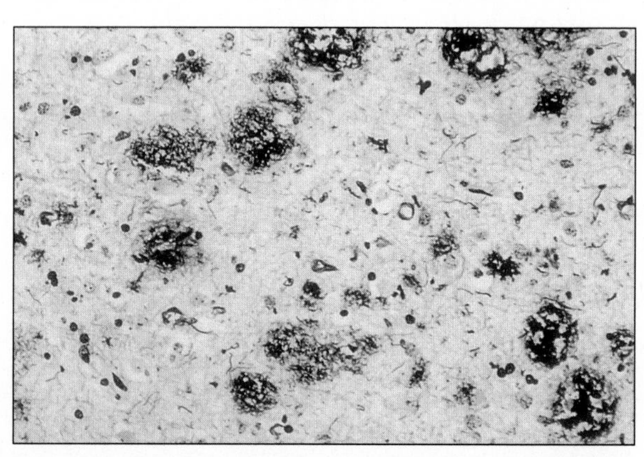

Fig. 4.56 As Fig. 4.55, but with methenamine silver staining. Note that occasional cored deposits are present. *(× 100.)*

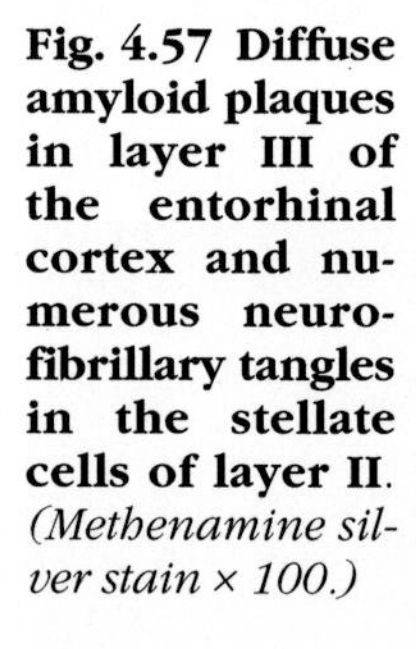

Fig. 4.57 Diffuse amyloid plaques in layer III of the entorhinal cortex and numerous neurofibrillary tangles in the stellate cells of layer II. *(Methenamine silver stain × 100.)*

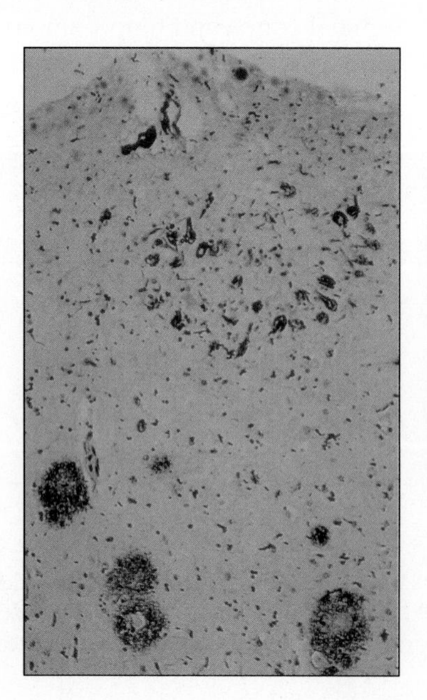

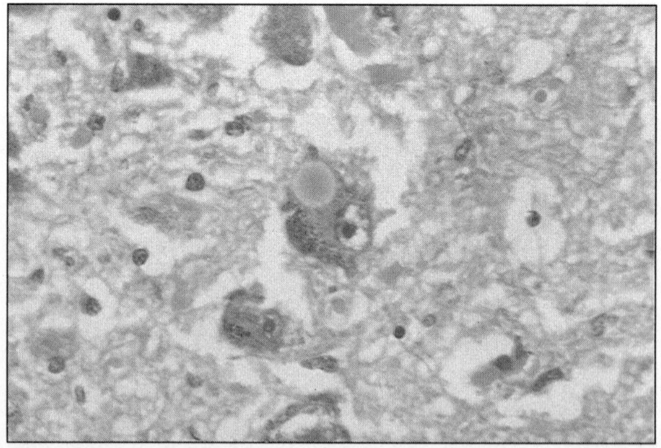

Fig. 4.58 Alzheimer's disease. Lewy body in a nerve cell of the substantia nigra in Alzheimer's disease. *(Haematoxylin–eosin × 400.)*

It is clear that there is a wide overlap in pathological features such as plaques, tangles, and Lewy bodies between prototypical cases of Alzheimer's disease, Parkinson's disease, and other cases of Parkinsonism and dementia in which variable quantities of any or all these changes may be present (see pages 164–166).

Other demented patients with Parkinson's disease show neither a significant Alzheimer-type nor a Lewy body-type of pathology in the cerebral cortex. In these patients a more severe loss of cells from regions such as the locus caeruleus, raphe and nucleus basalis has been reported and their dementia may reflect a lack of 'activation' due to a loss of these diffusely projecting cortical afferent systems. Alternatively, a loss of dopamine-containing cells in the ventral tegmental area, a region medial to the substantia nigra, which projects via the mesolimbic and mesocortical tracts to the hippocampus and frontal lobes, may contribute.

At present it seems that dementia in Parkinson's disease cannot be linked entirely to the degeneration of any one particular nerve cell group or neural pathway: the cause is pathologically heterogeneous. Co-existence of Alzheimer's disease or the presence of cortical Lewy body disease must be excluded. Demented and non-demented patients with 'pure' forms of Parkinson's disease need to be carefully compared to define the pathological cause of the dementia.

Pathogenesis

The cause of Parkinson's disease is still unknown. Its presence as an inherited disorder in a few families points to a genetic cause in some instances, but in the great majority of patients the disease appears to arise spontaneously. The genetic defect in question may involve a polymorphism in the cytochrome P450 CYP2D6 debrisoquine hydroxylase gene, thereby conferring a poor capacity for metabolism of potentially neurotoxic compounds. Possession of this polymorphism (as a recessive trait) by 5–10% of the population increases the risk of developing Parkinson's disease by 2.5 fold. The identification of a Parkinson disease-type of pathology in certain toxic scenarios, notably manganese poisoning in industrial workers or 1-methyl-4-phenyl 1,2,3,6 tetrahydropyridine (MPTP) injection in drug abusers, further implies an environmental cause. It is probable that a combination of both types of aetiology is responsible. An outside (common or uncommon) toxic agent, either taken directly into the brain from the environment or one that is inadequately handled or modified into a more toxic species by the body's detoxification system, might interplay with genetic factors in susceptible individuals.

How such a putative exogenous or endogenous agent might act on the (possibly genetically vulnerable) cells of the substantia nigra and locus caeruleus is not known. It seems possible that 'oxidative stress' induced by damage to the respiratory chain (electron transport) system of the mitochondria, and specifically damage to complex 1 (NADH CoQ_1 reductase) of that system, might be responsible. Production of toxic radicals (hydroxyl, superoxide) by reduced complex 1 activity, not adequately 'scavenged' by the cell's protective systems, could aggravate the damage and promote metabolic failure.

How such physiological changes relate to the formation of Lewy bodies is not clear, but a 'collapse' of the cytoskeleton could occur as part of a wider breakdown in the functional integrity of the cell due to failing ATP production.

Why the pigmented cells of the brain should be preferentially affected is not clear. It is possible that any damaging factor could access these cell types via their neurotransmitter reuptake system. Such a mechanism appears to explain the neuronal selectivity behind MPTP neurotoxicity.

5. Cortical–subcortical encephalopathies

Cortical–subcortical encephalopathies show clinical features characteristic of both a cortical and a subcortical type of encephalopathy and have patterns of brain pathology that involve both cortical and subcortical regions. Two major neurodegenerative conditions represent this group: cortical Lewy body disease and cortico-basal degeneration.

The effects of cerebrovascular diseases, which can involve blood vessels in any part of the brain, produce clinical profiles that share variable aspects of cortical and subcortical encephalopathies depending on the part of the brain targetted by the vascular disorder. Vascular dementia is therefore included in this chapter.

CORTICAL LEWY BODY DISEASE

Demographic features

Although first reported about 20 years ago and then described in a series of isolated case reports as an atypical Parkinsonian dementia, cortical Lewy body disease has only become recognised in its own right as an important cause of dementia with Parkinsonian features within the last few years. It is suggested that cortical Lewy body disease may be the second most common cause of dementia (after Alzheimer's disease) among the very elderly, accounting for perhaps as many as 20% of cases.

The various eponyms that been used to describe conditions that are probably all the same disorder are cortical Lewy body disease, diffuse Lewy body disease, and senile dementia of Lewy body type. Cortical Lewy body disease is the term used here and includes all others.

Usually the dementia comes first, with Parkinsonism appearing later in the course of the disease; some (mainly younger) patients may present with Parkinsonism, but quickly become demented. Familial cases among the elderly have not been recorded,but a family history seems possible for some patients with early onset disease. As in idiopathic Parkinson's disease slightly more men are affected than women.

Neurological symptoms and signs
Akinesia, rigidity and tremor

Psychological symptoms
Fluctuating confusion, hallucinations and secondary delusions
Aphasia, amnesia, perceptuo-spatial disorder

Investigations
SPET: posterior hemisphere abnormality

Pathological features

A CT scan shows no distinctive features except for a mild or moderate diffuse cortical atrophy with some ventricular enlargement. SPET imaging (**Fig. 5.1**) reveals a patchy reduction in uptake of tracer in the cerebral cortex, particularly in the posterior hemisphere.

Externally, the brain shows only a mild to moderate diffuse atrophy (**Fig. 5.2**), though sometimes the frontal, and particularly the temporal lobes, are more affected. A mild ventricular dilatation is present (**Fig. 5.3**) and substantia nigra and locus caeruleus are often depigmented. All other brain regions appear normal.

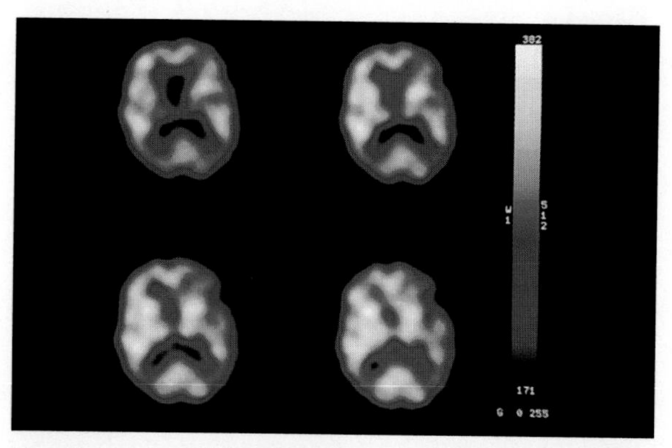

Fig. 5.1 A patchy reduction in brain metabolism, particularly in the posterior hemisphere. SPET imaging in a 74-year-old man.

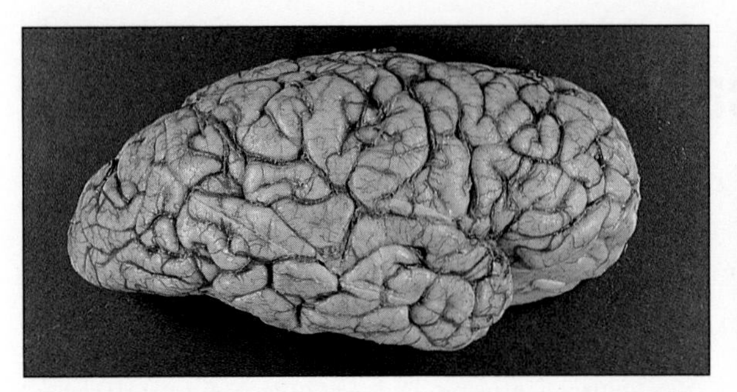

Fig. 5.2 Mild and generalised atrophy. Lateral view of the right hemisphere of the brain of a 71-year-old woman.

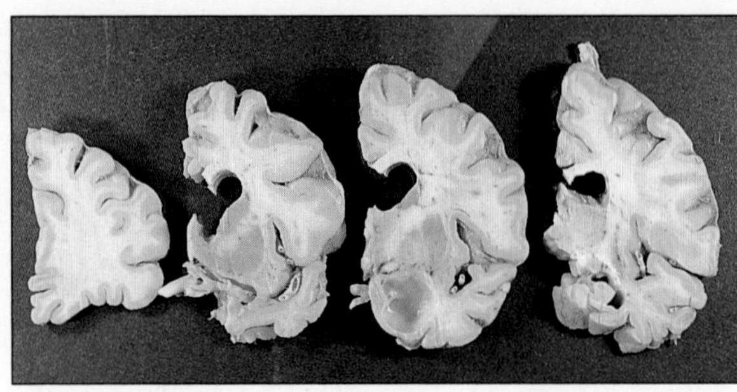

Fig. 5.3 Mild cortical atrophy and moderate ventricular dilatation, especially within the temporal horn. Coronal sections of the brain of a 70-year-old woman.

Age of onset
Any age after 40 years
Most common after 75 years.

Sex incidence
Affects males and females equally

Duration
Variable, usually a few years

Gross features
Mild generalized cortical atrophy
Depigmentation of substantia nigra

Histopathology
- Lewy inclusion bodies in cerebral cortical neurones, usually layers V and VI, mostly in cingulate and entorhinal cortex
- Ubiquitin protein
- Lewy bodies in substantia nigra
- Numerous cortical deposits of amyloid β/A4 protein in 40% of patients
- A few tangles present, more in the hippocampus and entorhinal cortex, and such patients have an amyloid angiopathy

Genetics
- Appears to be spontaneous; no confirmed familial cases yet reported

Histopathological changes

Histopathologically, the substantia nigra (**Fig. 5.4**) and locus caeruleus show a loss of pigmented neurones, with aggregates of residual neuromelanin lying freely within the neuropil or macrophages (**Fig. 5.5**). Lewy-type (**Fig. 5.6**) and 'pale' inclusion bodies are widely spread in surviving cells (see **Figs 4.47–4.52**).

These inclusions may also be present among other neuronal groups in the reticular substance and are widespread throughout the cerebral cortex (**Fig. 5.7**), favouring the anterior temporal, frontal, insular, cingulate and entorhinal (parahippocampal) regions. The actual density of cortical Lewy bodies is variable and age-dependent, with fewer in older patients, though with the same distribution. Such observations are analogous to those in Alzheimer's disease in which the densities of neuritic plaques and tangles are likewise age-dependant. As in Alzheimer's disease, there may, therefore, be a continuum of pathological changes between early and late onset disease.

Cortical Lewy bodies differ from those in the nigra and other subcortical regions. Usually, they do not show the same concentric laminated structure typical

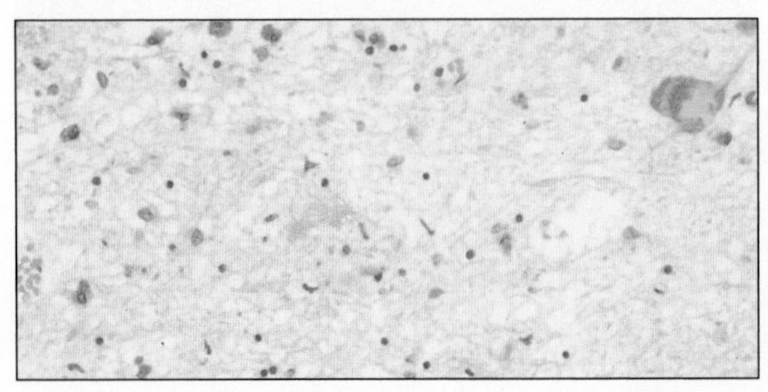

Fig. 5.4 Loss of nerve cells from the substantia nigra. *(Haematoxylin–eosin × 200.)*

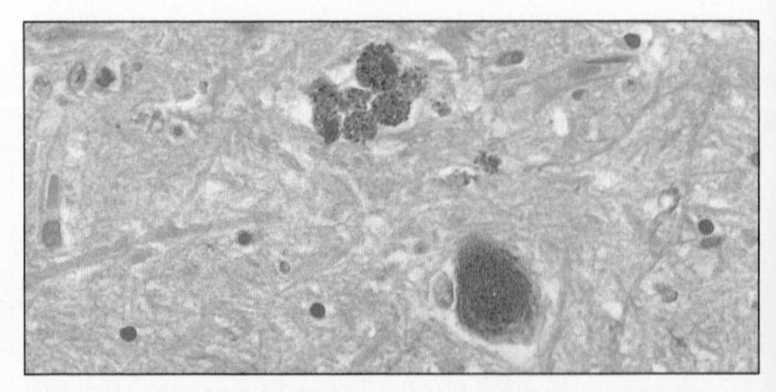

Fig. 5.5 Pigment aggregates within the substantia nigra. These mark the site of nerve cell death. *(Haematoxylin–eosin × 400.)*

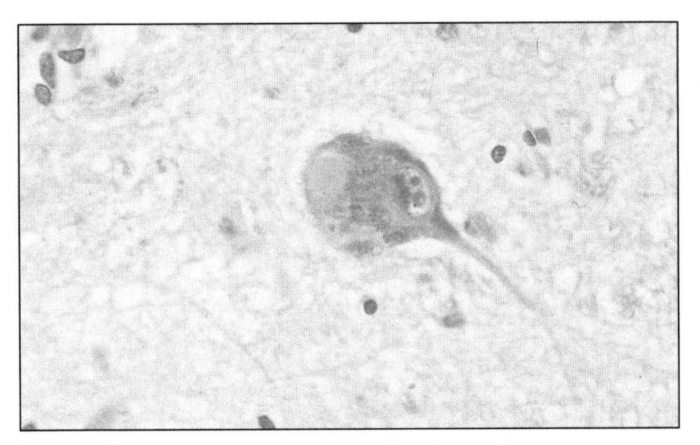

Fig. 5.6 Lewy body. A Lewy body within a surviving nerve cell in the substantia nigra. *(Haematoxylin–eosin × 400.)*

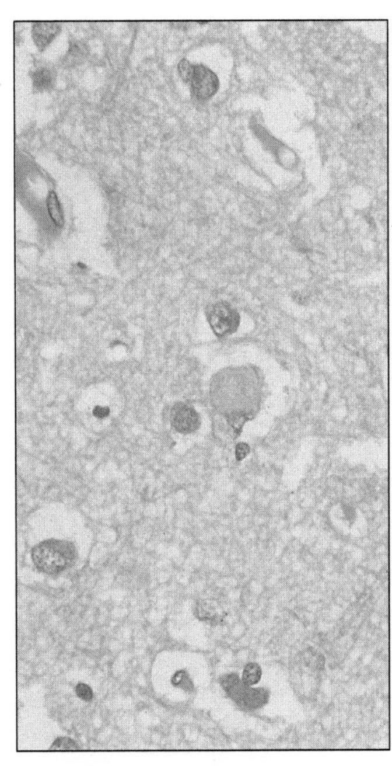

Fig. 5.7 Lewy body. Lewy inclusion body in a nerve cell of layer V of the cingulate cortex. *(Haematoxylin–eosin × 400.)*

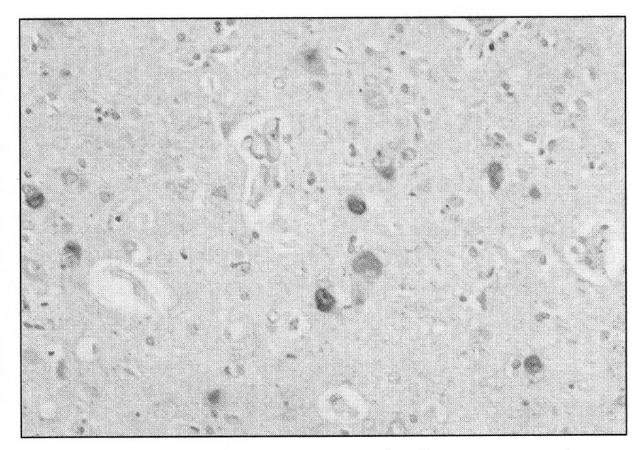

Fig. 5.8 Lewy bodies in the cerebral cortex are ubiquitinated. *(Anti-ubiquitin × 200.)*

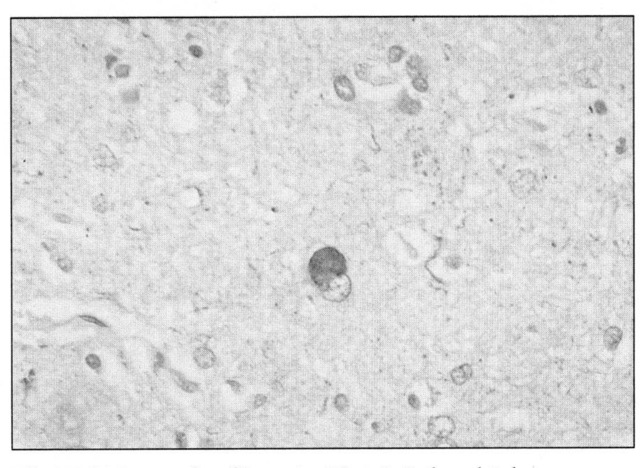

Fig. 5.9 Lewy bodies. As **Fig. 5.8**, but higher power. *(× 400.)*

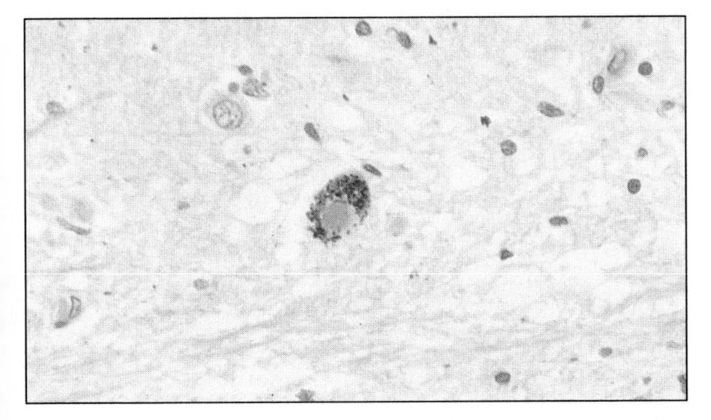

Fig. 5.10 Lewy bodies in the substantia nigra are also ubiquitinated. *(Anti-ubiquitin × 400.)*

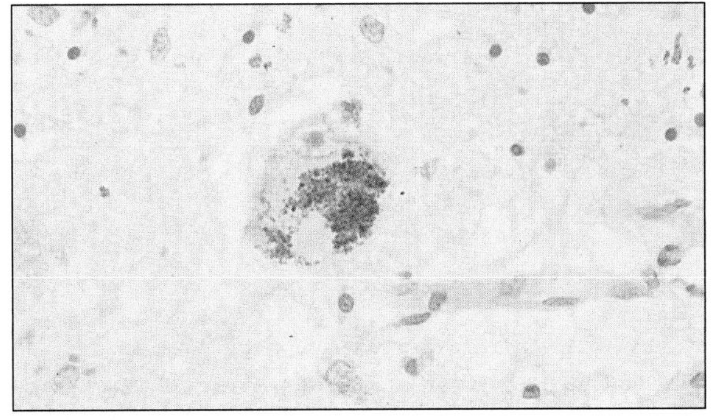

Fig. 5.11 Lewy bodies in substantia nigra are not tau-immunoreactive. *(Anti-tau × 400.)*

of those in the substantia nigra. They are commonly smaller, less well defined, irregular in shape, and diffusely and homogeneously stained (see **Fig. 5.7**). This makes them less easy to detect with a conventional haematoxylin-eosin stain (see **Fig. 5.7**), but they are strongly stained by antibodies against ubiquitin protein (**Figs 5.8** and **5.9**) as are those within the substantia nigra (**Fig. 5.10**). This method is therefore recommended for their routine detection.

Unlike Lewy bodies in the substantia nigra, which react with ubiquitin (see **Fig. 5.10**) but not tau (**Fig. 5.11**), cortical Lewy bodies are sometimes immunoreactive for tau antibodies and also label with anti-neurofilament antibodies. They can occur in neurones in any cortical layer, but are present mainly in layers V and VI. A gross loss of neurones, a significant accompanying astrocytosis, and loss of myelin from the white matter are not usually apparent.

In about 50% of patients there is a widespread deposition of amyloid β/A4 protein (see **Figs 5.12** and **5.13**), mainly as diffuse deposits (see **Fig. 5.13**). Usually, this is excessive for the age of the patient. While only a few of these amyloid deposits contain neurites, as defined by silver (**Fig. 5.14**) or anti-paired helical filament (anti-PHF) immunostaining, most are mildly reactive with tau antibodies, displaying thread-like profiles (**Fig. 5.15**), which are also widespread throughout the neuropil (see **Fig. 5.15**). Anti-ubiquitin staining shows a large amount of par-

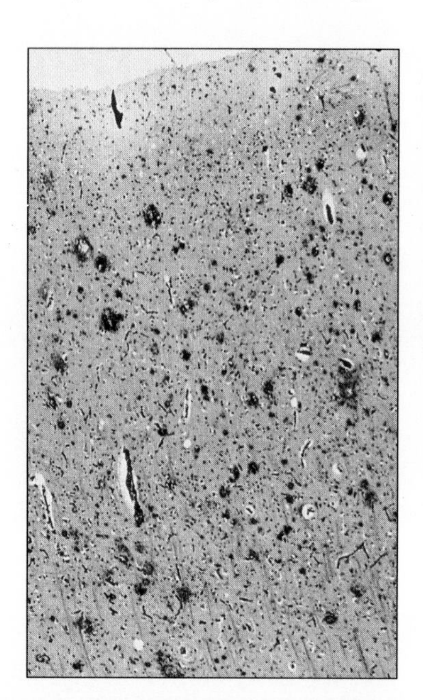

Fig. 5.12 Widespread deposition of amyloid β/A4 protein in the cerebral cortex in the form of diffuse plaques. *(Methenamine silver stain × 100.)*

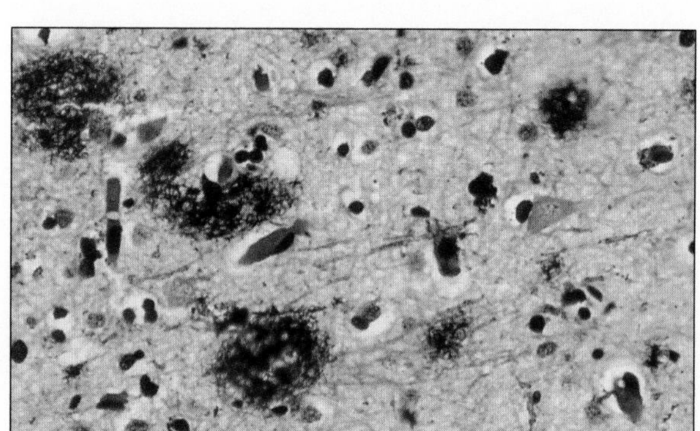

Fig. 5.13 Widespread deposition of amyloid β/A4 protein in the cerebral cortex in the form of diffuse plaques. *(Methenamine silver stain × 200.)*

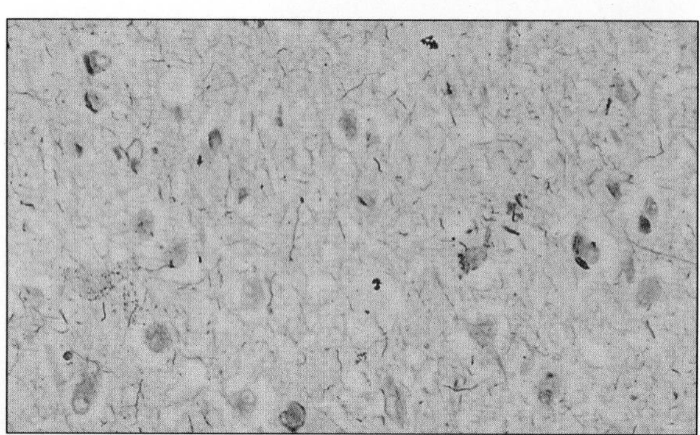

Fig. 5.14 The diffuse amyloid plaques do not contain neurites. Same field as **Fig. 5.13**. *(Palmgren silver stain × 200.)*

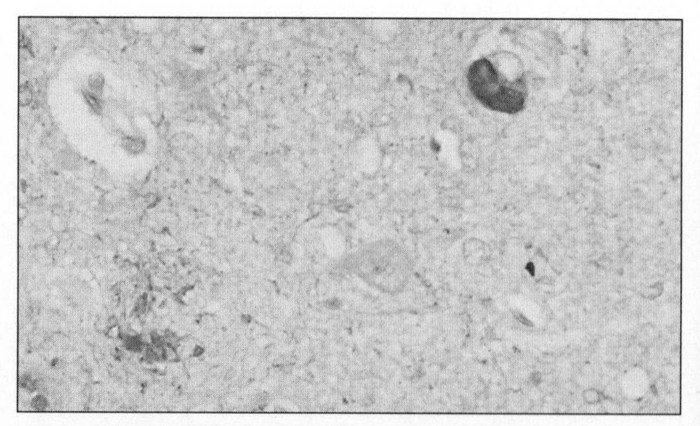

Fig. 5.15 Tau-immunoreactive neurites within amyloid plaques, and in the neuropil as 'threads', in the temporal cortex. *(Anti-tau × 200.)*

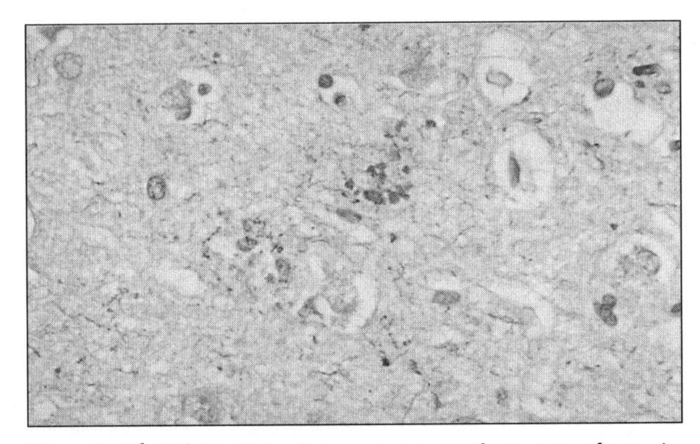

Fig. 5.16 Ubiquitin-immunoreactive neurites in amyloid plaques and in neuropil threads in the temporal cortex. *(Anti-ubiquitin × 200.)*

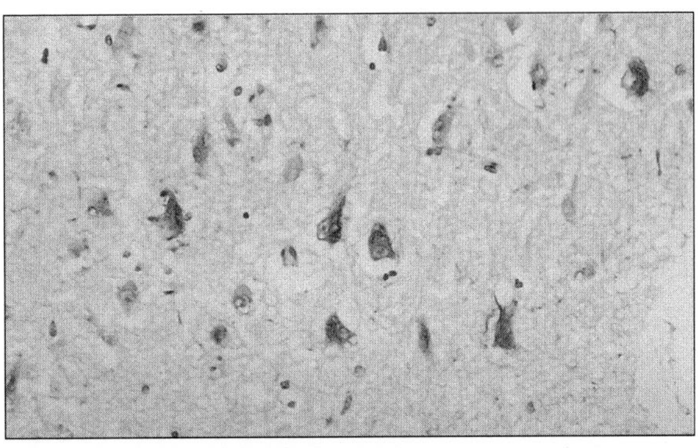

Fig. 5.17 Neurofibrillary tangles in pyramidal cells of CA1 region of the hippocampus. *(Anti-tau × 200.)*

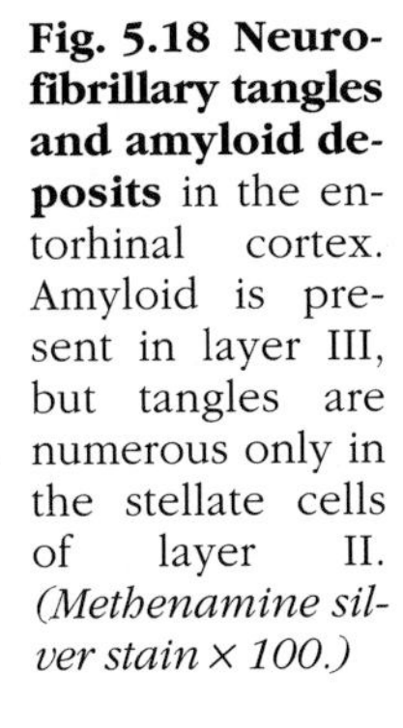

Fig. 5.18 Neurofibrillary tangles and amyloid deposits in the entorhinal cortex. Amyloid is present in layer III, but tangles are numerous only in the stellate cells of layer II. *(Methenamine silver stain × 100.)*

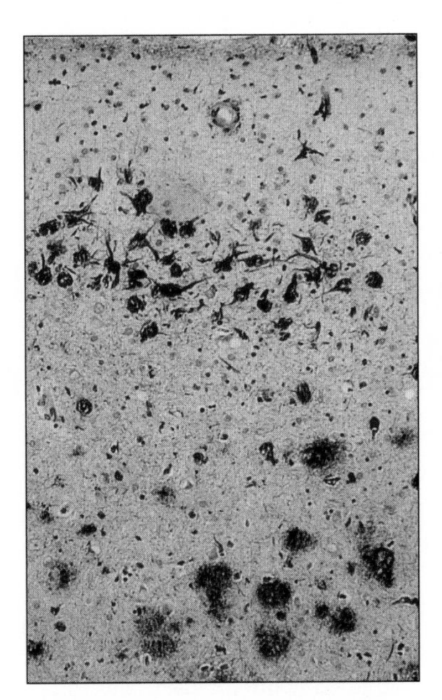

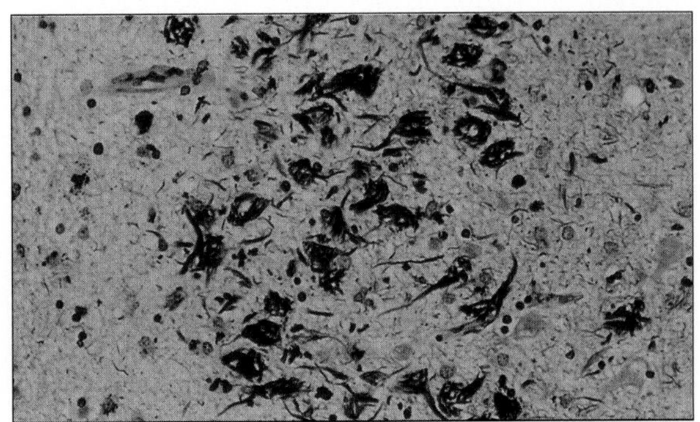

Fig. 5.19 Neurofibrillary tangles in the entorhinal cortex are numerous only in the stellate cells of layer II. *(Methenamine silver stain × 200.)*

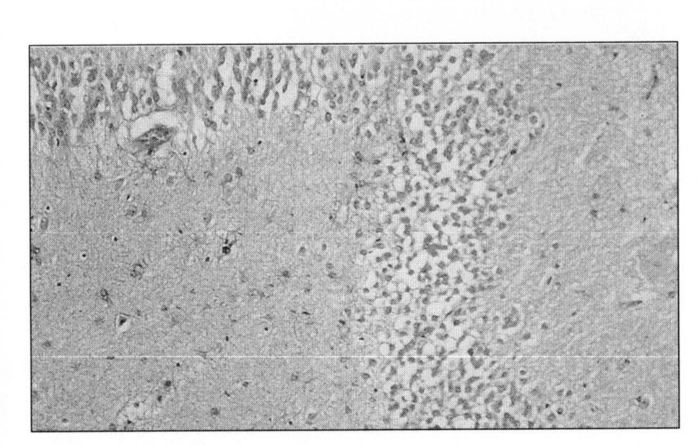

Fig. 5.20 Reactive astrocytosis in the end-folium of the Ammon's horn region of the hippocampus. *(Phosphotungstic acid–haematoxylin × 100.)*

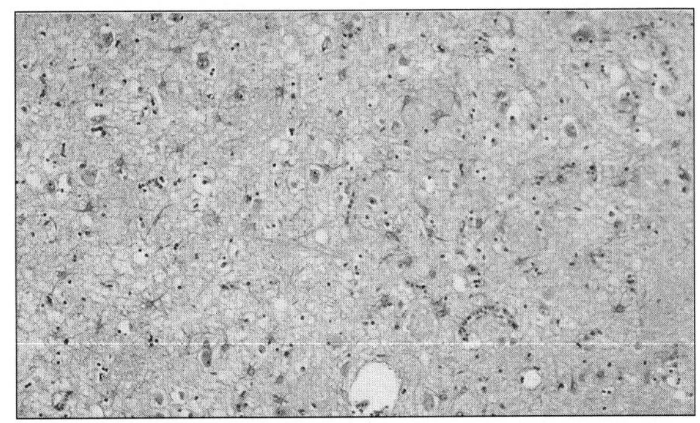

Fig. 5.21 Reactive astrocytosis in the subiculum of the hippocampus. *(Phosphotungstic acid–haematoxylin × 100.)*

ticulate material within the amyloid deposits (**Fig. 5.16**) and the threads (see **Fig. 5.16**), and within white matter. Both silver and anti-tau immunostaining detect occasional neurofibrillary tangles within the neocortex, but these may be much more extensive in the subiculum and CA1 region of the hippocampus (**Fig. 5.17**), and particularly in the entorhinal cortex (**Figs 5.18** and **5.19**). There may be a moderate astrocytosis within the CA4/5 (**Fig. 5.20**), CA1 and subicular (**Fig. 5.21**) regions of the hippocampus.

Many leptomeningeal and intraparenchymal arteries show a deposition of amyloid β/A4 protein within their walls, particularly in patients who have severe parenchymal deposits of β/A4 protein and neurofibrillary tangles. There appears to be no difference in terms of Lewy body density between patients showing numerous Alzheimer-type features and those who do not.

At present it is not clear whether the former patients have co-existing Alzheimer's and Lewy body disease (the basic pathologies of each disorder become increasingly common in old age), or whether cortical Lewy body disease with plaques and tangles (sometimes referred to as the cortical Lewy body variant of Alzheimer's disease) represents a 'point' on a spectrum of disease with typical Alzheimer's disease and typical Lewy body disease occupying each pole (see pages 164–166).

CORTICO-BASAL DEGENERATION

Demographic features

In 1968, Rebeiz and colleagues described the clinical and pathological features of three patients with a disorder they termed 'cortico dentato nigral degeneration with neuronal achromasia'. About 40 other patients with a similar disorder have since been mentioned in the literature, though it is likely that the disorder is more prevalent than this paucity of reported cases would suggest. It is probable that other cases are 'hidden' under the rubric of 'atypical Parkinsonism', 'Parkinsonism-plus', 'akinetic-rigid syndrome' or 'multisystem atrophy', or have been misdiagnosed as progressive supranuclear palsy, with which the condition shares many features.

The age of onset of this disorder is 50–75 years and its duration is 5–10 years. It appears to be more common in men than in women, the ratio being 2:1. No familial cases have been reported.

Neurological symptoms and signs
Asymmetrical akinesia and rigidity
Dyskinesia
Psychological symptoms
Apraxia
Alien limb
Cortical sensory loss
Mental slowness and inefficient memory
Investigations
SPET: asymmetrical fronto-parietal abnormality

Pathological features

On CT scan (**Fig. 5.22**) the brain may show a mild to moderate diffuse symmetrical atrophy, but sometimes there is an asymmetrical atrophy, which is most severe on the side contralateral to the side of greatest clinical involvement. In other instances the CT scan is normal.

Age of onset
40–65 years
Sex incidence
Males and females affected equally
Duration
5–10 years.
Gross features
- Mild cerebral atrophy, asymmetrically affecting thalamo-parietal cortex on the side contralateral to that showing greatest clinical change
- Depigmentation of the substantia nigra

Histopathology
- Basophilic 'whorled' inclusions in substantia nigra, locus caeruleus, nucleus basalis of Meynert, and other subcortical areas
- Inclusions are tau, but not ubiquitin positive
- Nerve cell loss. Parietal cortex shows severe nerve cell loss, neuronal swelling, and achromasia.
- Heavy astrocytosis
- Tau positive cells in other parts of the neocortex
- Swollen cells react with antibodies against αB crystallin

Genetics
- No inherited cases reported

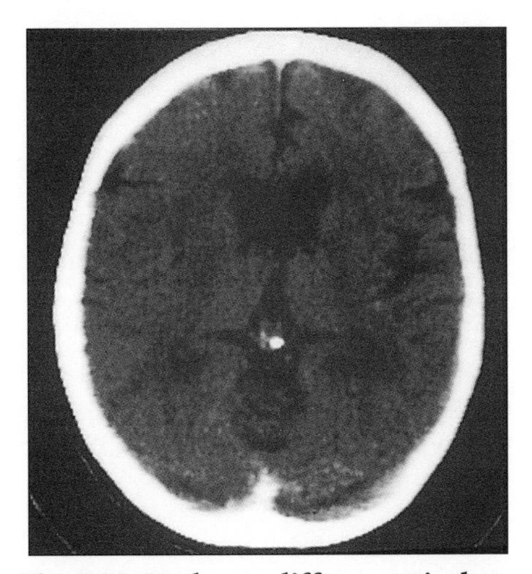

Fig. 5.22 Moderate diffuse cortical atrophy with greater involvement of the left perisylvian region. CT scan of the brain of a 63-year-old woman. The lateral ventricles are moderately, though symmetrically, enlarged.

SPET imaging (**Fig. 5.23**) demonstrates a marked asymmetrical thalamo-parietal metabolic decline contralateral to the side of greatest clinical involvement. At autopsy the brain is usually mildly and diffusely atrophic, and this affects mainly frontal regions. Its weight is only slightly reduced. The lateral ventricles are dilated (**Fig. 5.24**) and the substantia nigra is often grossly depigmented. Sometimes, there is an obvious and focal loss of grey and white matter from the parietal lobe (parasylvian region), at the level of the thalamus (see **Fig. 5.24**). Otherwise, the brain is macroscopically normal.

Histologically, the substantia nigra is always severely affected, showing an intense loss of neurones (**Fig. 5.25**) with some astrocytosis. There is a large amount of residual melanin pigment extra-cellularly or within macrophages. Lewy bodies are occasionally present in some surviving cells, particularly in more elderly patients, but these are thought to be age-associated rather than indicative of Parkinson's disease. The characteristic change in this region is

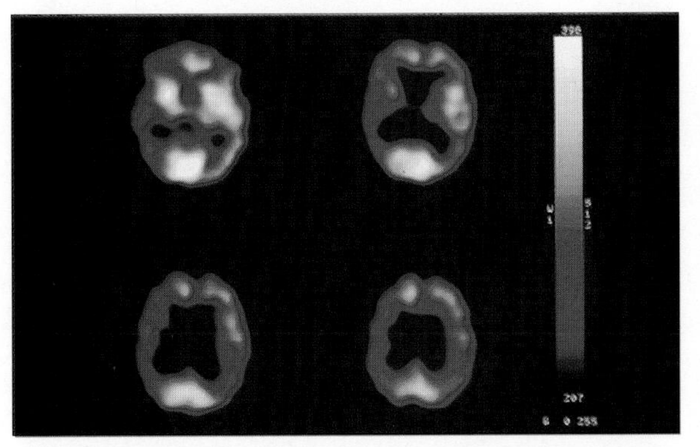

Fig. 5.23 Asymmetrical (left-sided) reduction in brain metabolism involving the posterior cortex and thalamus. SPET imaging in a 65-year-old man.

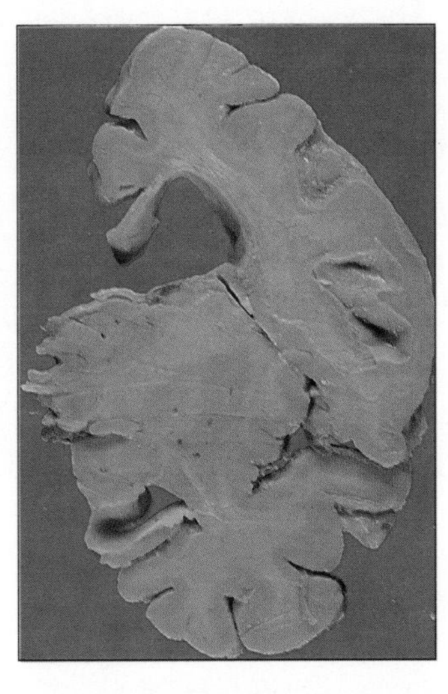

Fig. 5.24 Atrophy of the posterior parietal cortex with preservation of the temporal lobe. Coronal section of the brain of a 60-year-old man. The lateral ventricle is dilated and the corpus callosum thinned.

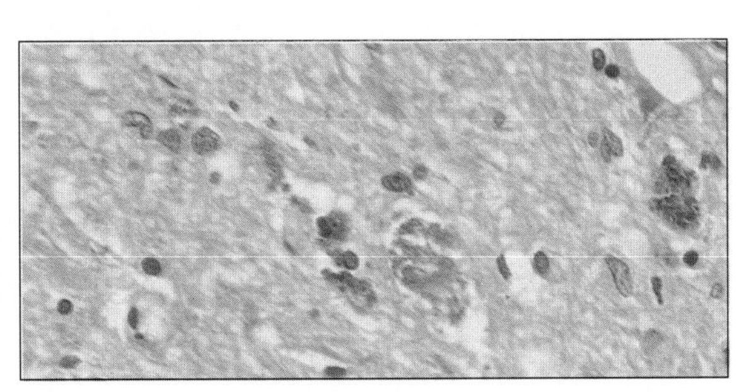

Fig. 5.25 Loss of nerve cells from the substantia nigra with accumulations of free pigment in the neuropil. *(Haematoxylin–eosin × 400.)*

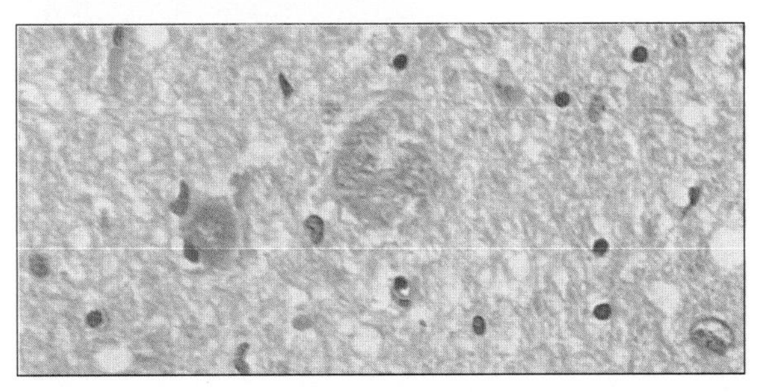

Fig. 5.26 A surviving nerve cell in the substantia nigra containing a basophilic whorled inclusion. *(Haematoxylin–eosin × 400.)*

the presence of rounded or whorled, weakly basophilic inclusions reminiscent of neurofibrillary tangles within nigral cells (**Figs 5.26** and **5.27**; see also **Fig. 5.29**). Cells showing such changes are also widespread through other basal structures, such as the nucleus basalis (**Fig. 5.28**; see also **Fig. 5.30**), thalamus, subthalamic nucleus, globus pallidus, red nucleus, dorsal raphe and locus caeruleus. Such inclusions are weakly argyrophilic (**Figs 5.29** and **5.30**) and strongly positive with antisera against tau proteins (**Figs 5.31** and **5.32**), but lack immunoreactivity with ubiquitin antisera (see NFT of Alzheimer's disease). Swollen, achromatic (i.e. weakly basophilic) cells are seen in the parietal cortical regions (**Figs 5.33** and **5.34**). Immunostaining reveals that these (**Fig. 5.35**) and other scattered cells throughout the cerebral cortex, especially the frontal regions (**Fig. 5.36**), and the dentate gyrus of the hippocampus (**Fig. 5.37**) are also tau-positive. Tau-positive 'threads' are widely present in grey and white matter areas, and the white matter shows widespread, though moderate, astrocytosis. The dentate gyrus of the hippocampus is also moderately gliosed (**Figs 5.38** and **5.39**).

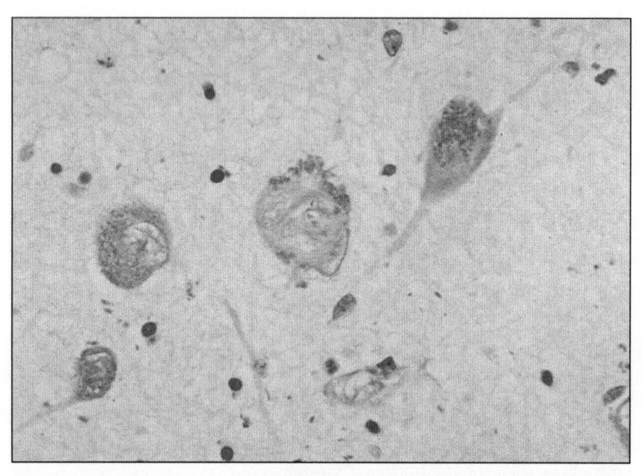

Fig. 5.27 A whorled inclusion in the substantia nigra. *(Nissl stain × 400.)*

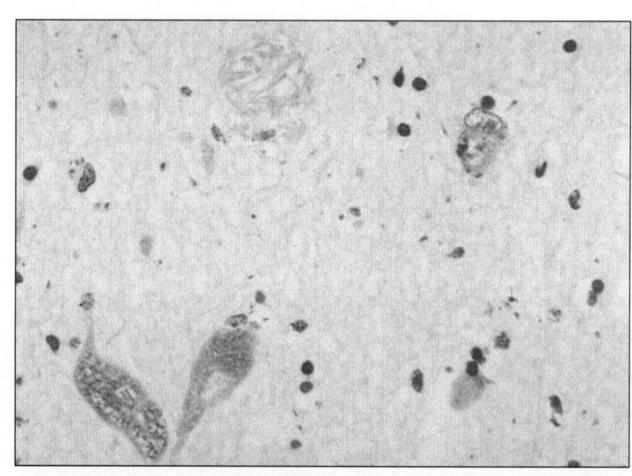

Fig. 5.28 A whorled inclusion in the nucleus basalis of Meynert. *(Nissl stain × 400.)*

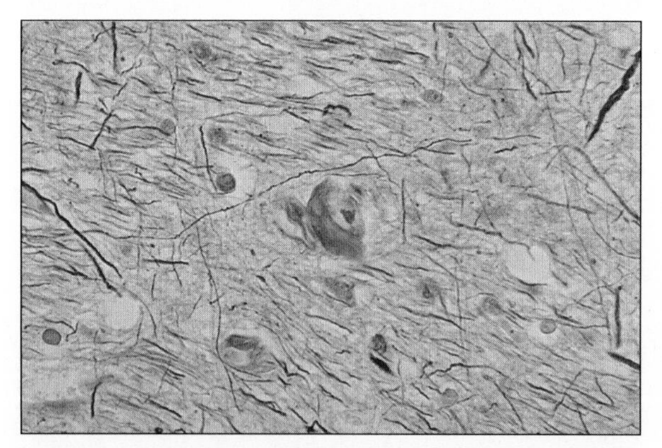

Fig. 5.29 Whorled inclusions in the substantia nigra are only weakly argyrophilic. *(Palmgren silver stain × 400.)*

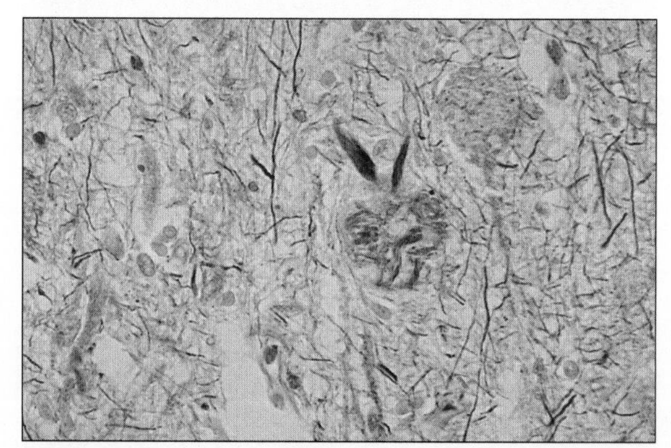

Fig. 5.30 Whorled inclusions in the nucleus basalis of Meynert are also only weakly argyrophilic. *(Palmgren silver stain × 400.)*

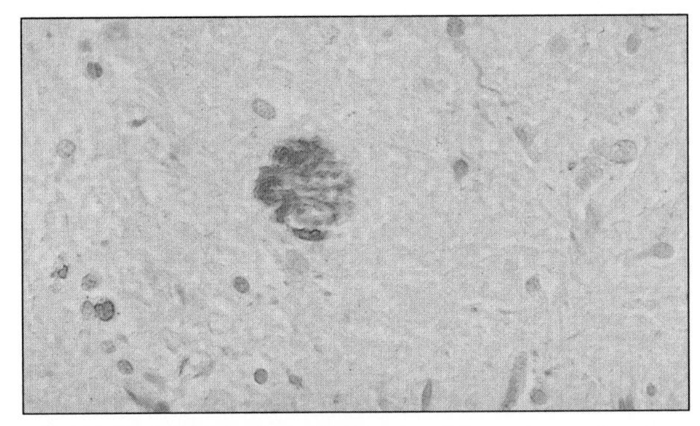

Fig. 5.31 Whorled inclusions in the substantia nigra containing tau proteins. *(Anti-tau × 400.)*

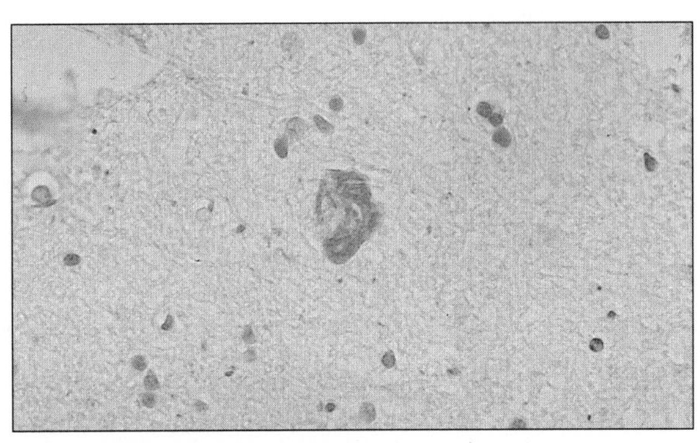

Fig. 5.32 Whorled inclusions in the nucleus basalis of Meynert also containing tau proteins. *(Anti-tau × 400.)*

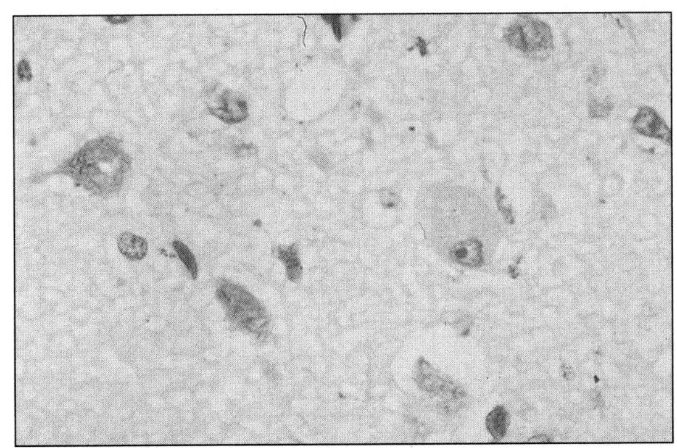

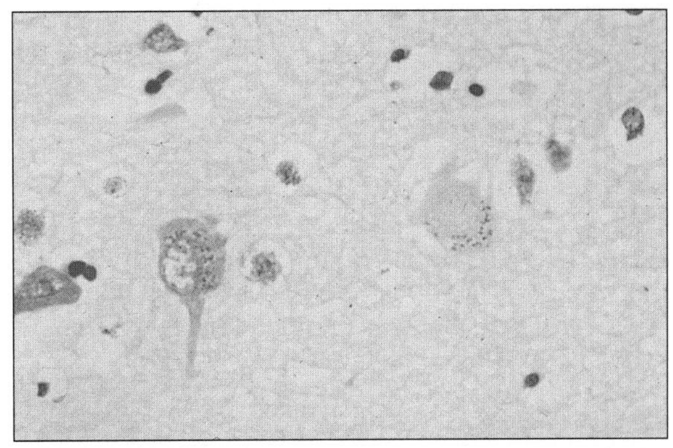

Fig. 5.33 and 5.34 Swollen achromatic nerve cells in the posterior parietal cortex. There is a loss of Nissl substance and nuclear disintegration. Lipofuscin appears as stained granules. *(Nissl stain × 400.)*

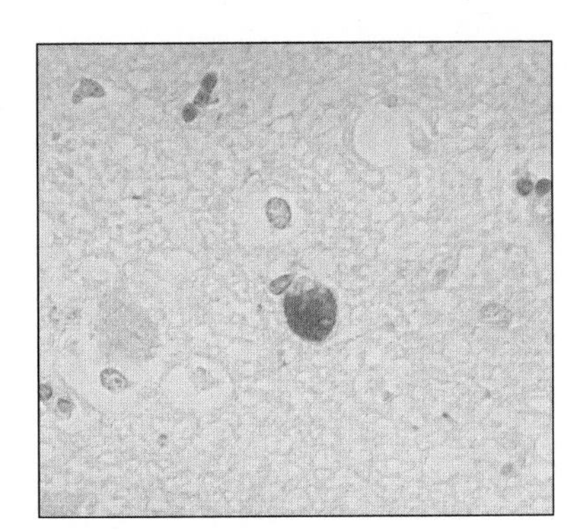

Fig. 5.35 Swollen neurones of the parietal cortex are also tau-reactive. *(Anti-tau × 400.)*

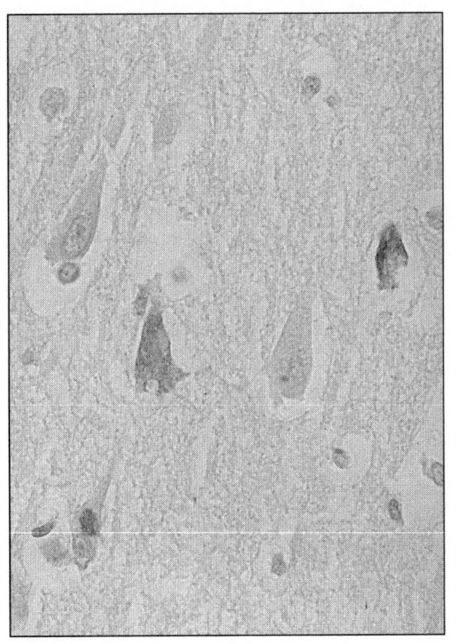

Fig. 5.36 Tau-reactive cells in the frontal cortex. *(× 400.)*

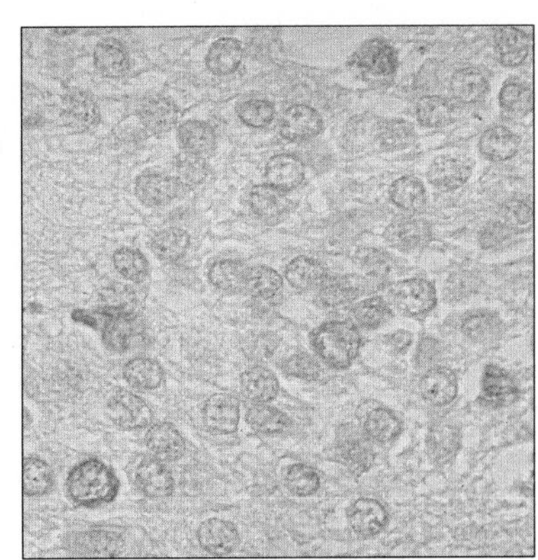

Fig. 5.37 Tau-reactive cells in the dentate gyrus of the hippocampus. *(× 400.)*

Within the parietal cortex, and usually on the side contralateral to the more severe clinical involvement, an asymmetrical and quite focal region of cortex shows extreme neuronal loss (**Fig. 5.40**) with florid astrocytosis (**Figs 5.41** and **5.42**), mainly in the grey matter rather than the white matter.

The swollen, achromatic neurones (see **Figs 5.33** and **5.34**) are reactive with antibodies against αB crystallin (**Fig. 5.43**). Similarly, immunoreactive astrocytes are present in subpial regions (**Figs 5.44** and **5.45**). Typical Pick-type inclusions, neurofibrillary tangles or Lewy bodies are absent.

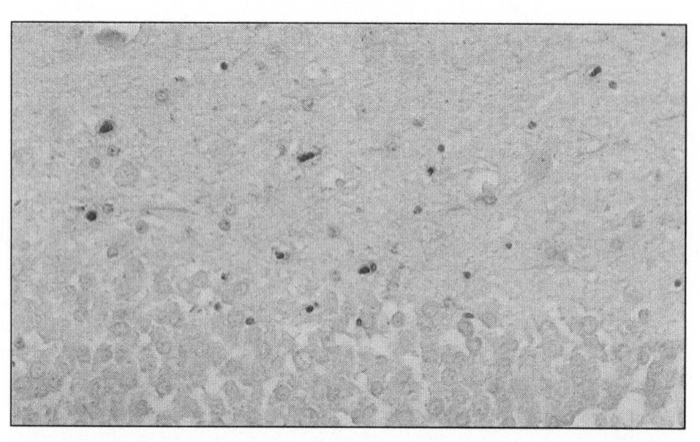

Fig. 5.38 Reactive astrocytosis in the end-folium region of Ammon's horn of the hippocampus. *(Phosphotungstic acid–haematoxylin × 200.)*

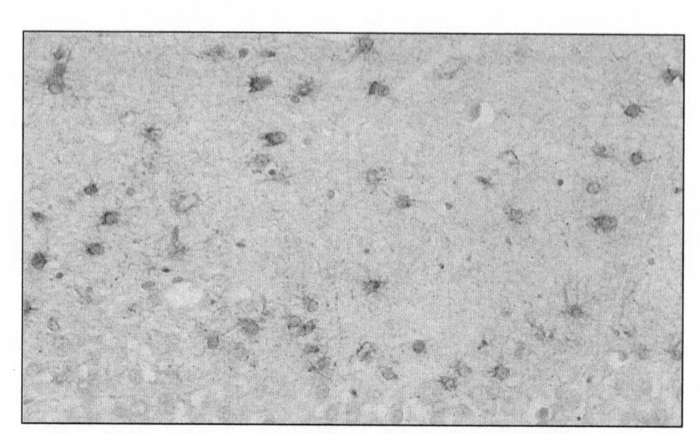

Fig. 5.39 As Fig. 5.38, but anti-GFAP. *(× 200.)*

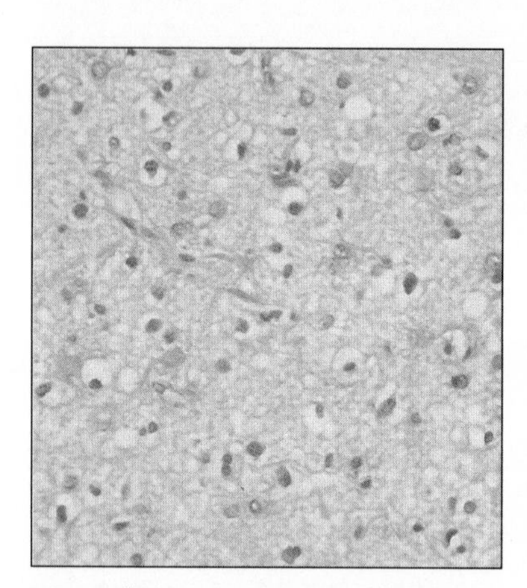

Fig. 5.40 Loss of nerve cells from the posterior parietal cortex. *(Haematoxylin–eosin × 200.)*

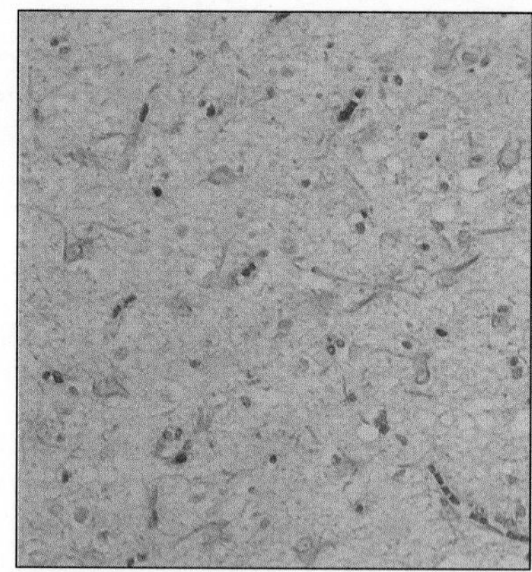

Fig. 5.41 Florid astrocytosis within the posterior parietal cortex. *(Phosphotungstic acid–haematoxylin × 200.)*

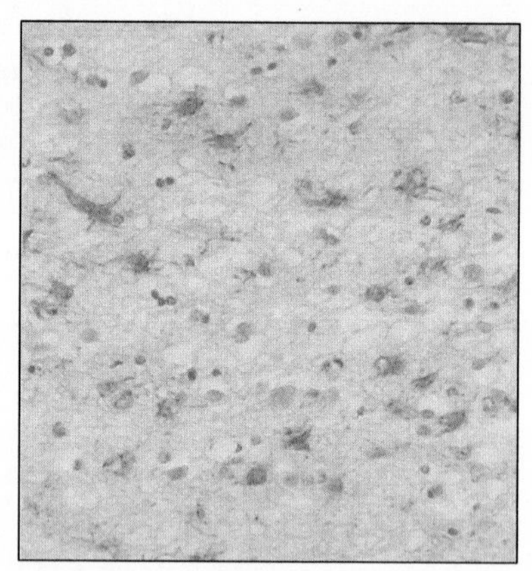

Fig. 5.42 As Fig. 5.41, but anti-GFAP.

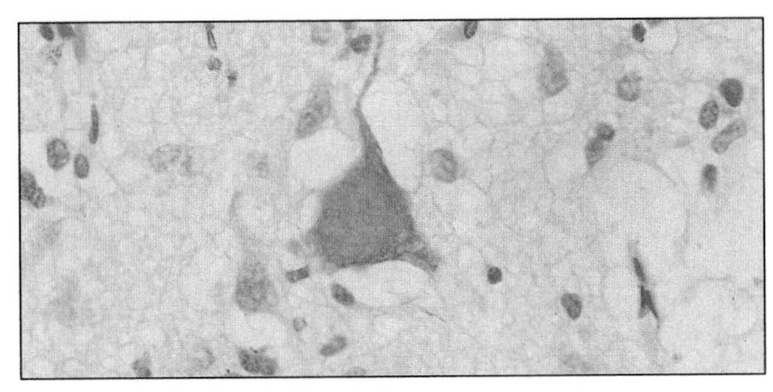

Fig. 5.43 αB crystallin reactivity. The swollen achromatic pyramidal cell in layer V of the posterior parietal cortex is strongly immunoreactive with αB crystallin. *(Anti-αB crystallin × 400.)*

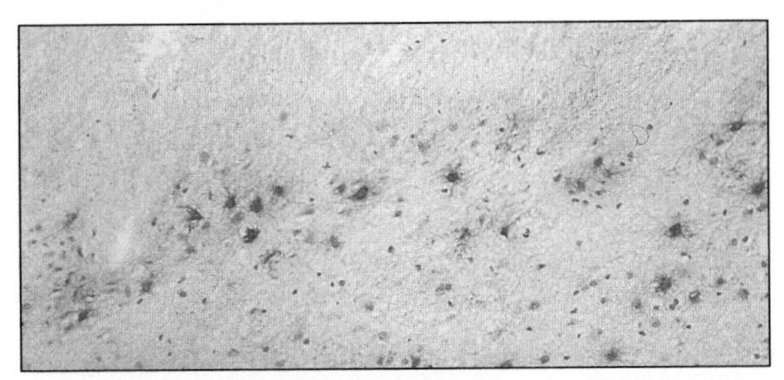

Fig. 5.44 αB crystallin reactivity. Astrocytes in layer I of the posterior parietal cortex are strongly reactive with αB crystallin antibody. *(Anti-αB crystallin × 200.)*

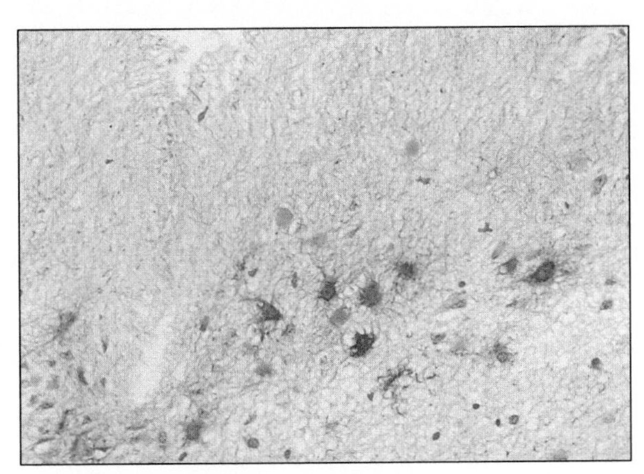

Fig. 5.45 αB crystallin reactivity. Astrocytes in layer I of the posterior parietal cortex are strongly reactive with αB crystallin antibody. *(Anti-αB crystallin × 400.)*

Relationship to other Parkinsonian conditions

The clinical syndromes of progressive supranuclear palsy, Parkinson's disease, cortical Lewy body disease and cortico-basal degeneration share many clinical features. This is due mainly to the involvement of the substantia nigra, an aspect of the pathology common to all of them. A diversity of pathological changes underlies the disorders and it is by no means clear whether any of them share any aetiological or pathogenetic features.

VASCULAR DEMENTIA

Introduction

Fluctuations in cardiac output due to various heart disorders can cause a (transient) hypoperfusion of the brain, as can disease within, or affecting, the main arteries supplying the brain (for example, atherosclerosis within carotid and vertebral arteries, cervical spondylosis). Perfusional fluctuations like these can cause global clinical changes such as a transient loss of consciousness or more focal and lasting functional deficits. The latter relate to ischaemic/hypoxic events within the brain, affecting, for example, the 'watershed' areas between the anterior and middle cerebral artery territories and the middle and posterior cerebral artery territories, or the penetrating arteries of the cerebellum, brain stem or basal ganglia. Ischaemic infarcts, large or microscopic, can therefore occur in regions such as the occipital pole (**Fig. 5.46**) or cerebellar hemispheres (**Figs 5.47–5.49**). Such changes may be insufficient in themselves to cause intellectual or cognitive decline, but may complicate the clinical picture of a dementia due to neurodegeneration in an elderly person.

The term 'vascular dementia' can be used to describe cerebrovascular lesions of various types that cause cerebral injury and impair multiple cognitive functions, thereby leading to dementia. Different and confusing titles have been applied to these pathologies in the past, and some remain in current use. Indeed, the term 'multi-infarct' dementia has been used clinically to describe the dementia that can result from ischaemic, anoxic, or even haemorrhagic damage to the brain, irrespective of cause. It is, however, not always appropriate in a strict pathological sense to apply this term to each and every process that results in such a compromise of the blood supply to the brain with consequent loss of cognitive or memory function.

Cerebral haemorrhage, or infarction due to focal thromboembolic phenomena (i.e. stroke) and leading to localised neuropsychological deficits, is common in middle-aged and elderly persons. Repeated complete strokes due to infarction result in a progressive neuropsychological decline (multiple (cortical and subcortical) infarct dementia). In contrast, routine autopsies on elderly people commonly reveal the presence of small softenings, which are sometimes numerous, due to thromboembolism within any part of the brain. These are not associated with any previously discernible decline in cognition or memory . However, clinically 'silent' infarction in the white matter may lead to progressive dementia (subcortical arteriosclerotic dementia).

Given its age-related prevalence, it is only to be expected that cerebrovascular disease should represent a significant cause of dementia in the elderly, providing the cerebral lesions are sufficiently large

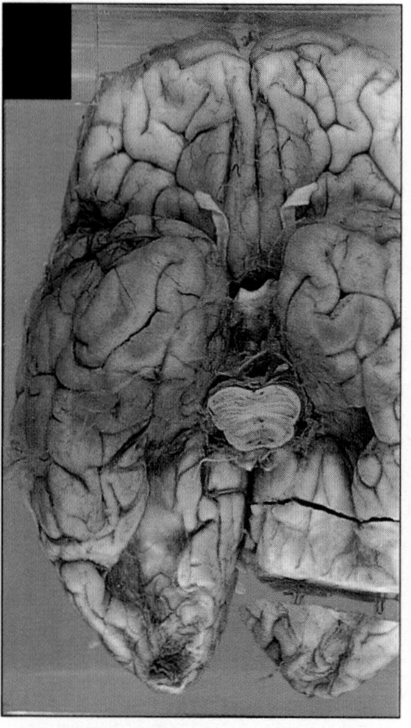

Fig. 5.46 Bilateral infarction of the medial parts of the occipital lobe following cardiac hypoperfusion.

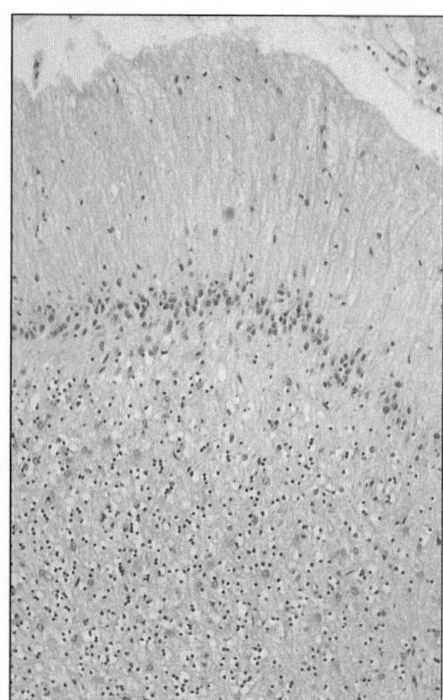

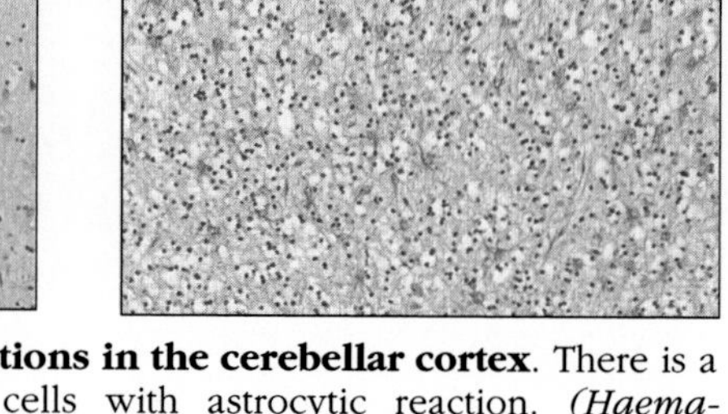

Figs 5.47 and 5.48 Microinfarctions in the cerebellar cortex. There is a loss of Purkinje and granule cells with astrocytic reaction. *(Haematoxylin–eosin × 100.)*

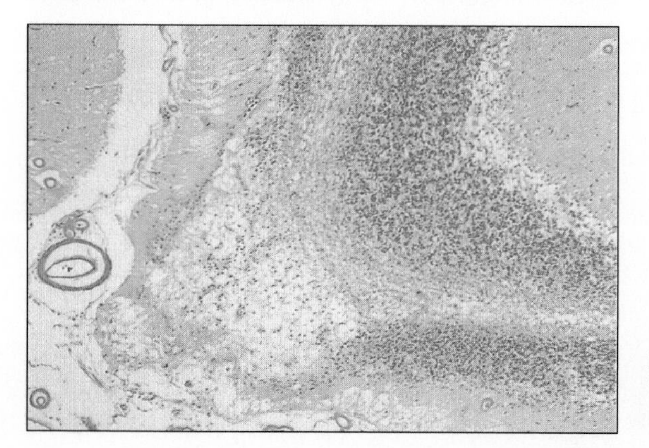

Fig. 5.49 Microinfarctions in the cerebellar cortex. There is a loss of Purkinje and granule cells. *(Phosphotungstic acid–haematoxylin × 100.)*

Neurological symptoms and signs (early)
Pseudobulbar palsy
Corticospinal signs
Parkinsonism
Ataxia

Psychological symptoms
Mental slowness
Inefficient memory

Investigations
SPET: frontal lobe abnormality
CT. MRI multiple periventricular white matter lesions

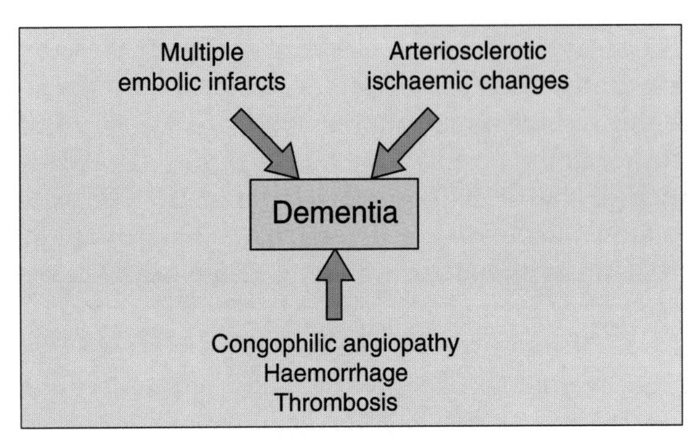

Fig. 5.50 Vascular causes of dementia.

enough and appropriately placed. Epidemiological studies seem to confirm this. Cerebrovascular disease is perhaps the second most common cause of, or contributor, to dementia after Alzheimer's disease.

The main pathological causes of vascular dementia are shown in **Fig. 5.50**.

- Multiple (cortical and subcortical) infarct dementia is due to the cumulative effects of thromboembolisation of cerebral blood vessels. It is associated with *atherosclerotic* changes in the major *extracranial* and *extracerebral* arteries supplying the brain.
- Subcortical arteriosclerotic dementia is related to the effects of long-standing *hypertension* on large and small *intraparenchymal* arteries causing a chronic cerebral ischaemia.
- Congophilic angiopathy is due to the deposition of an *amyloid* protein within the walls of *extracerebral* and *intraparenchymal* arteries leading to haemorrhagic or thrombotic changes.

Age of onset
Any age after 40 years
More common over 70 years of age

Sex incidence
Males affected more often than females

Duration
Variable, up to 10 years

Gross features
- Multiple completed infarcts in cerebral cortical and subcortical grey matter and internal capsule

Or
- White matter demyelination, often with lacunae, usually in frontal and temporal cortex. Incomplete infarction

Histopathology
- Completed infarcts, many cases with histopathology of Alzheimer's disease

Or
- Fibrous and hyaline degeneration of arteries. Stenosis of lumen. Microcystic degeneration around blood vessels, sometimes confluent leading to incomplete infarction of white matter. Reactive astrocytosis

Genetics
- Spontaneous (associated with atherosclerosis of extracerebral arteries or hypertension and cigarette smoking)

Pathological changes

Subcortical arteriosclerotic encephalopathy

The patient is usually male and the vascular damage is nearly always associated with heavy cigarette smoking and long-standing hypertension. The clinical picture is a subcortical encephalopathy.

A CT scan (**Fig. 5.51**) reveals widespread lucency (leuko-araiosis) of the deeper white matter, particularly around the ventricles, but sparing the immediate subcortical white matter.

Usually, the brain is of normal weight and external appearance, although sometimes there is evidence of atrophy and an occasional cortical infarction. The large extracerebral arteries, particularly the internal carotid and basilar arteries, show severe atherosclerosis with irregular dilations and tortuosity (ectasia) (**Figs 5.52–5.54**). Such changes are, however, not in themselves the cause of the dementia: damage of this kind to the basal vessels is rare in the absence of degenerative disease within the intracerebral branches of the main distributive arteries, particularly those of the middle, and sometimes the posterior, cerebral artery.

Slicing the brain reveals dilatation of the lateral ventricles and numerous, sometimes confluent, foci of softening and fragmentation within the deep white matter of the cerebral cortex (**Fig. 5.55**), particularly that of the frontal, temporal or parietal lobe, and often with a preferential periventricular distribution. Such areas of damage within the white matter of the cortex correspond to the regions of 'leukoaraiosis' – areas of translucency – detected on CT (see **Fig. 5.51**) scanning. Other lesions may be seen around the blood vessels within the basal ganglia and these relate to a cystic change known as 'etat lacunaire' (**Figs 5.56–5.58**). As with ectasia of the extracerebral arteries, etat lacunaire of the larger penetrating arteries is not in itself the cause of the dementia, but the tissue microinfarction that surrounds such affected vessels obviously contributes to the overall deficits.

The most important histopathological changes are seen within the damaged white matter areas where the small arteries show the characteristic changes of arteriosclerosis. These comprise a fibrous thickening ('onion-skinning') and hyalinisation (**Figs 5.59–5.65**), resulting in their stenosis or necrosis (see **Fig. 5.65**).

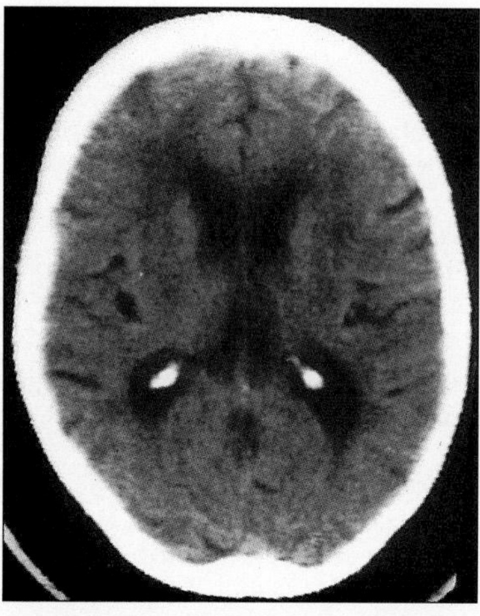

Fig. 5.51 Periventricular lucencies, dilatation of the lateral ventricles and diffuse cerebral atrophy. CT scan of the brain of an 82-year-old woman.

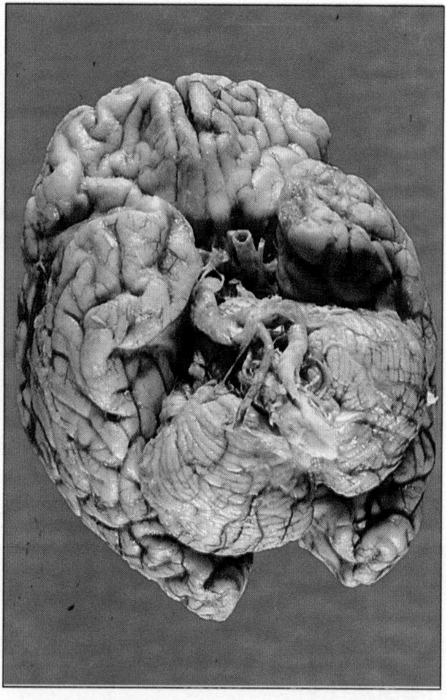

Fig. 5.52 Ectasia of the basilar artery associated with severe systemic atherosclerosis in an 83-year-old woman.

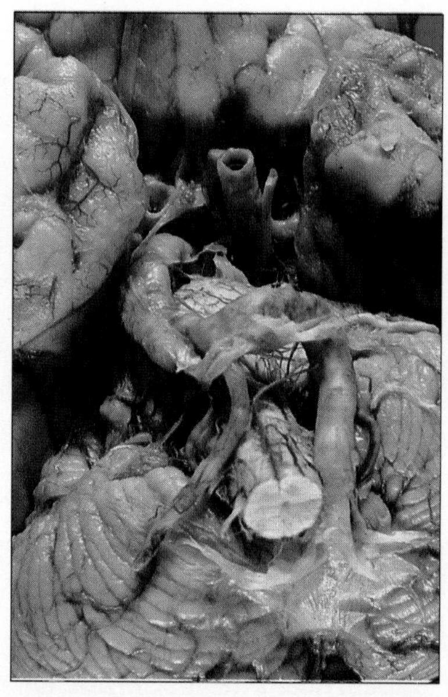

Fig. 5.53 Ectasia of the basilar artery associated with severe atherosclerosis in an 83-year-old woman. Higher power view.

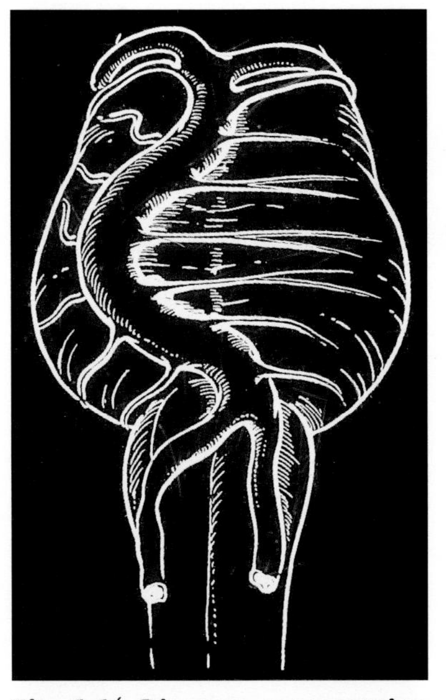

Fig. 5.54 Diagram representing ectasia of the basilar artery. Note the stretching of arteries penetrating the brain stem.

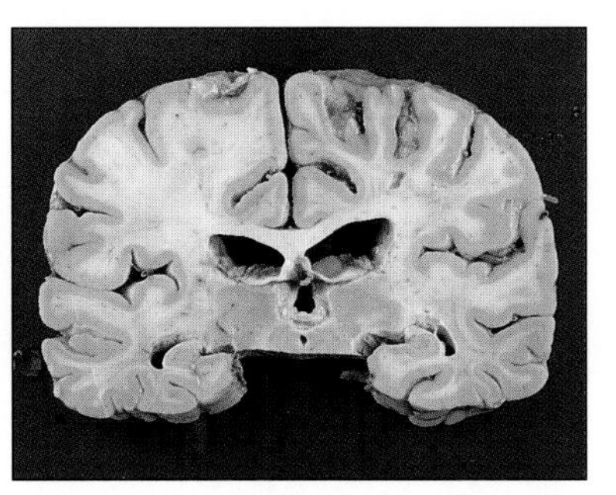

Fig. 5.55 Softening within the deep white matter of the parietal cortex, with the presence of 'lacunes'. Coronal slice of the brain of a 71-year-old man.

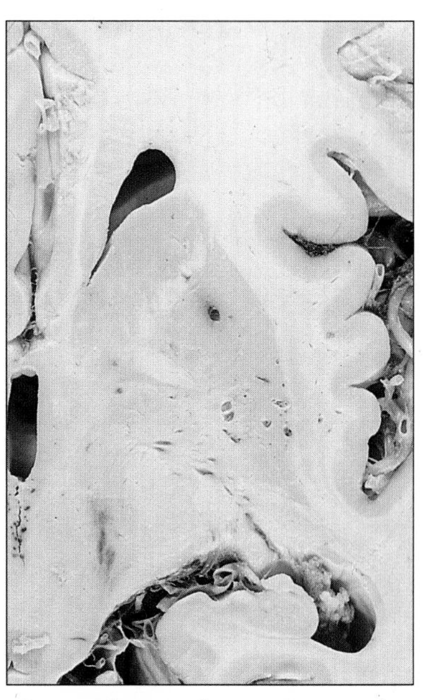

Fig. 5.56 'Etat lacunaire' within the basal forebrain region in a 72-year-old man.

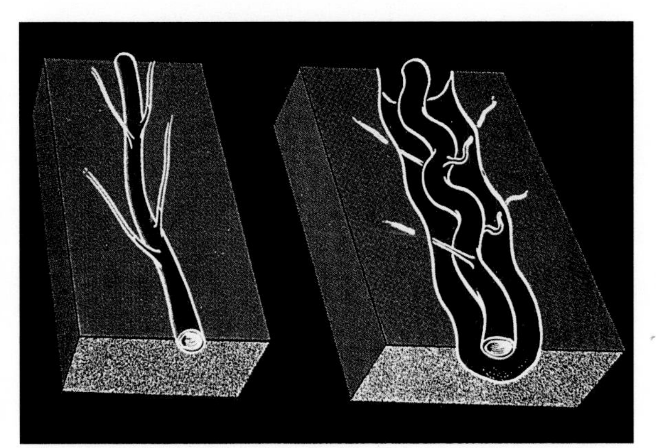

Fig. 5.57 Diagram depicting etat lacunaire. Note the loss of contact between brain tissue and blood vessel.

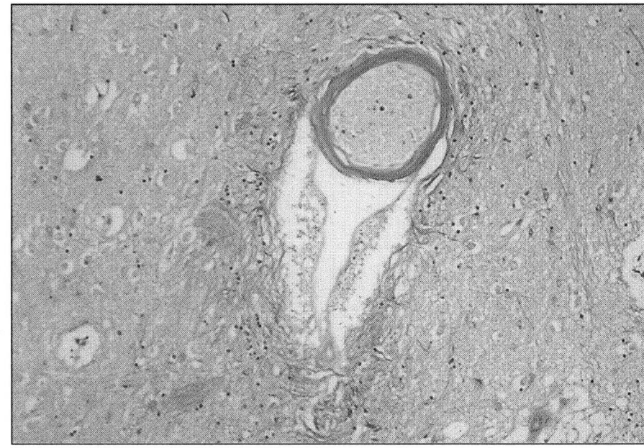

Fig. 5.58 Small artery within the basal forebrain region showing etat lacunaire. Note the astrocytic reaction in surrounding brain tissue, due to local micro-infarction. *(Phosphotungstic acid–haematoxylin × 400.)*

Such narrowing results in local and chronic underperfusion of brain tissue with the formation of multiple, small, and sometimes incomplete, areas of ischaemic necrosis. Alternatively, they may present as larger and more complete infarctions if the involved vessel becomes thrombosed. These changes lead to extensive 'honeycombing' (**Figs 5.66** and **5.67**) of the white matter and produce

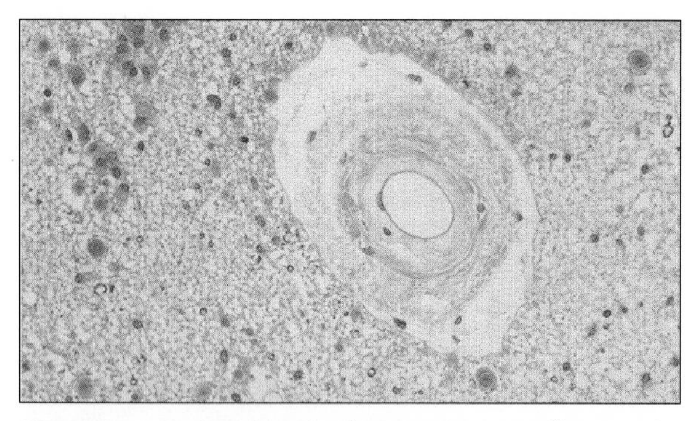

Fig. 5.59 Arteriosclerotic changes in a small artery in the white matter. There is a loss of elastic tissue with proliferation of collagen causing 'onion-skinning' of the vessel wall. The lumen is reduced. *(Haematoxylin–eosin × 400.)*

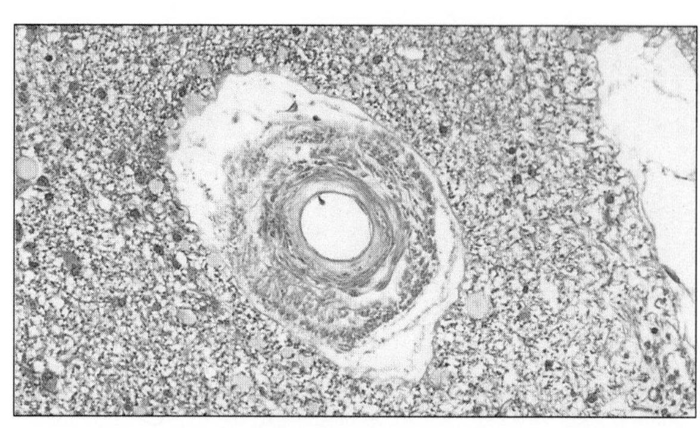

Fig. 5.60 Arteriosclerotic changes in a small artery in the white matter. Same vessel as in **Fig. 5.59.** *(Phosphotungstic acid–haematoxylin × 400.)*

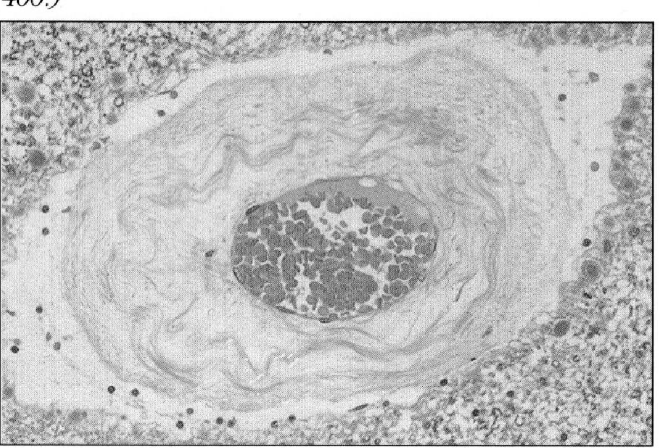

Fig. 5.61 Fibrous proliferation in the wall of a small artery, with surrounding microcystic degeneration. *(Haematoxylin–eosin × 400.)*

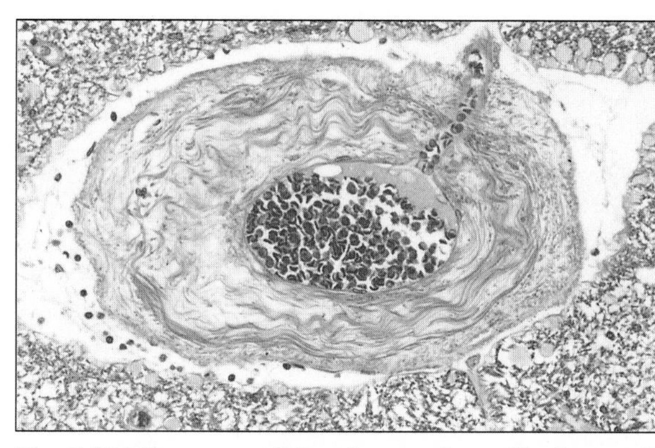

Fig. 5.62 Fibrous proliferation in the wall of a small artery with surrounding microcystic degeneration. Same vessel as in **Fig. 5.61**. *(Phosphotungstic acid–haematoxylin × 400.)*

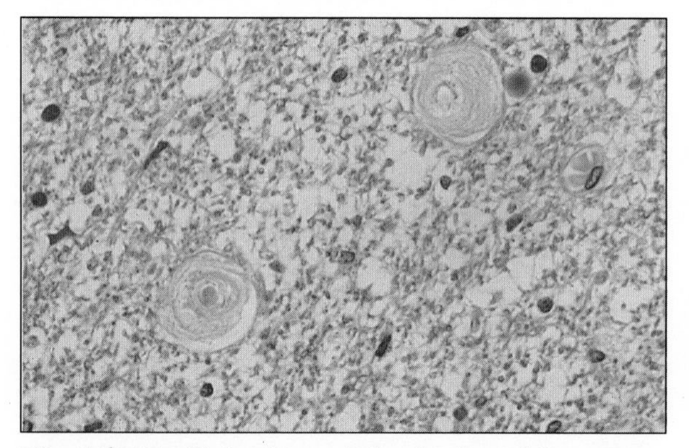

Fig. 5.63 Hyalinised arterioles in the white matter of the temporal cortex. *(Haematoxylin–eosin × 400.)*

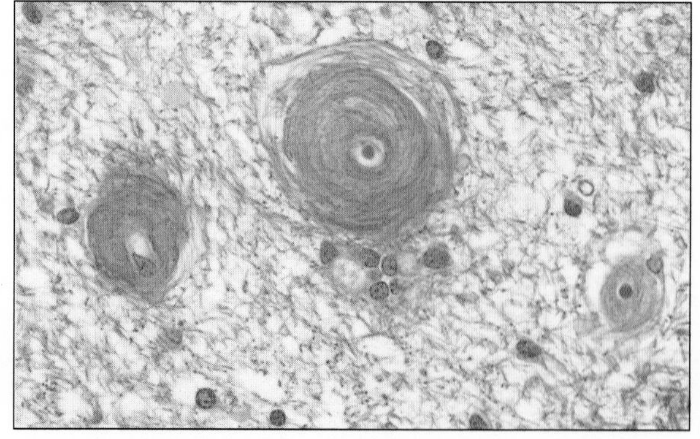

Fig. 5.64 Hyalinised arterioles in the white matter of the temporal cortex. Same vessels as in **Fig. 5.63**. *(Phosphotungstic acid–haematoxylin × 400.)*

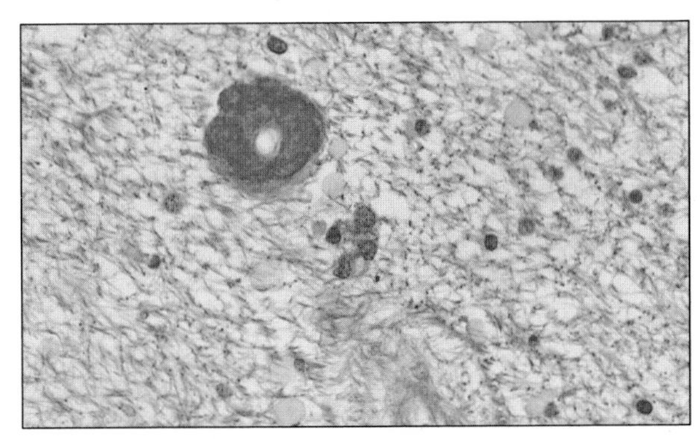

Fig. 5.65 Wall of a small artery undergoing necrosis. *(Phosphotungstic acid–haematoxylin × 400.)*

widespread demyelination and axonal loss (**Figs 5.68** and **5.69**). The area of damage can extend from the ventricle towards the grey matter, but usually leaves this and the subjacent arcuate fibres intact (see **Figs 5.68** and **5.69**).

In addition to loss of axons and myelin, there is a reactive astrocytosis (**Figs 5.70** and **5.71**). Arteries in the grey matter may also be affected (**Figs 5.72** and **5.74**), some of which may become 'leaky' to plasma proteins (**Fig. 5.73**), and are associated with a pronounced astrocytic reaction of the gemistocytic type (**Fig. 5.73**). In both grey and

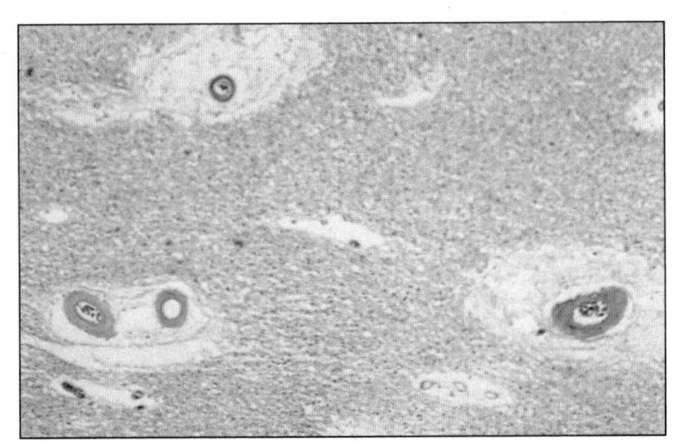

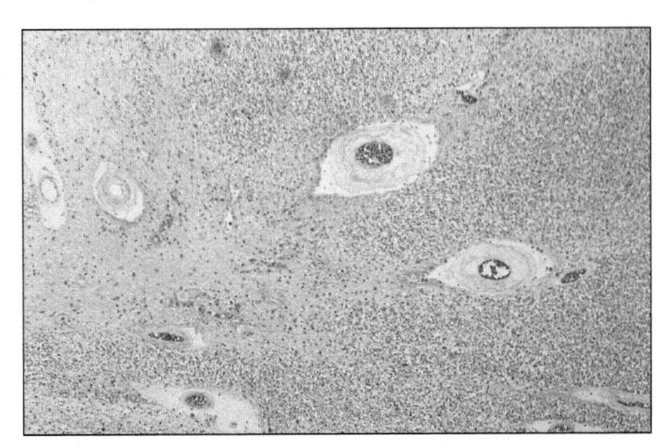

Figs 5.66 and 5.67 'Honeycombing' of the white matter, causing local microinfarction and loss of myelin. *(Haematoxylin–eosin × 200.)*

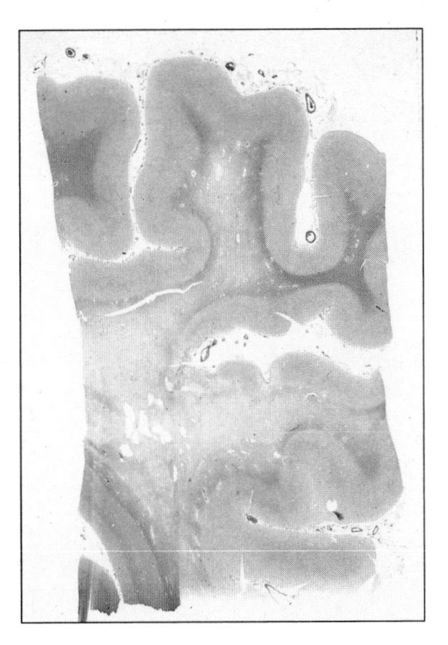

Fig. 5.68 (left) Gross loss of myelin from the deep white matter of the occipital cortex due to ischaemia causing an incomplete infarction. The arcuate fibres are relatively preserved. *(Phosphotungstic acid–haematoxylin–eosin × 0.5.)*

Fig. 5.69 (right) Loss of axons from the periventricular white matter in the occipital lobe. *(Palmgren silver × 0.5.)*

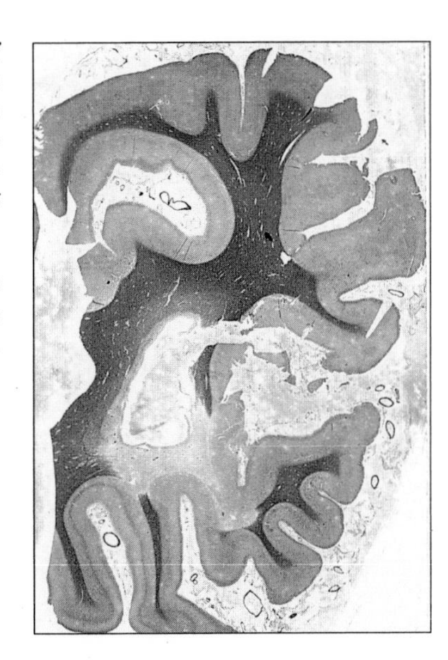

be present around affected vessels (see **Fig. 5.64**), and haemosiderin deposition (**Fig. 5.75**) marks the presence of extravasated red cells or actual haemorrhage. Microaneurysm formation may also occur (**Fig. 5.76**).

This pattern of damage has been described as a 'subcortical arteriosclerotic encephalopathy' or 'Binswanger's disease'.

Multi-infarct dementia (cortical and subcortical)

In patients with 'multi-infarct dementia', as defined pathologically, the vascular damage preferentially affects grey matter areas and involves the cortex rather than the subcortex. The onset of disease may be sudden and focal and progression can sometimes be 'stepwise' as further episodes of tissue damage occur. Such a course is, however, not

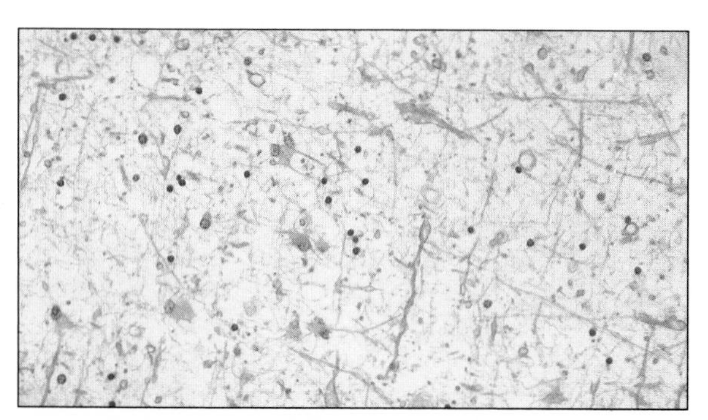

Fig. 5.70 Loss of myelin and axons from deeper white matter. *(Haematoxylin–eosin × 100.)*

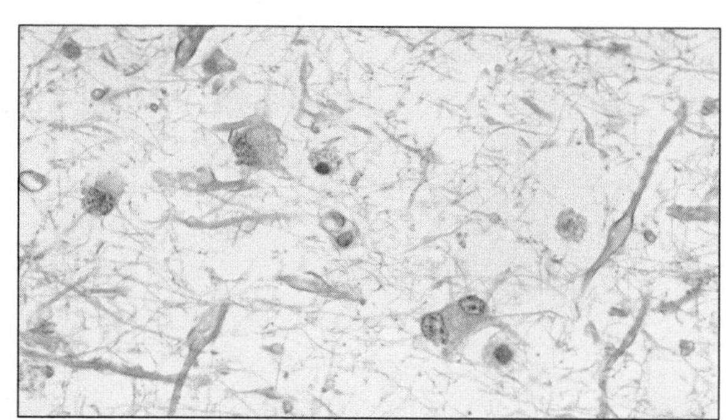

Fig. 5.71 Higher power view of Fig. 5.70, showing reactive astrocytosis. *(Haematoxylin–eosin × 400.)*

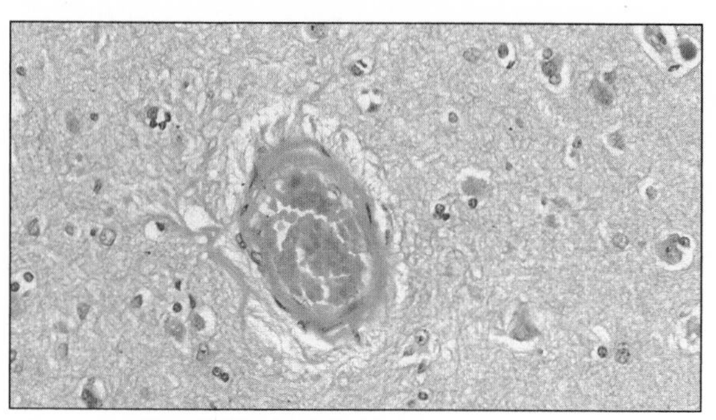

Fig. 5.72 Hyalinised blood vessel in the temporal cortex. *(Haematoxylin–eosin × 200.)*

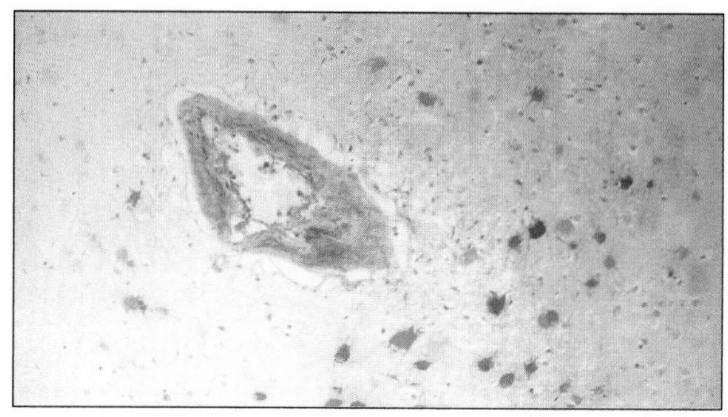

Fig. 5.73 Hyalinised artery in the temporal cortex showing leakage of plasma proteins. Note the reactive astrocytes containing a large amount of plasma protein. *(Anti-IgG × 100.)*

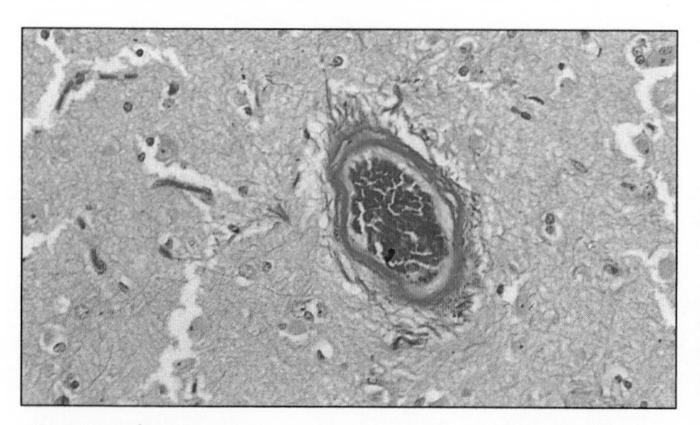

Fig. 5.74 Reactive astrocytosis surrounding a hyalinised vessel. *(Phosphotungstic acid–haematoxylin × 200.)*

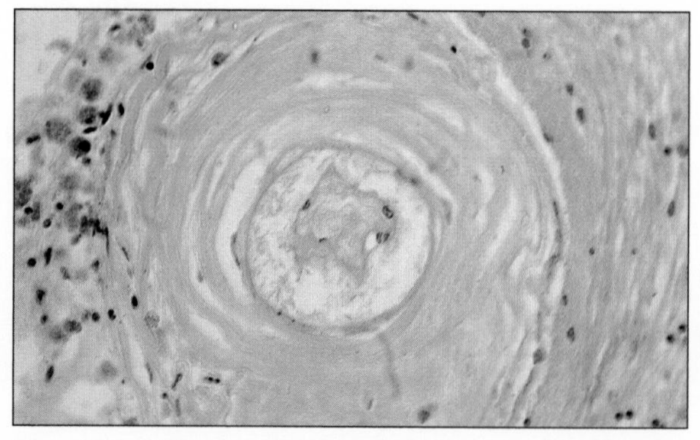

Fig. 5.75 Old microhaemorrhage around a fibrosed artery. *(Haematoxylin–eosin × 400.)*

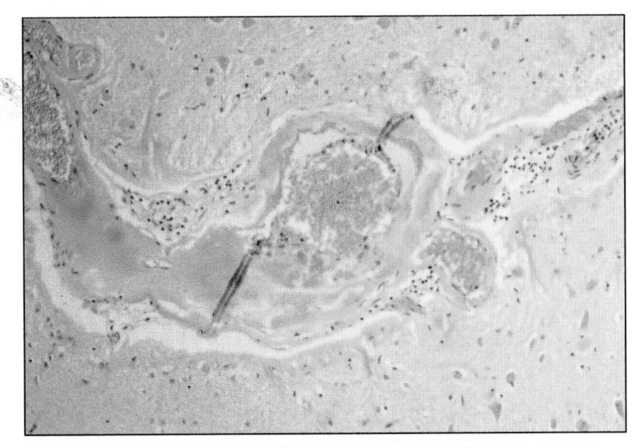

Fig. 5.76 A hyalinised artery in the hippocampus showing microaneurysm formation. *(Haematoxylin–eosin × 400.)*

definitive as more progressive exist, particularly when the grey matter infarction is combined with white matter lesions or with Alzheimer's disease.

By definition, 'multi-infarct dementia' is associated with overt and often multiple regions of tissue infarction within the brain. These can be detected on CT scans (**Figs 5.77** and **5.78**) as focal regions of translucency around the margins of the brain. SPET imaging (**Fig. 5.79**) defines local areas of hypometabolism corresponding to these regions of reduced tissue density.

The brain may be of normal weight, without evidence of generalised atrophy. The basal vessels will show numerous patches of atheroma, often with some degree of ectasia. Externally, there may

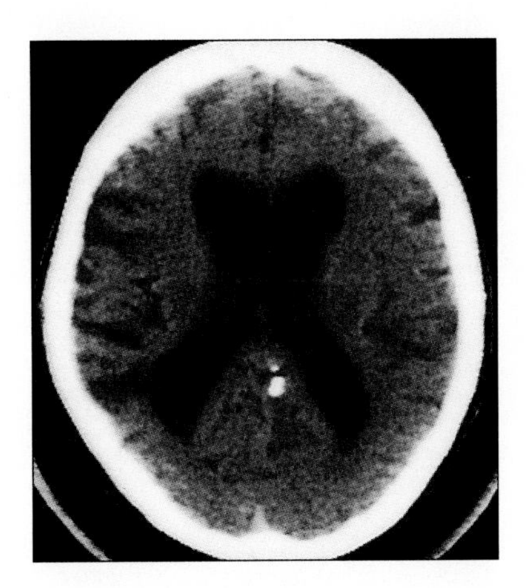

Fig. 5.77 (left) An old infarction in the right middle cerebral artery territory and the left posterior hemisphere. CT scan of the brain of a 63-year-old man.

Fig. 5.78 (right)An old infarction in the right middle cerebral artery territory and the cerebellum. CT scan of the brain of the 63-year-old man featured in **Fig. 5.77**.

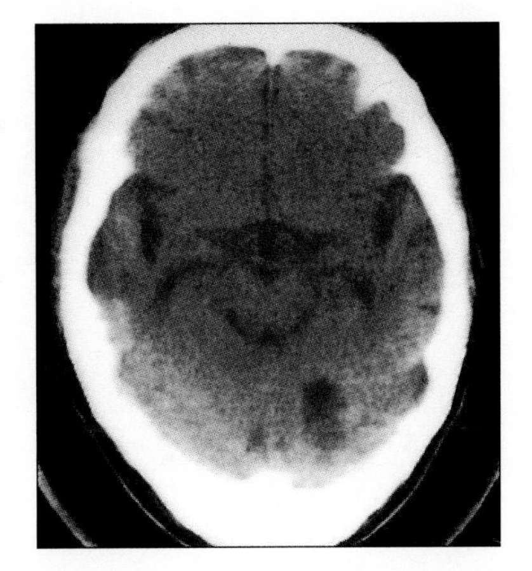

Fig. 5.79 Regions of hypometabolism due to tissue infarction within the right middle cerebral artery territory, right temporal lobe and cerebellum. SPET imaging of the brain of the 63-year-old man featured in **Figs 5.77** and **5.78**.

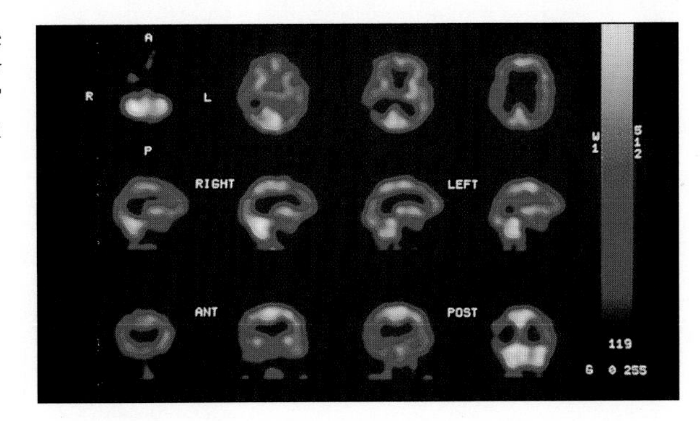

be evidence of old (**Fig. 5.80**) or more recent frank infarcts affecting the cortex, most often in the region of the middle cerebral artery, but also in that of the posterior cerebral artery. They range in size from a few mm to many cm in diameter depending on the site of vascular occlusion and the extent of collateral circulation. Occasionally, there is massive destruction of one hemisphere, but the lesions usually affect both hemispheres to some extent, commonly asymmetrically.

On coronal section, the ventricles are enlarged, again often asymmetrically (see **Fig. 5.82**) and unevenly, with one part of either ventricle being preferentially dilated, according to the distribution of the affected tissue. There are single, although usually multiple, softenings of varying sizes, recent (**Fig. 5.81**) or old (**Figs 5.82–5.89**) and involving both the cortical grey and white matter (see **Figs 5.82–5.89**), basal ganglia (see **Figs 5.82** and **5.85**) or thalamus. The largest lesions are normally within the middle cerebral artery territory or the temporo-occipital region (see **Figs 5.83** and **Fig. 5.86**). When the posterior cerebral artery is involved there may be lesions in the calcarine cortex (**Fig. 5.87**), the hippocampus and the hippocampal gyrus (see **Figs 5.88** and **5.89**).

The term 'multi-infarct dementia' has therefore been ascribed the clinical picture associated with the cumulative presence of large and small, presumably embolically derived, infarcts.

Tomlinson and colleagues have noted that the extent of the dementia is associated statistically

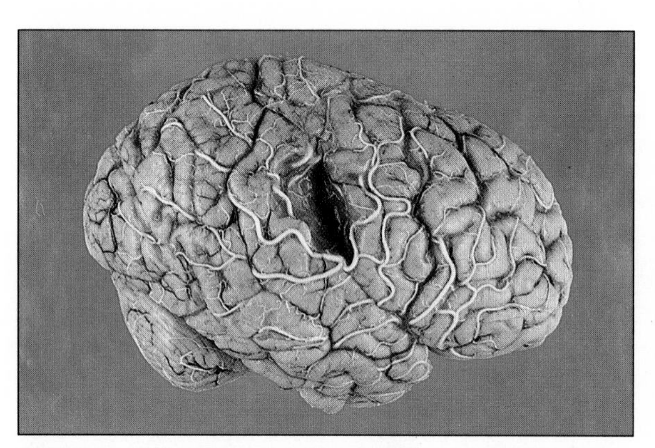

Fig. 5.80 Old cerebral infarct in the parietal cortex.

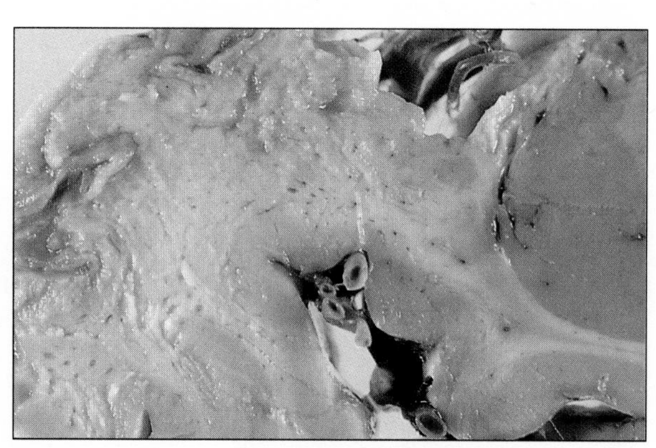

Fig. 5.81 Recent cerebral softening in the temporal lobe.

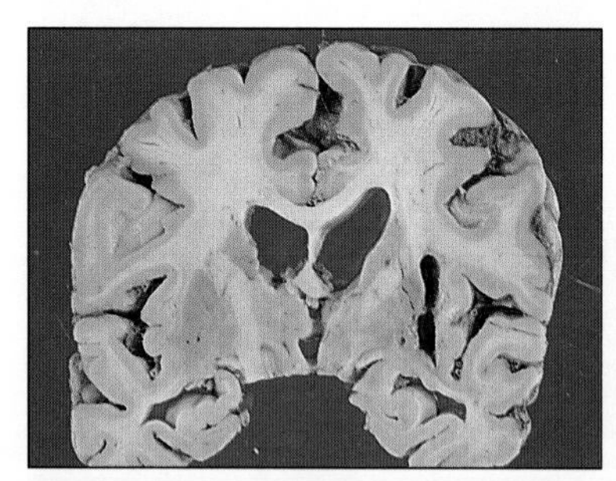

Fig. 5.82 Old cystic infarct in the claustrum.

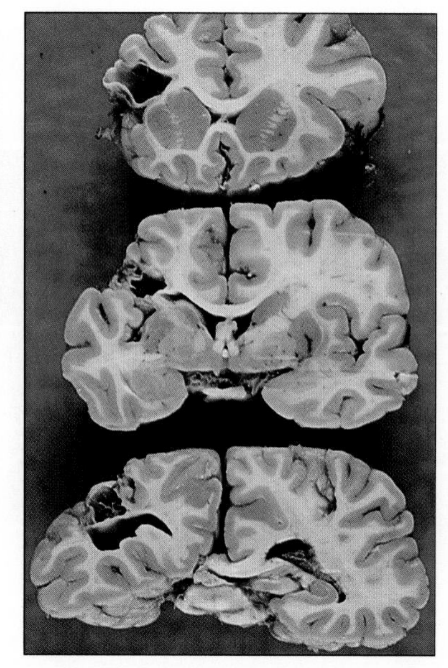

Fig. 5.83 Multiple old in the frontal and parietal cortex.

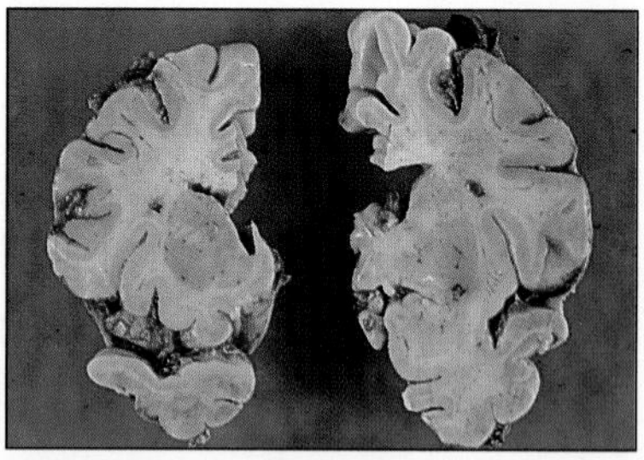

Fig. 5.84 Old infarcts in the white matter of the frontal and parietal cortex.

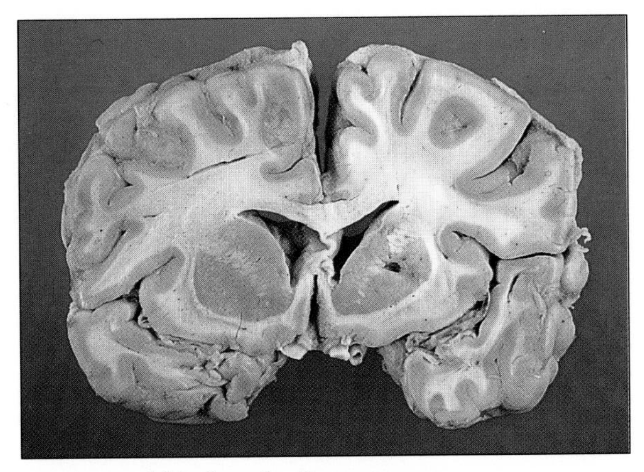

Fig. 5.85 Old infarct in the putamen.

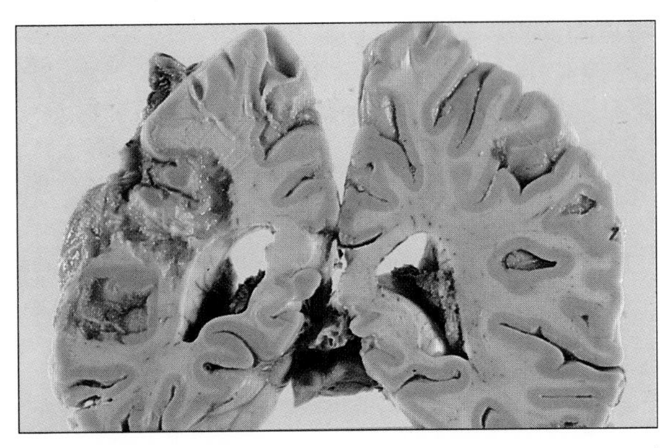

Fig. 5.86 Old infarction in the posterior parietal cortex.

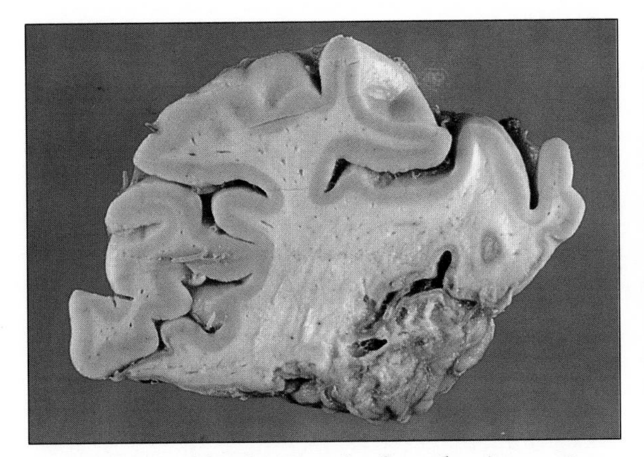

Fig. 5.87 An old infarction in the calcarine cortex.

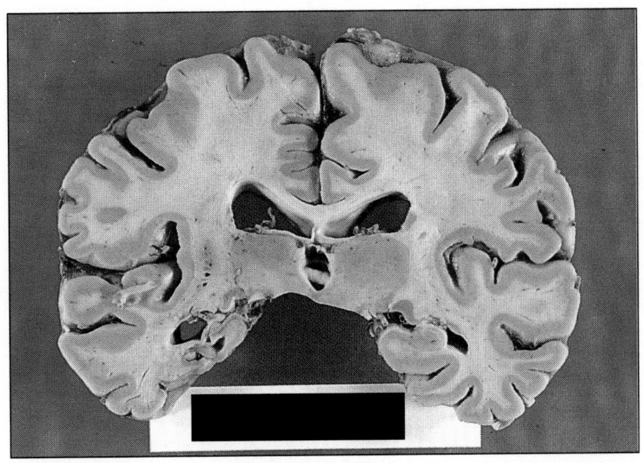

Fig. 5.88.An old infarction in the hippocampus and inferior temporal cortex.

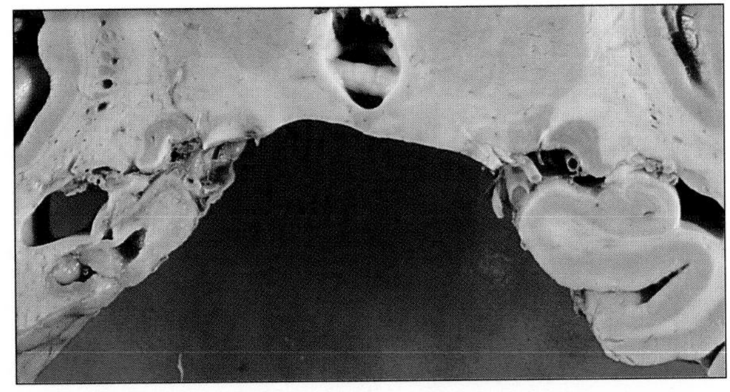

Fig. 5.89 Old infarction in the hippocampus and iinferior temporal cortex. Higher power view of **Fig.5.88.**

with increases in the volume of tissue destroyed. A 50–100 ml tissue loss represents the *threshold* to the *presence* of dementia. People with a tissue loss below this level do not display evidence of a cognitive decline. However, others dispute this. Erkinjuntii has reported demented patients in whom as little as 5 ml of tissue destruction has occurred.

Histologically, the infarcts vary in appearance according to age.

- Some, when complete, ultimately leave sharply defined fluid-filled cysts (see **Figs 5.82** and **5.83**), with residual and peripheral glial reaction.

- Others, if more recent or partial, lead to loss of neurones and myelin with a pronounced astrocytic and macrophagic response (**Figs 5.91–5.92**).

The embolised vessel may show organisation (**Fig. 5.93**) or even eventual recanalisation (**Fig. 5.94**).

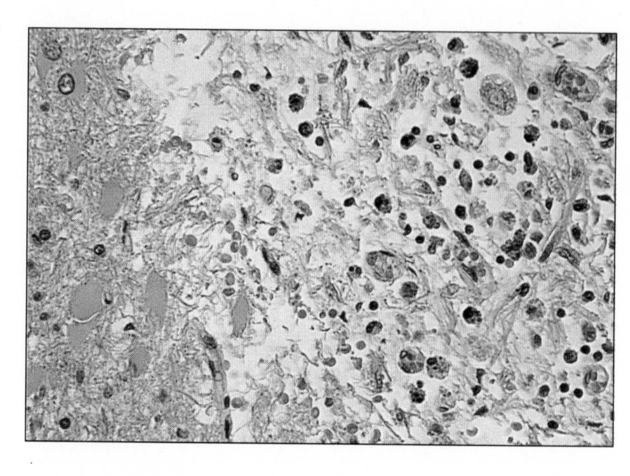

Fig. 5.90 Histological appearance of brain infarction with reactive astrocytosis and macrophage infiltration. *(Haematoxylin–eosin × 100.)*

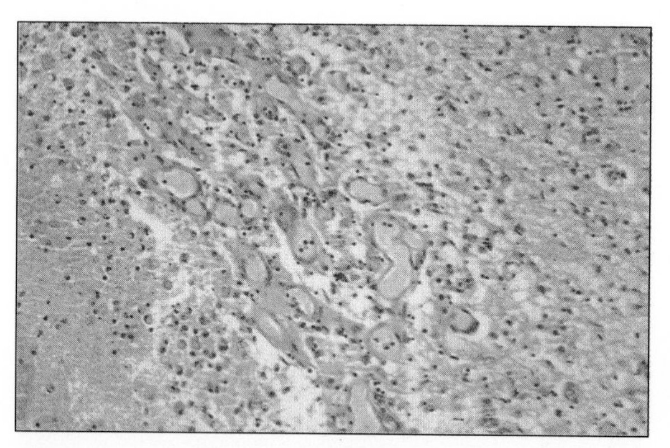

Fig. 5.91 An old infarction showing organisation of the thrombus. *(Haematoxylin–eosin × 200.)*

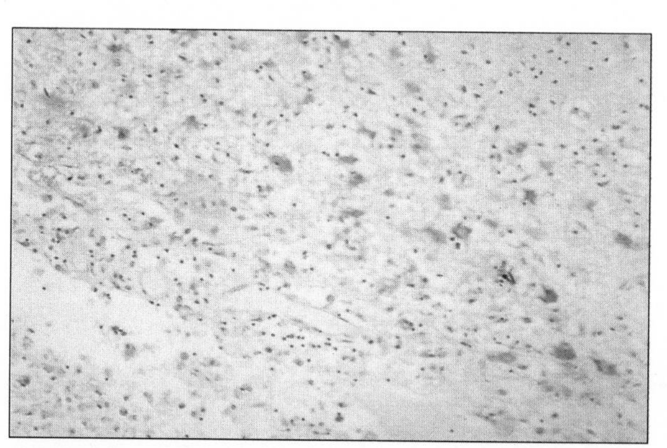

Fig. 5.92 Reactive astrocytosis surrounding the organising infarction, as in **Fig. 5.92**. *(Anti-GFAP × 100.)*

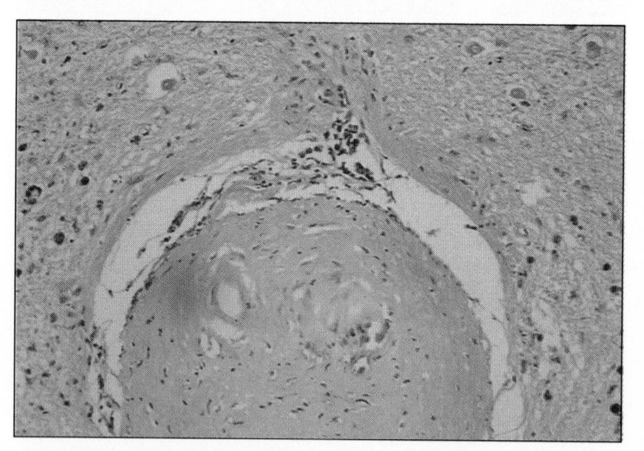

Fig. 5.93 Old thrombosis. Note the organisation and recanalisation. *(Haematoxylin–eosin × 200.)*

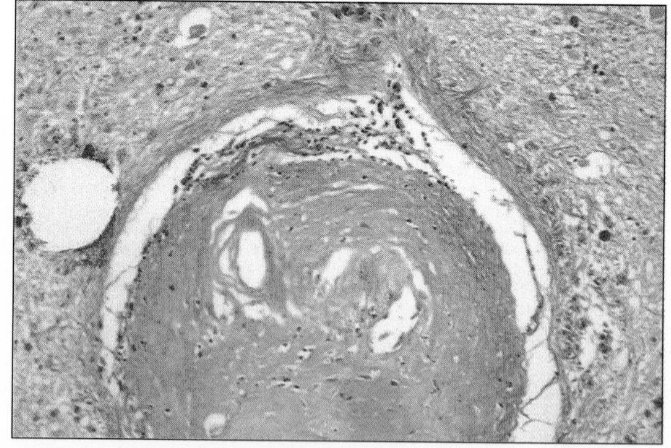

Fig. 5.94 Old thrombosis. Again, note the organisation and recanalisation. *(Phosphotungstic acid–haematoxylin × 200.)*

Combined dementia of vascular and Alzheimer types

Because of the the increasing prevalence of both cerebrovascular disease and Alzheimer's disease with age, there is a large number of (usually very) elderly people (10–25% of all elderly demented people) who display a dementia that can be attributed pathologically to the combined presence of Alzheimer's disease and cerebrovascular lesions. These people have typical Alzheimer-type pathological changes (see pages 26–46) and either grey and white matter infarcts (as seen in multi-infarct dementia: vide supra) or periventricular translucencies (leukoaraioses, of the kind associated with subcortical arteriosclerotic encephalopathy.

Such an association between these incomplete white matter infarcts and Alzheimer's disease has often been noted. It is probable, however, that they represent separate, but coincidental, pathologies, and do not imply that the white matter lesions are an integral part of the Alzheimer's disease process.

Other causes

Other less common causes of vascular dementia, associated with multiple infarctions but not due to thrombo-embolic phenomena, are as follows:

- Rupture of intracranial aneurysms.
- Collagen vascular disease.
- Meningo-vascular syphilis in which cerebral infarction may be associated with vasculitis or end-arteritis obliterans. It is also possible that an obstructive hydrocephalus secondary to meningeal fibrosis may be a contributory, or even the sole, cause.
- The inherited diseases of hereditary cerebral haemorrhage with amyloidosis, Dutch (HCHWA-D) (**Fig. 3.158**, page 59) and Icelandic types, in which an amyloid protein (β/A4 protein and cystatin C, respectively) is deposited in vessel walls. This may lead to haemorrhagic infarction and dementia in the long term.

Cerebral congophilic angiopathy

Cerebral congophilic angiopathy (CAA) may accompany Alzheimer's disease in a mild form (see page 47, **Figs 3.113–3.118**). Alternatively, a more severe form can exist in the absence of typical Alzheimer's disease. A β/A4 protein, similar to that of the senile plaque amyloid is deposited extracellularly within the adventitia of extracerebral (**Fig. 5.95**) and intraparenchymal (**Fig 5.96**) arteries.

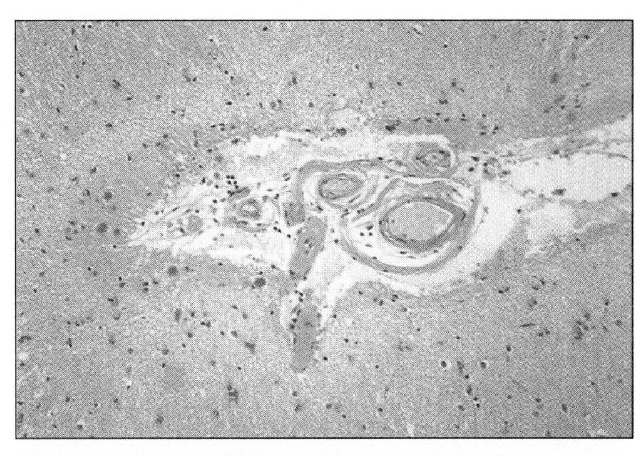

Fig. 5.95 Congophilic amyloid angiopathy. Note the thickened and eosinophilic wall of affected leptomeningeal arteries. *(Haematoxylin–eosin × 100.)*

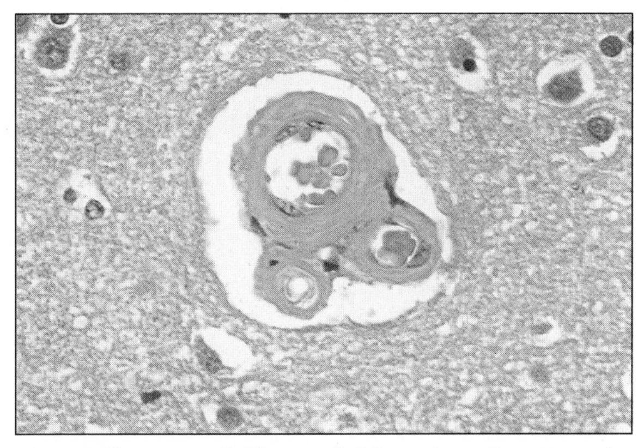

Fig. 5.96 Congophilic amyloid angiopathy. Note the thickened and eosinophilic wall of affected intraparenchymal arteries. *(Haematoxylin–eosin × 400).*

The amyloid, like that of plaque amyloid, can be detected by Congo red staining (**Figs 5.97** and **5.98**) and displays birefringence under cross-polarised light (**Fig. 5.99**).

Massive cerebral haemorrhage is rare in CAA, but the affected vessels, both leptomeningeal (**Figs 5.100–102**) or intraparenchymal (**Figs 5.103–5.105**), are often associated with less severe haemorrhage into the subarachnoid space or brain tissue. Amyloidotic vessels may also thrombose (**Figs 5.106–5.108**) leading to extravasation and subsequent breakdown of red blood cells and haemosiderin deposition in perivascular macrophages. Fibrinoid necrosis may also occur. Damaged areas around either haemorrhagic, thrombosed or stenosed vessels show reactive astrocytosis and a loss of nerve cells (see **Fig 5.108** and **5.109**).

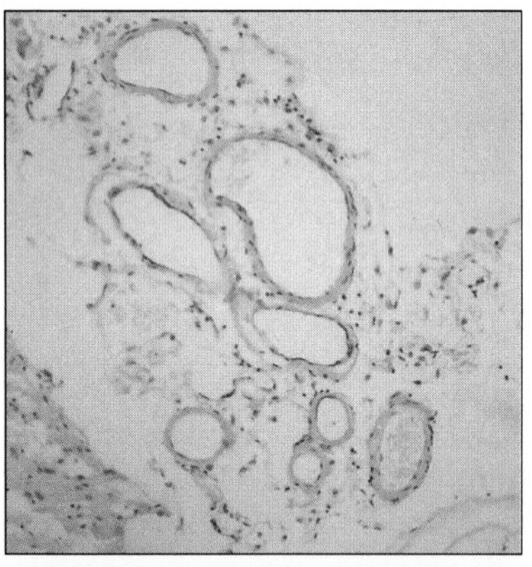

Fig. 5.97 Congo red staining of leptomeningeal arteries. *(Congo red × 100.)*

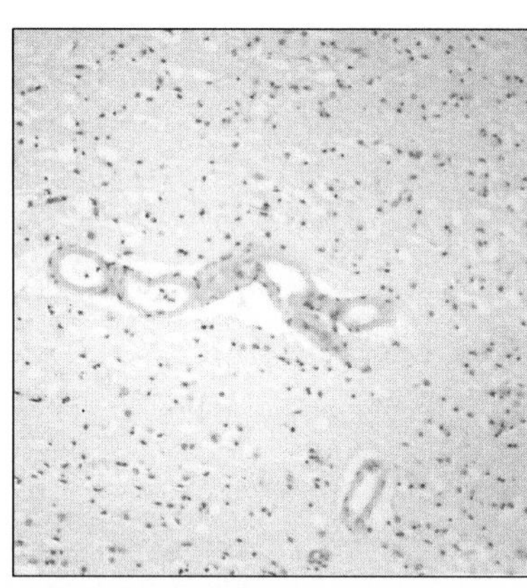

Fig. 5.98 Congo red staining of intracerebral arteries. *(Congo red × 100.)*

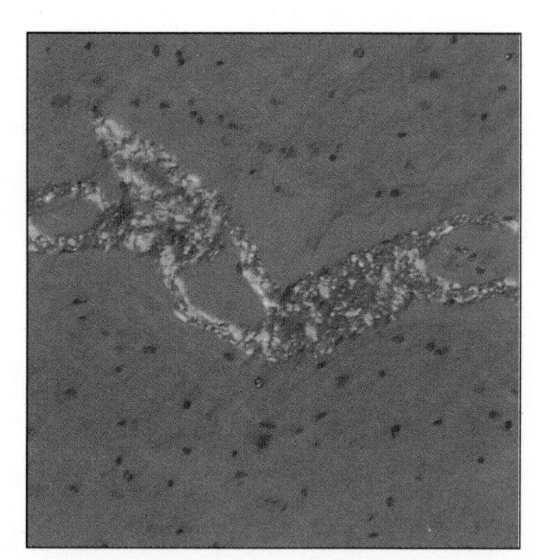

Fig. 5.99 Congophilic vessels showing characteristic yellow-green birefringence after viewing through cross-polarised light. *(Congo red × 200.)*

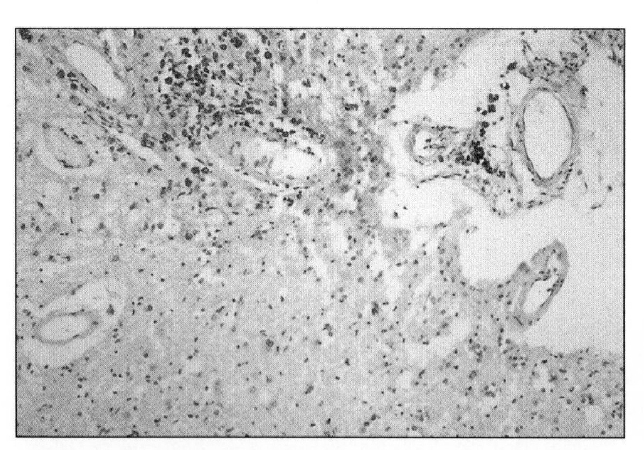

Fig. 5.100 Old microhaemorrhage around congophilic leptomeningeal arteries. *(Congo red × 200.)*

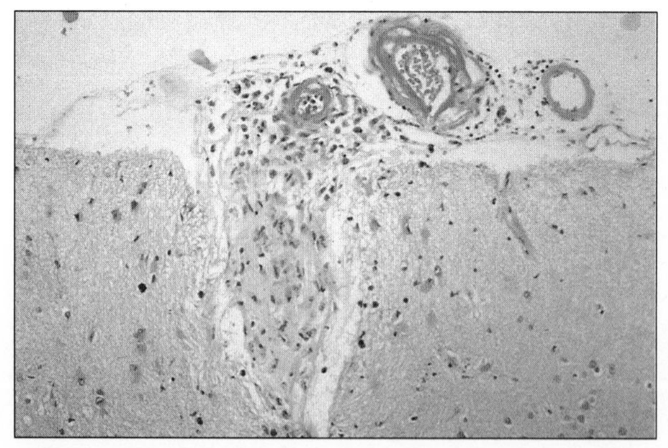

Fig. 5.101 Old microhaemorrhage around congophilic leptomeningeal arteries. *(Haematoxylin–eosin × 200.)*

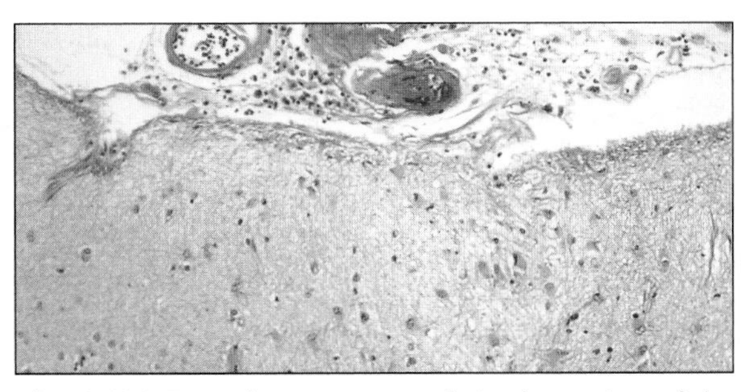

Fig. 5.102 Reactive astrocytosis in the region of the brain affected by haemorrhage from a congophilic artery. *(Phosphotungstic acid–haematoxylin × 200.)*

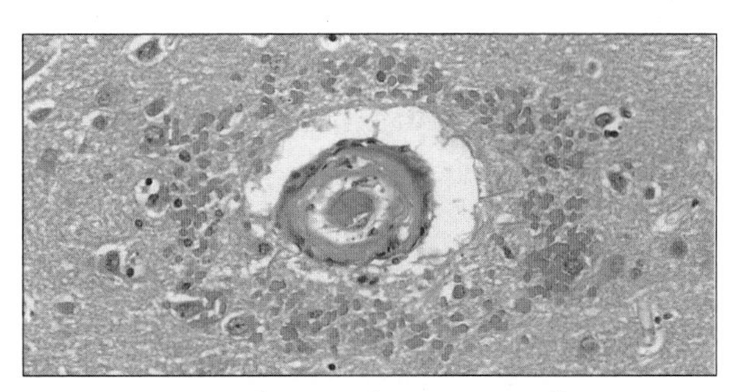

Fig. 5.103 Recent haemorrhage surrounding a congophilic artery. *(Haematoxylin–eosin × 400.)*

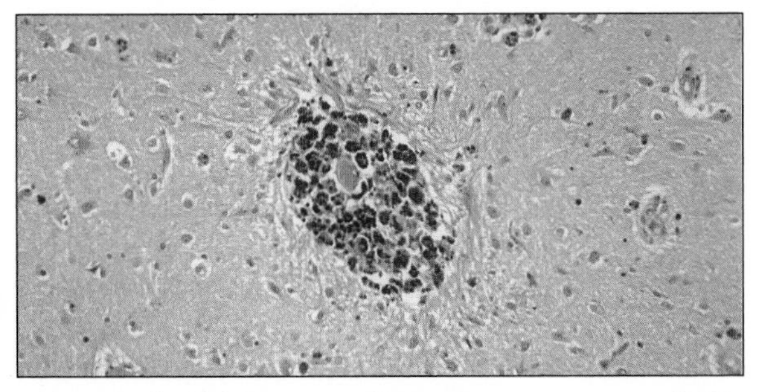

Fig. 5.104 Old haemorrhage from a congophilic artery. *(Haematoxylin–eosin × 400.)*

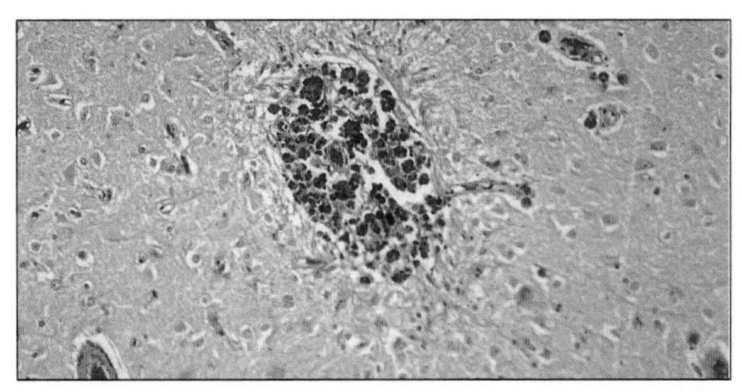

Fig. 5.105 Old haemorrhage with surrounding reactive astrocytosis in the brain tissue. *(Phosphotungstic acid–haematoxylin × 400.)*

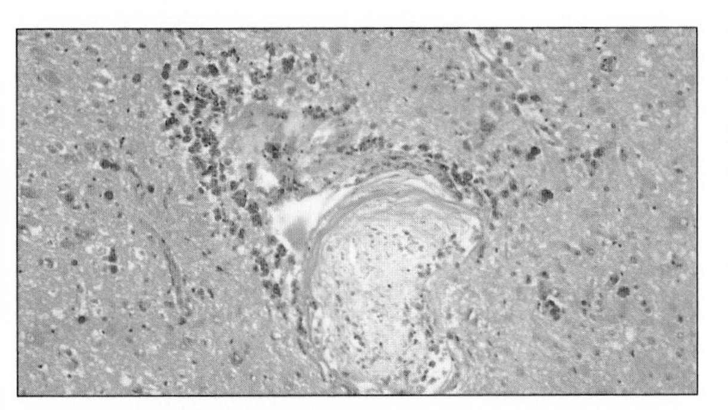

Fig. 5.106 Arterial thrombosis and haemorrhage into surrounding tissue. Note the severe astrocytic reaction. *(Haematoxylin–eosin × 100.)*

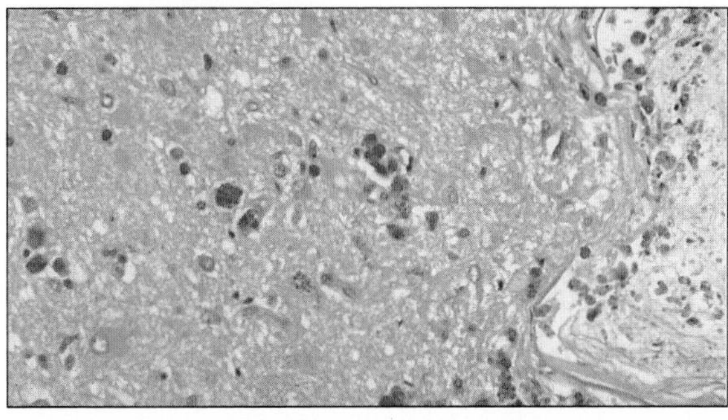

Fig. 5.107 Arterial thrombosis and haemorrhage into surrounding tissue. Higher power view of **Fig. 5.106.** *(× 200.)*

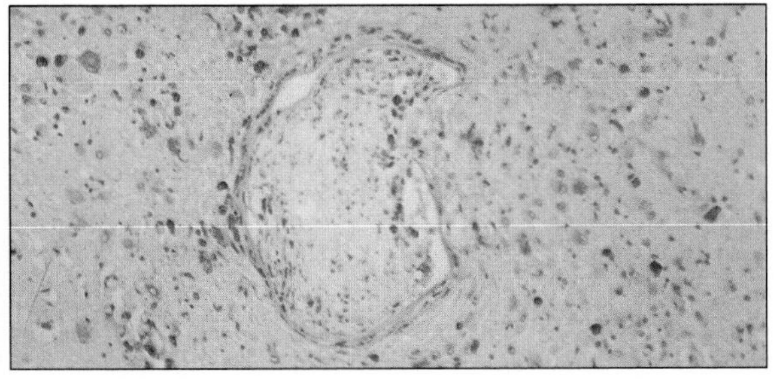

Fig. 5.108 Microhaemorrhage, loss of nerve cells, and reactive astrocytosis around a congophilic artery. *(Nissl stain × 100.)*

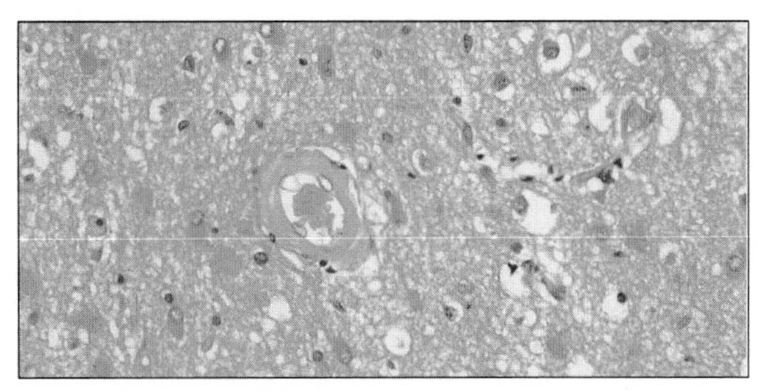

Fig. 5.109 A region of ischaemic infarction with astrocytosis surrounding a congophilic artery. *(Haematoxylin–eosin × 400.)*

A moderate number of, or even many, diffuse and cored parenchymal deposits of β/A4 protein can occur throughout the neocortex (**Figs 5.110** and **5.111**), but they are not found in the cerebellum.

Subpial deposits of amyloid are seen (**Fig. 5.112**) and often the amyloid appears to surround or stream away from affected arteries (**Fig. 5.113**). Although the cored plaques can be detected by haematoxylin–eosin staining (**Fig. 5.114**) they do not contain neurites (see Alzheimer's disease, page 27) (**Fig. 5.115**).

Neurofibrillary tangles are rare or absent in the neocortex, but are occasionally numerous in the hippocampal region, particularly involving layer II stellate cells of the entorhinal cortex (**Figs 5.116** and **5.117**).

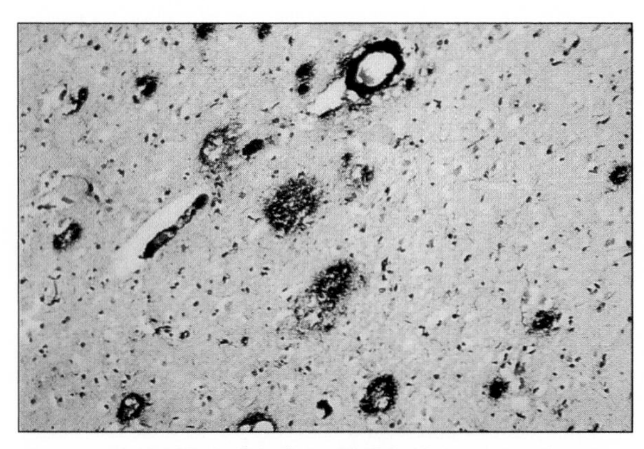

Fig. 5.110 Diffuse β/A4 amyloid plaques in the temporal cortex. *(Methenamine silver × 200.)*

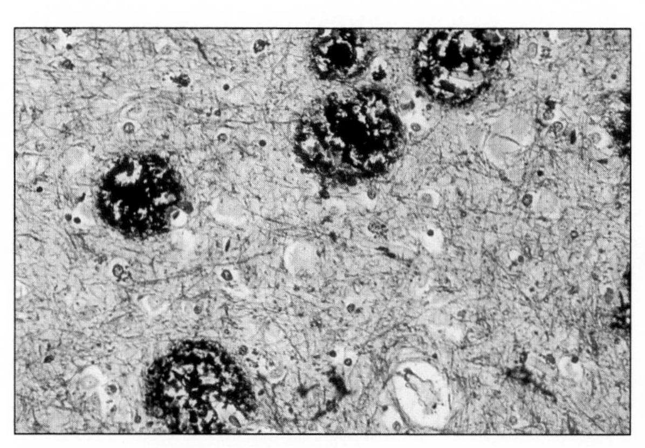

Fig. 5.111 Cored amyloid plaques in the occipital cortex. *(Methenamine silver × 200.)*

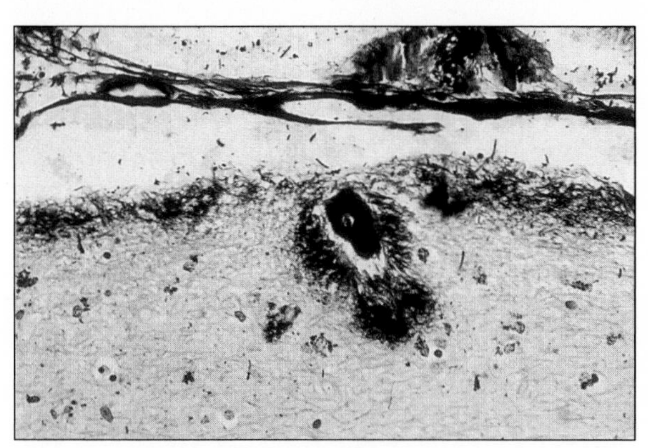

Fig. 5.112 Subpial amyloid deposits in the occipital cortex. *(Methenamine silver × 200.)*

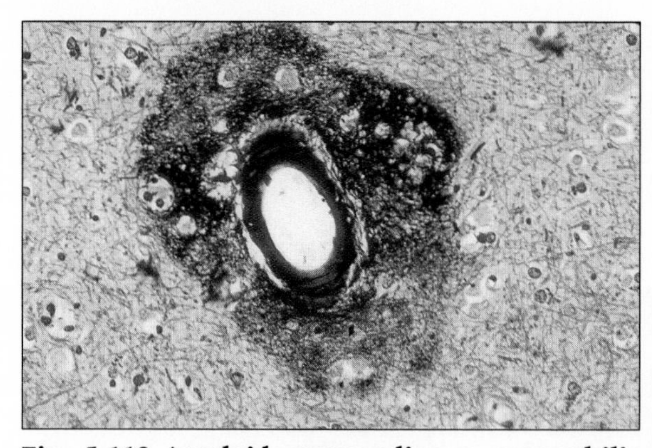

Fig. 5.113 Amyloid surrounding a congophilic artery in the occipital cortex. *(Methenamine silver × 200.)*

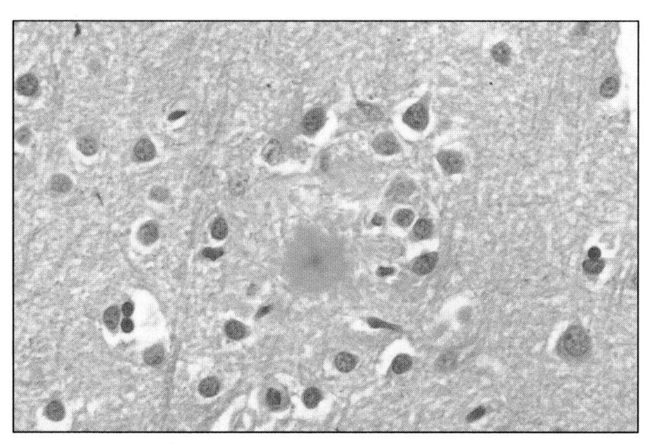

Fig. 5.114 Cored amyloid plaque in the occipital cortex. *(Haematoxylin–eosin × 400.)*

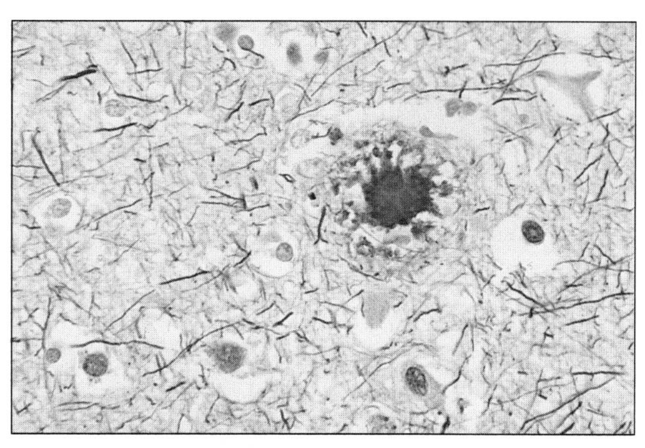

Fig. 5.115 Cored plaques do not contain neurites. *(Palmgren silver stain × 400.)*

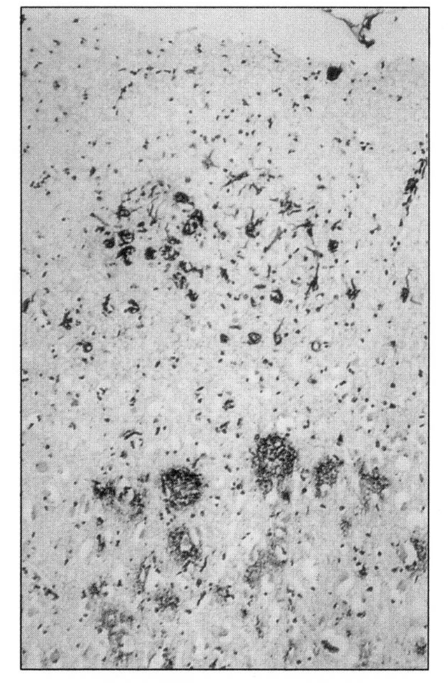

Fig. 5.116 Diffuse amyloid plaques in entorhinal cortex layer III with neurofibrillary tangles in layer II stellate cells. *(Methenamine silver × 100.)*

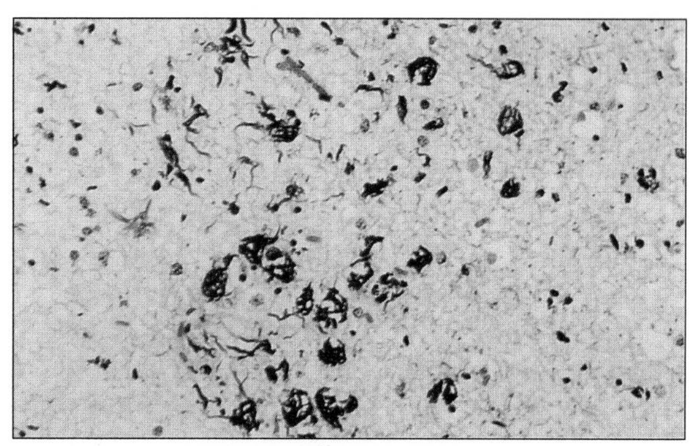

Fig. 5.117 Neurofibrillary tangles in layer II stellate cells of the entorhinal cortex. *(Methenamine silver × 200.)*

Whether CAA is a disorder in its own right or is one that forms part of the Alzheimer's disease spectrum of pathology with an emphasis on vascular changes is not known. However, it is clear that in the inherited condition of HCHWA-D, β/A4 protein deposition in plaques and blood vessel walls relates to a mismetabolism of APP due to mutations on the APP gene at codons 692 and 693 (see **Fig. 3.158**, page 59). This, like Alzheimer's disease itself, may belong to a group of disorders resulting from faulty APP metabolism. Collectively, these conditions could be called β-amyloidopathies.

Epidemiology

It has been estimated that as many as 35% of all elderly demented people may have a significant or sole vascular component to their dementia, but how common the various forms of dementia are relative to each other is uncertain. Tomlinson emphasises that the multi-infarct pattern of pathology is the most common. Binswanger's disease has been less frequently reported, but it may be more common with clinically milder cases, presenting with only minimal cognitive impairment but displaying numerous periventricular lucencies on CT scanning, being less often identified at post mortem.

It is likely that *all* vascular dementia can be placed on a continuum of pathological change, with clinically advanced and pathologically well-defined 'multi-infarct dementia' due to grey and white matter infarctions at one end and established Binswanger's disease at the other end.

The presence of extensive Alzheimer-type changes in the combined vascular-Alzheimer's disease group may pose diagnostic problems clinically, because advanced Alzheimer's disease may mask or blunt the presence of any additional vascular insults. Vascular defects can be detected clinically with confidence only in early stages. As the extent of overt tissue infarction or leukoaraiosis may be less in the combined vascular–Alzheimer group than in the vascular dementia group alone, it is likely that the Alzheimer's disease pathology is largely responsible for producing the clinical impairment, with any vascular lesions contributing less or no further functional deficiency.

Congophilic angiopathy is a common, if not fundamental, part of the Alzheimer's disease pathology, but occurs only infrequently as a disease entity alone. The approximate contribution pathological form of vascular dementia makes the total number of cases as illustrated in **Fig. 5.118**.

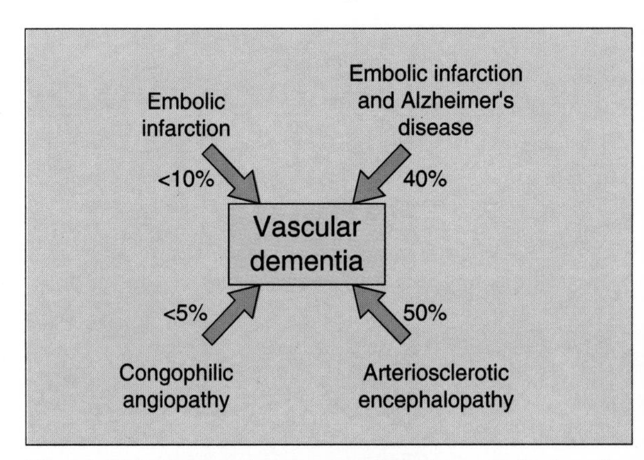

Fig. 5.118 Percentage contribution made by the various causes of vascular dementia.

6. Multifocal encephalopathies

Some neurodegenerative disorders affect both the grey and white matter areas of the cerebral cortex, and multiple subcortical and non-cortical regions. No well-defined 'boundaries' to disease seem to occur. Functional systems are widely damaged and a plethora of neuropsychological and neurological disturbances can be invoked. The prion diseases (spongiform encephalopathies) typically produce this type of brain disorder.

PRION DISEASES

Demographic features

Prion diseases, otherwise known as the transmissible spongiform encephalopathies, are fatal neurodegenerative diseases that affect both humans and animals. The disorders of scrapie in sheep and goats, transmissible mink encephalopathy, chronic wasting disease in deer, bovine and feline spongiform encephalopathies and exotic ungulate encephalopathy all have their human counterparts in kuru, Creutzfeldt–Jakob disease (CJD), fatal familial insomnia (FFI), and Gerstmann–Sträussler– Sheinker syndrome (GSS). The human prion diseases manifest three aspects of degeneration of the CNS:

- Infectiveness
- Inheritance
- Sporadic occurrence

Neurological symptoms and signs
Cortical blindness
Ataxia
Paresis
Myoclonus
Psychological symptoms
Periodic akinetic mutism
Aphasia
Frontal lobe syndrome
Investigations
EEG: abnormal and phasic
SPET: multifocal cerebral deficits

Kuru

Kuru used to be common only among the Foré tribesmen of the eastern highlands of Papua New Guinea. It affected mainly women and young children, and resulted from a ritualistic cannibalism in which the 'contaminated' remains of the deceased were handled or consumed, thereby passing the condition along generations. Such practices are now prohibited and the incidence and prevalence of kuru has fallen dramatically. Only occasional new cases are reported, and are probably due to a prolonged incubation period.

Ataxia is the predominant feature of kuru, the term 'kuru' being a local word meaning 'trembling with cold or fear'. It is possible that the disorder originated from a sporadic case of CJD in this population occurring earlier in the century.

Creutzfeldt–Jakob disease

Creutzfeldt–Jakob disease is a subacute disorder found throughout the world being first described in the 1920s. It occurs in males and females equally, and its onset is usually during the sixth or seventh decade. It occurs worldwide with a prevalence of about 1 death/2 million of the population/year. However, clusters of the disease have been reported in central Europe, Israel, and North and South America, where the prevalence is several times higher.

Clinically, most patients have a multifocal encephalopathy, which usually presents with dementia and myoclonus. Death is common within 3–12 months of onset. The presenting feature of about 10–20% of patients is ataxia, with a dementia occurring later.

The disorder is usually sporadic, but 10–15% of patients have a family history, sometimes showing a clear inheritance as a fully penetrant autosomal dominant condition. Such inherited disease may account for geographical clustering.

Fatal familial insomnia

Fatal familial insomnia is an inherited condition characterised by untreatable insomnia and dysautonomia, and in which there is a selective degeneration of certain regions of the thalamus. It is sometimes known as the 'thalamic type' of CJD.

Gerstmann–Sträussler–Sheinker syndrome

Gerstmann–Sträussler–Sheinker syndrome (GSS) was first described between 1928 and 1936. It is much rarer than CJD with an incidence of 1–10 cases/hundred million population.

The presenting feature is usually ataxia with dementia occurring later. It progresses appreciably more slowly than CJD, with a duration averaging 5 years or more.

The disease usually appears to to be familial, being inherited in an autosomally dominant fashion. Most patients are confined to a relatively small number of well-documented pedigrees.

Pathology of prion diseases

CT scans (**Fig. 6.1**) of patients with CJD show no unusual changes, except sometimes a mild ventricular enlargement. The pattern of brain metabolism is likewise undistinctive when viewed by SPET imaging (**Fig. 6.2**), showing multiple patchy reductions in tracer uptake in cortical regions.

Age of onset
Usually 40–65 years

Sex incidence
Males and females affected equally

Duration
Subacute; usually up to 3 years, often less than 1 year. Some forms over 5 years

Gross features
Brain appears normal in most cases, though may show generalized atrophy in longer durations

Histopathology
- Spongiform degeneration of cerebral cortex. Loss of nerve cells. Severe astrocytosis. All areas of cortex affected; all laminae involved. Occipital cortex most frequently and severely affected
- Caudate nucleus and putamen usually affected
- Cerebellum and thalamus often involved
- Deposits of prion protein, as plaques, in the cerebellum and cerebral cortex in 15% of patients

Genetics
- Mainly sporadic
- 15% of patients inherit the disorder either due to a mutation or insertion in the prion gene present on the short arm of chromosome 20
- Can be transmitted through ingestion or inoculation of affected tissues

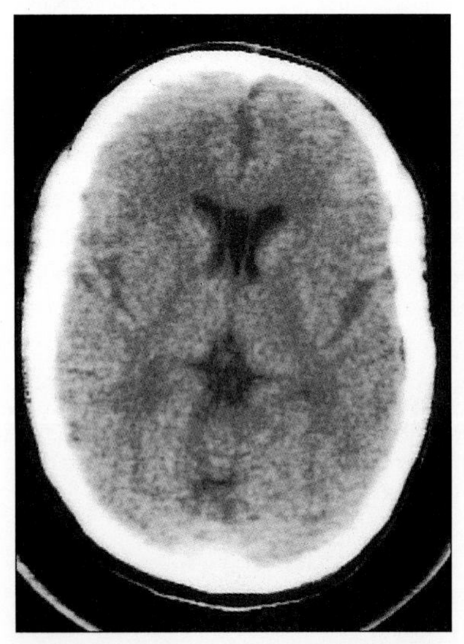

Fig. 6.1 Creutzfeldt–Jakob disease. This CT scan of the brain of a 40-year-old man with Creutzfeldt–Jakob disease is normal.

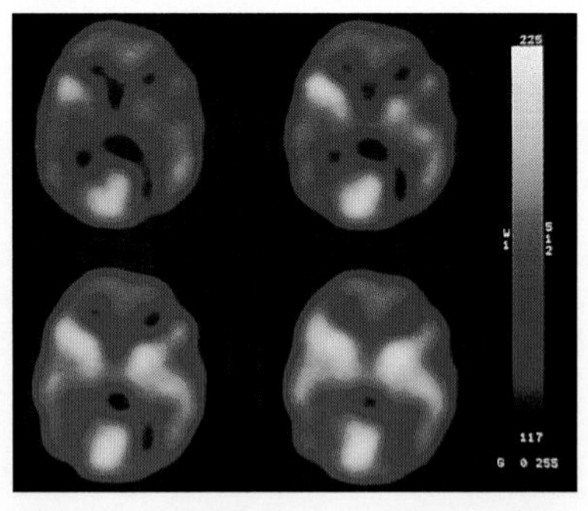

Fig. 6.2 Multiple, patchy reductions in brain metabolism. SPET imaging of a 51-year-old man.

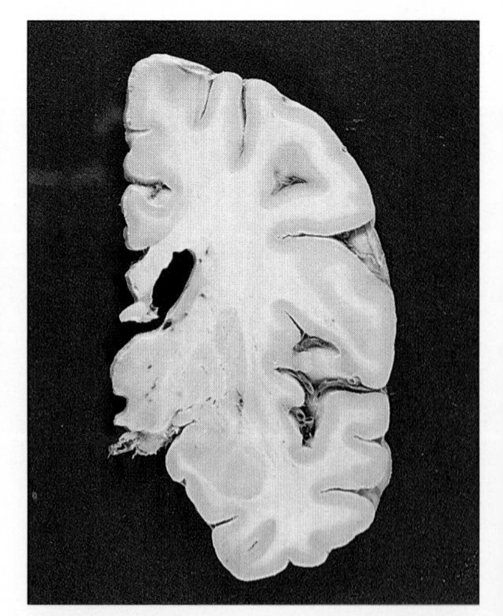

Fig. 6.3 No specific abnormality. Coronal slice of the brain of a 60-year-old woman, showing a lack of specific abnormality. The lateral ventricle is slightly enlarged.

At autopsy, if survival has been short, brain weight is usually normal and demonstrates little or no macroscopic change, though some mild ventricular enlargement may be seen (**Fig. 6.3**). If survival has been longer, and especially in cases GSS, a considerable amount of atrophy may be evident, with the brain weight sometimes being reduced to less than 1000 g.

Histopathological changes

As well as showing overlapping clinical symptomatology, the various prion disorders share many aspects of neuropathology. Typically, the brain shows the classic histopathological triad of spongiform change, neuronal loss and gliosis. Within this constellation of change there is extensive individual patient variation, possibly relating to the aetiology or the duration of illness.

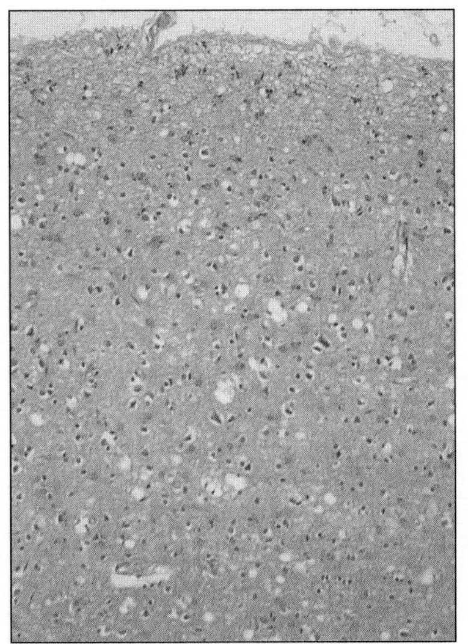

Fig. 6.4 Spongiform degeneration with reactive astrocytosis in the temporal cortex. *(Haematoxylin–eosin × 100.)*

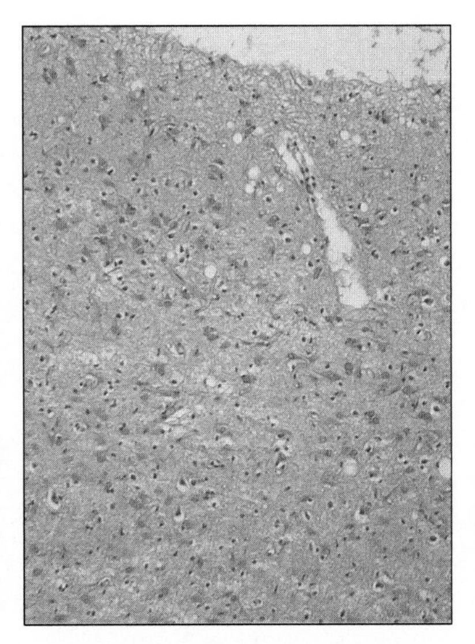

Fig. 6.5 Spongiform degeneration with reactive astrocytosis in the occipital cortex. *(Haematoxylin–eosin × 100.)*

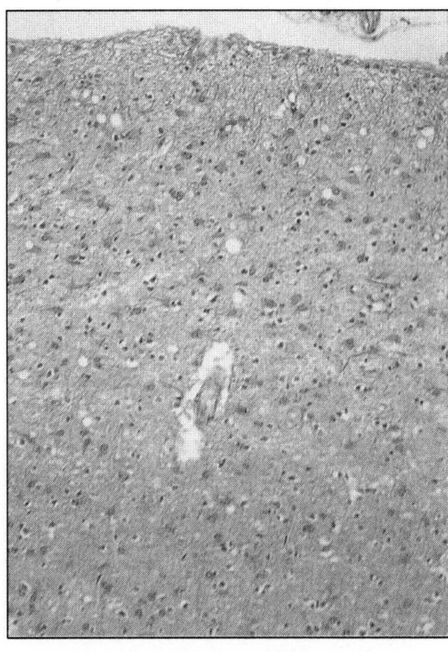

Fig. 6.6 Reactive astrocytosis in the temporal cortex. *(Phosphotungstic acid–haematoxylin × 100.)*

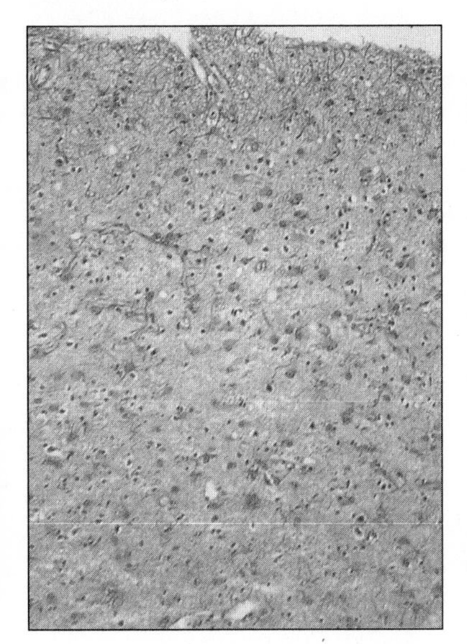

Fig. 6.7 Reactive astrocytosis in the occipital cortex. *(Phosphotungstic acid–haematoxylin × 100.)*

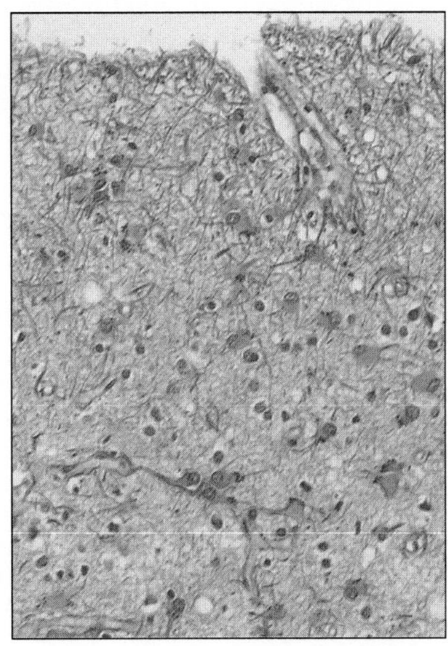

Fig. 6.8 Reactive astrocytosis in the occipital cortex. *(Phosphotungstic acid–haematoxylin × 200.)*

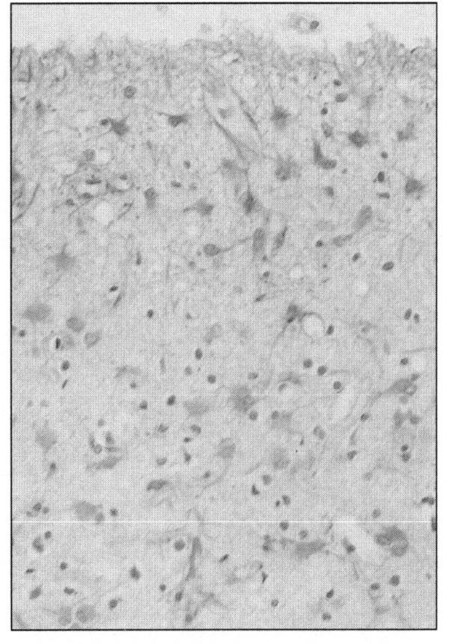

Fig. 6.9 Reactive astrocytosis in the occipital cortex. As **Fig. 6.8,** but anti-GFAP. *(× 200.)*

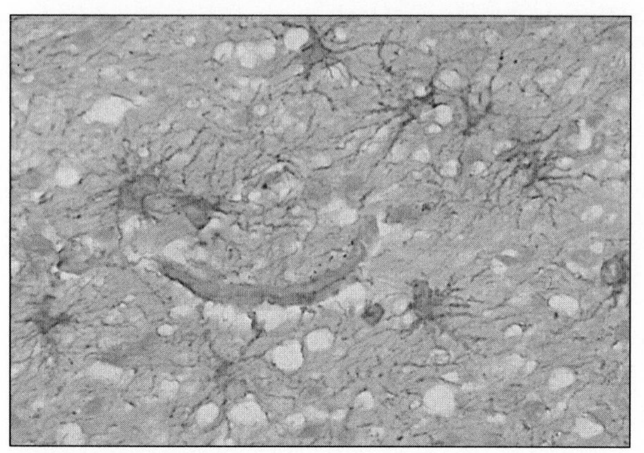

Fig. 6.10 Reactive astrocytosis within the white matter of the cerebral cortex. *(Anti-GFAP counterstained with periodic acid–Schiff × 200.)*

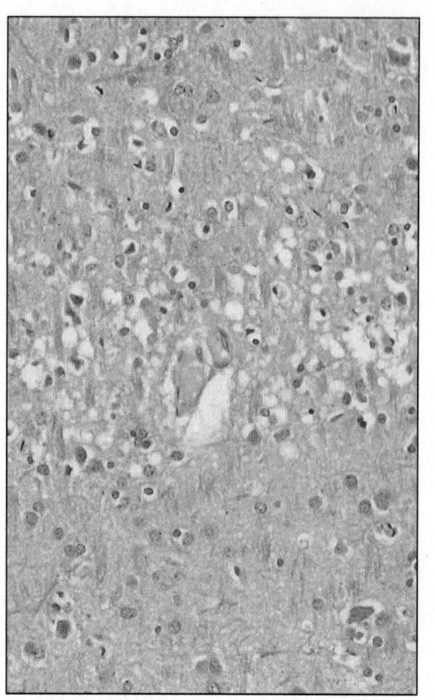

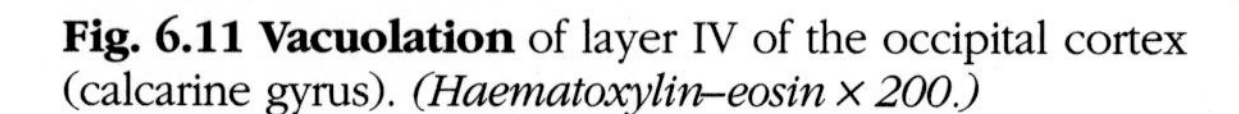

Fig. 6.11 Vacuolation of layer IV of the occipital cortex (calcarine gyrus). *(Haematoxylin–eosin × 200.)*

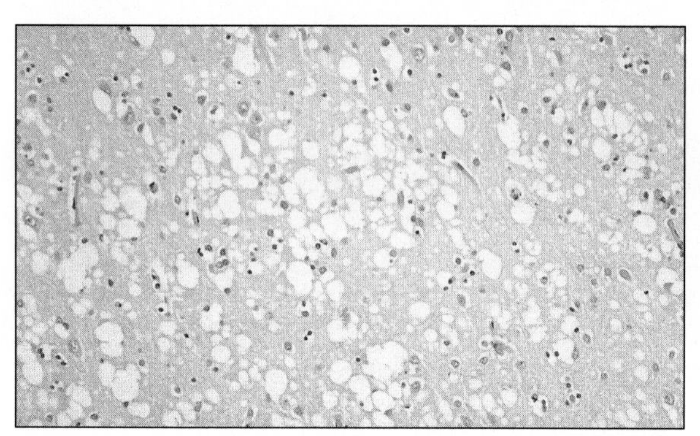

Fig. 6.12 Severe spongiform degeneration without gliosis in the cerebral cortex. *(Haematoxylin–eosin × 200.)*

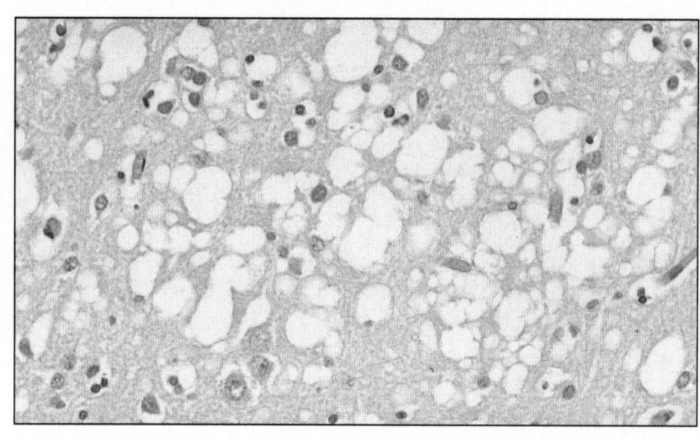

Fig. 6.13 Severe spongiform degeneration without gliosis in the cerebral cortex. As **Fig. 6.12**, but higher power view. *(× 400.)*

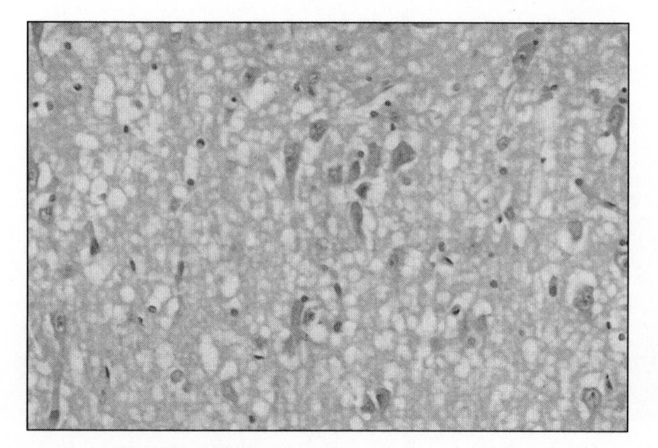

Fig. 6.14 Severe spongiform degeneration in the subiculum of the hippocampus. *(Haematoxylin–eosin × 200.)*

As the name implies, the brain typically, but not always, shows a spongiform type of degeneration that can affect the grey matter of the cerebral cortex (**Figs 6.4–6.13**), hippocampus (**Fig. 6.14**), and amygdala, basal ganglia (**Fig. 6.15**) and thalamus (**Figs 6.16** and **6.17**), and sometimes, though usually to a much lesser extent, the cerebellar cortex (**Fig. 6.18**). Although not apparent to the naked eye, this spongy change is comprised microscopically of a multitude of small, rounded or oval, vacuoles within the neuropil of the grey matter. Each vacuole measures 1–2 micrometres in diameter, and up to more than 50 micrometres where they have coalesced (see **Figs 6.12** and **6.13**). Any area of cortex, and all layers within the cortex, can be affected, usually equivalently, though often there is a preference for the occipital lobe, and sometimes particularly layer IV of this region (see **Fig. 6.11**).

Electron microscopy reveals that these vacuoles, to be membrane bound and to occur *within* the processes of neurones and glia. This change is quite distinct from the spongy-type that typically occurs in the fronto-temporal dementias (page 79), and sometimes in Alzheimer's disease or Huntington's disease (page 106), where the tissue cavitation is due to an enlarged *extracellular* space caused by neuronal atrophy and loss.

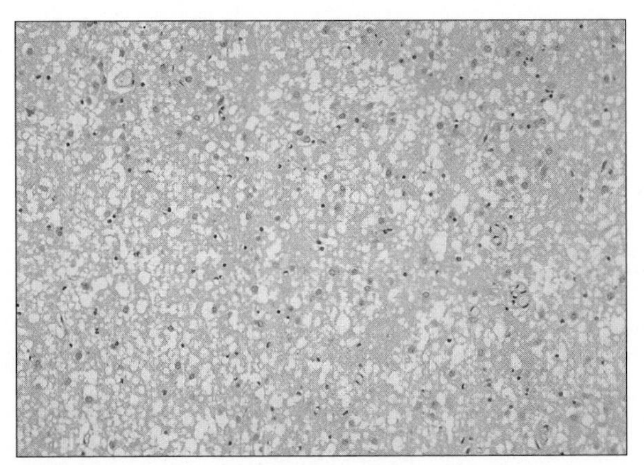

Fig. 6.15 Severe spongiform degeneration in the putamen. *(Haematoxylin–eosin × 100.)*

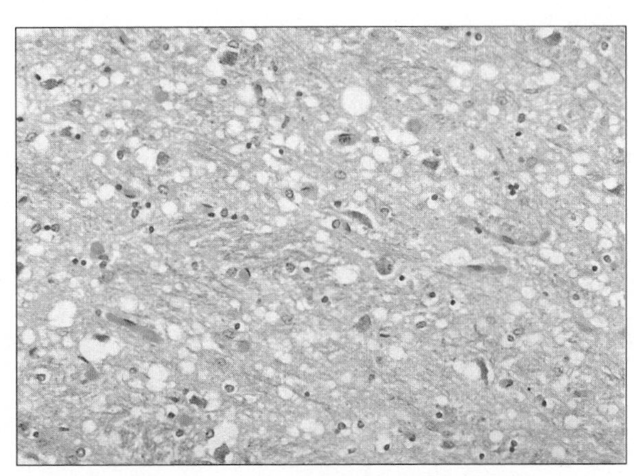

Fig. 6.16 Moderate spongiform degeneration in the medial thalamus. *(Haematoxylin–eosin × 100.)*

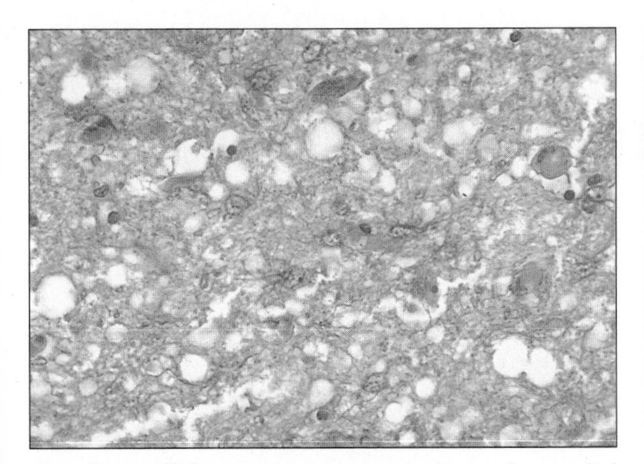

Fig. 6.17 Mild reactive astrocytosis in the medial thalamus. *(Haematoxylin–eosin × 200.)*

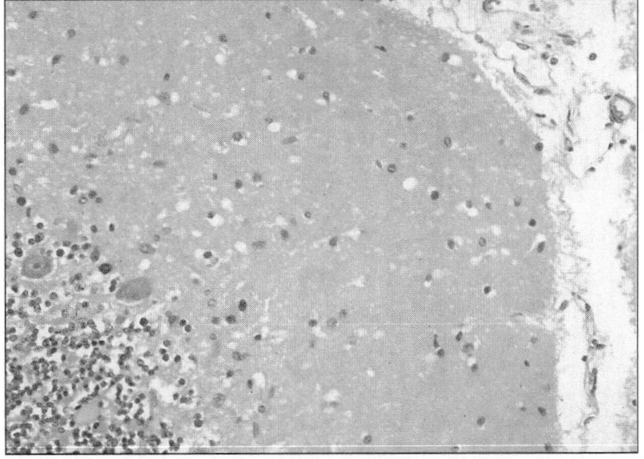

Fig. 6.18 Mild spongiform degeneration within the molecular layer of the cerebellum. *(Haematoxylin–eosin × 100.)*

Usually there is a variable loss of nerve cells in CJD, ranging from severe (see **Figs 6.4, 6.7, 6.15** and **6.17**) to slight and difficult to detect (see **Figs 6.32** and **6.35**). This affects the cerebral cortex, (se **Figs 6.4** and **6.7**) striatum (see **Fig. 6.15**), and thalamus (see **Fig. 6.17**). Surviving cells often demonstrate cytoplasmic vacuolation (**Fig. 6.19**) or swelling (**Fig. 6.20**) ('ballooning') and stain strongly with antibodies against the protein αB crystallin (**Fig. 6.21**) (see page 166).

There may be an astrocytic proliferation, particularly if the disease has been long-standing (see **Figs 6.5, 6.7–6.10, 6.22** and **6.23**), but this is not always so (see **Figs 6.12, 6.13** and **6.24**), especially if there is a severe spongiform change. Astrocytosis can occur within both the grey and white matter of the

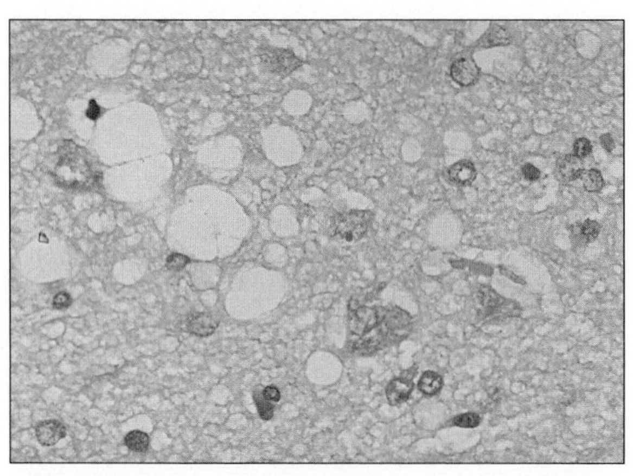

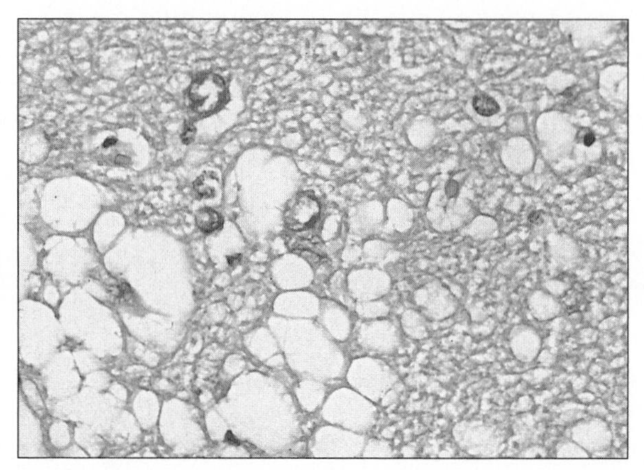

Figs 6.19 and 6.20 Vacuolation and swelling of nerve cells in the temporal cortex. *(Haematoxylin–eosin × 400.)*

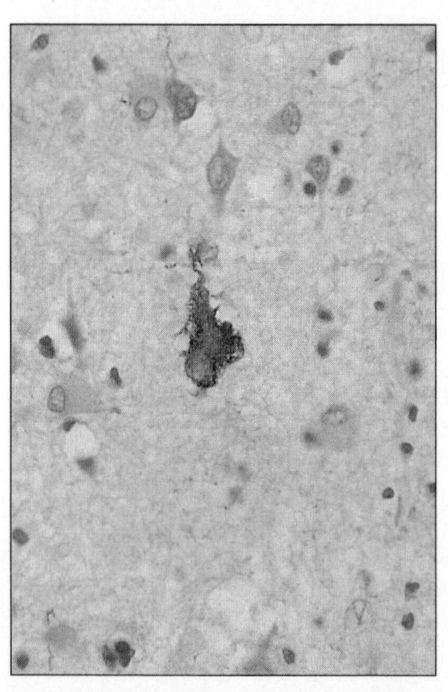

Fig. 6.21 Swollen nerve cells are reactive to αB crystallin antigen. *(Anti-αB crystallin × 400.)*

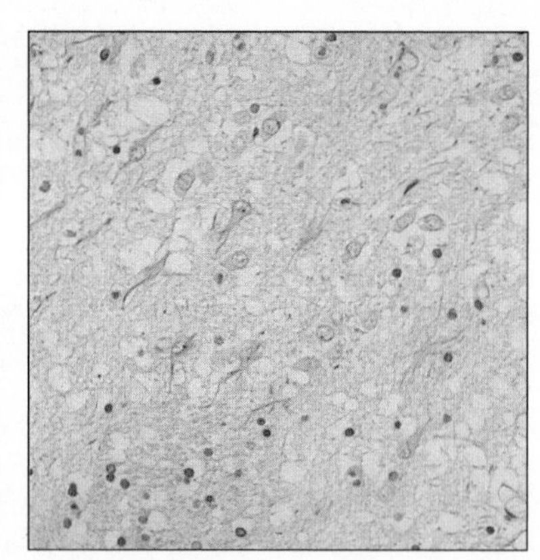

Fig. 6.22 Astrocytosis in the putamen. *(Phosphotungstic acid–haematoxylin × 200.)*

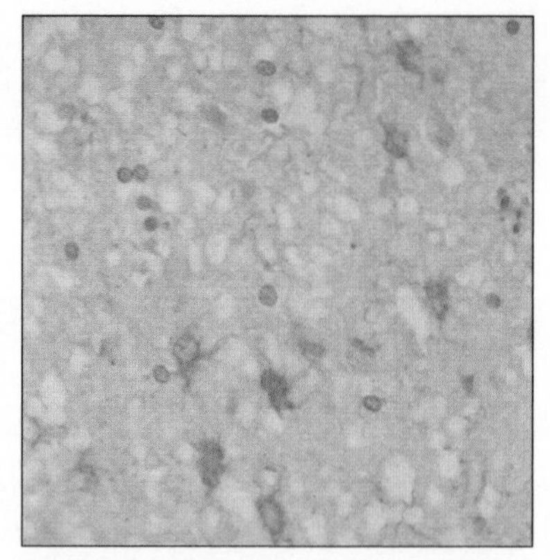

Fig. 6.23 Astrocytosis in the putamen. As **Fig. 6.22**, but anti-GFAP. *(× 400.)*

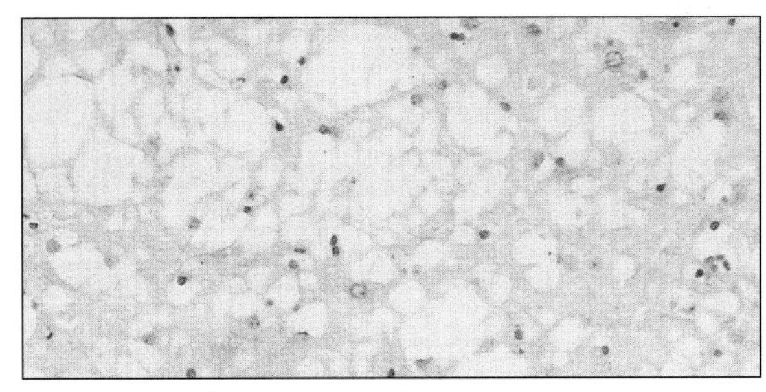

Fig. 6.24 Lack of reactive astrocytosis in a cerebral cortex displaying severe spongiform change. *(Phosphotungstic acid–haematoxylin × 400.)*

cerebral cortex (see **Figs 6.5, 6.6** and **6.8–6.10**), in the striatum (**Figs 6.22** and **6.23**), and in the long fibre tracts of the internal capsule and brain stem.

Within the cerebellum, there may be a partial to severe loss of Purkinje cells, with many of those surviving showing axonal torpedoes (**Figs 6.25** and **6.26**). Granule cells may also be lost, particularly if Purkinje cell loss is severe (see **Fig. 6.28**).

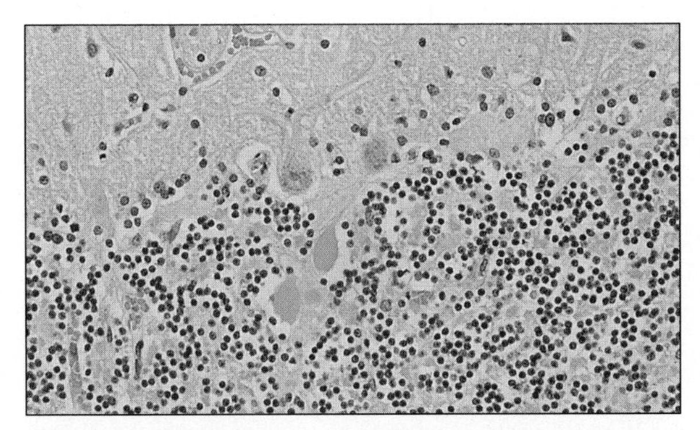

Fig. 6.25 Partial loss of Purkinje cells with axonal torpedoes present on surviving cells. *(Haematoxylin–eosin × 200.)*

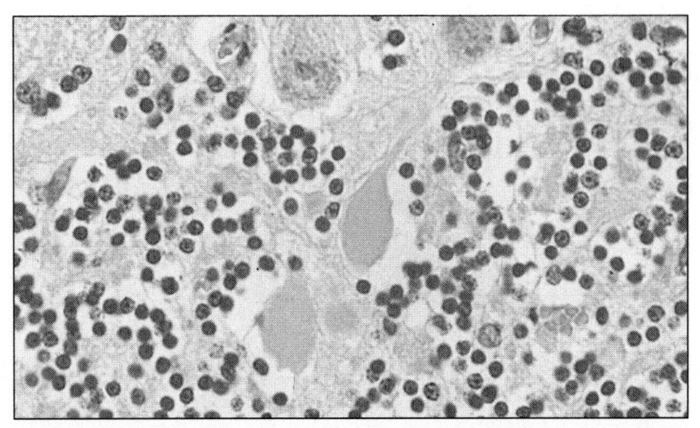

Fig. 6.26 Partial loss of Purkinje cells with axonal torpedoes present on surviving cells. *(Haematoxylin–eosin × 400.)*

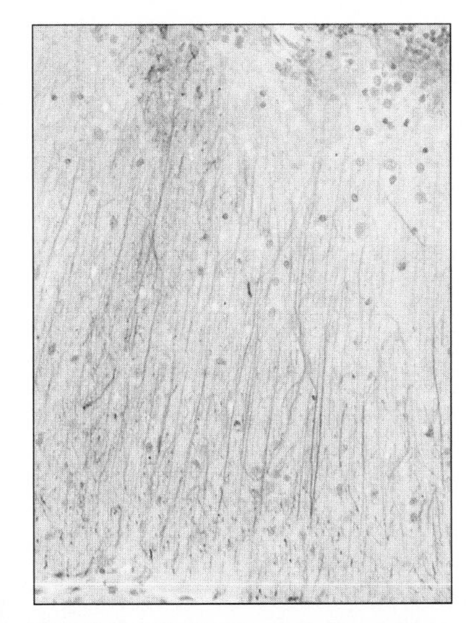

Fig. 6.27 Moderate reactive astrocytosis within the molecular layer of the cerebellum due to proliferation of the Bergmann glia. *(Anti-GFAP × 200.)*

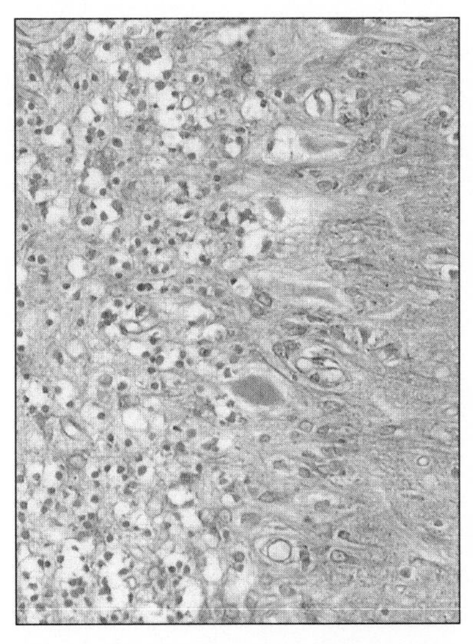

Fig. 6.28 Severe loss of granule cells in a disease in which many Purkinje cells are lost and where there is a marked reactive astrocytosis. *(Anti-GFAP counterstained with periodic acid–Schiff × 400.)*

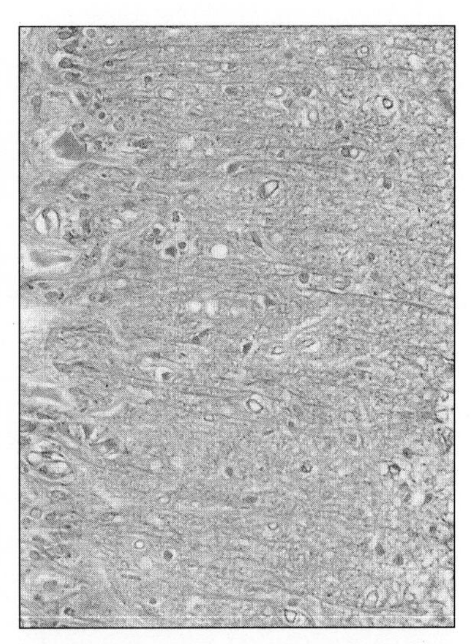

Fig. 6.29 Severe astrocytosis within the molecular layer of the cerebellum in a disease in which many Purkinje cells are lost. *(Anti-GFAP counterstained with periodic acid–Schiff × 400.)*

The Bergmann glia of the Purkinje cell layer proliferates (**Figs 6.27–6.29**), with the number of radiating fibrils increasing, again especially if Purkinje cell loss is severe (see **Figs 6.28** and **6.29**).

The cerebellar white matter shows gliosis (**Fig. 6.30**). A variable microglial reaction is common in both the cerebral and cerebellar cortex, particularly if there is extensive neuronal loss (**Fig. 6.31**).

The contribution any one of these three types of change (i.e. spongiform change, neuronal loss, and gliosis) makes to the overall pathology appears to be extremely variable, and may be aetiologically related or duration-dependent. Longer-standing disease is usually associated with a greater degree of change. In some cases of short-duration disease, tissue vacuolation is slight or absent, even in the cerebral (**Fig. 6.32**) and cerebellar (see **Fig. 6.38**) cortex or striatum (see **Fig. 6.35**), but a mild gliosis in the grey (**Fig. 6.33**) and white matter (**Fig. 6.34**) of the cerebral cortex and in the grey matter of the cerebellar cortex (see **Figs 6.38** and **6.39**) and striatum (**Figs 6.36** and **6.37**) can still be detected. Usually, there appears to be an inverse relationship between spongiform change and astrocytosis (com-

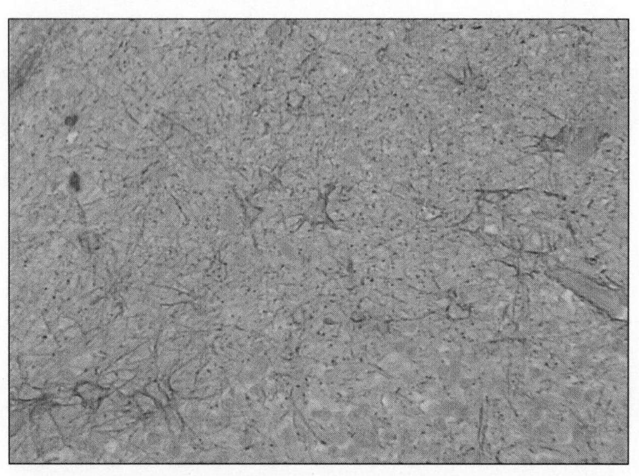

Fig. 6.30 Severe reactive astrocytosis in the white matter of the cerebellum. *(Anti-GFAP counterstained with periodic acid–Schiff × 400.)*

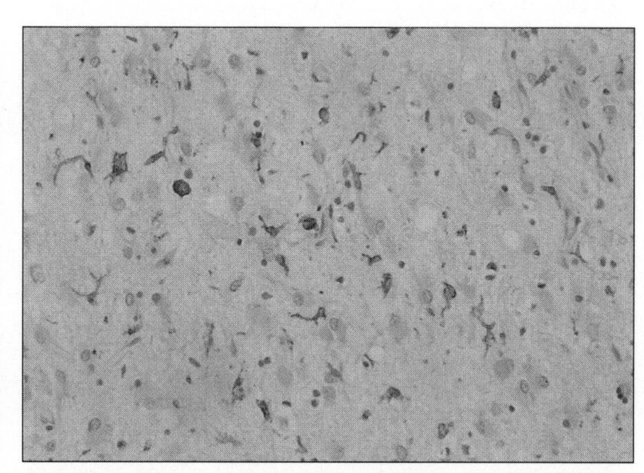

Fig. 6.31 Many activated microglial cells in an area of occipital cortex where neuronal loss is high. *(Anti-ferritin × 400.)*

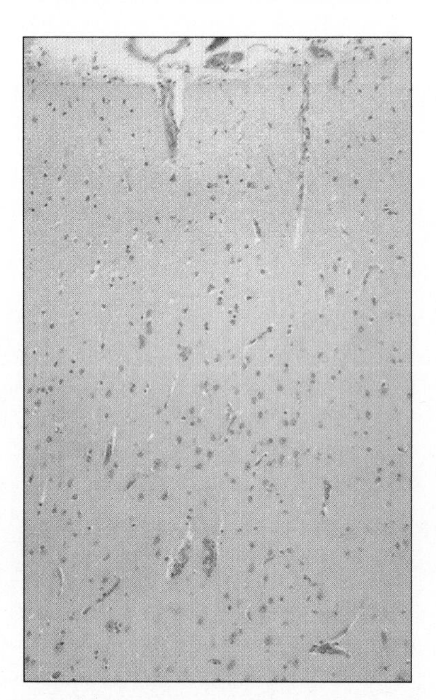

Fig. 6.32 (left) Lack of vacuolation in the cerebral cortex of a 51-year-old man. *(Haematoxylin–eosin × 200.)*

Fig. 6.33 (right) Reactive astrocytosis in the cortex of the patient featured in **Fig. 6.32**. *(Anti-GFAP × 200.)*

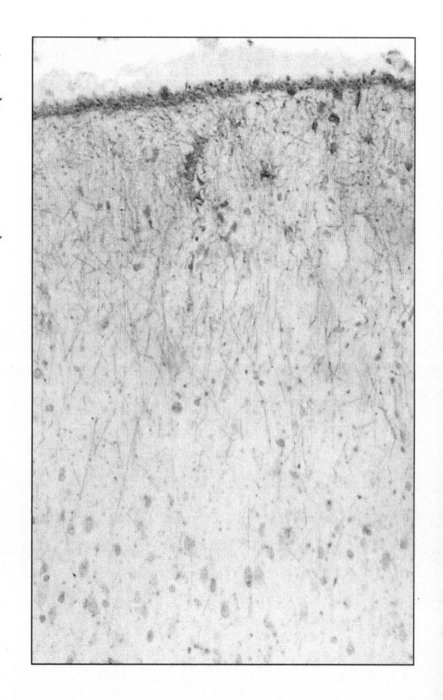

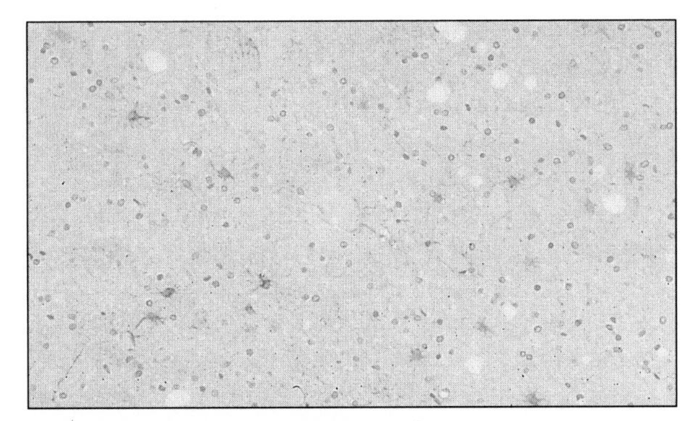

Fig. 6.34 Reactive astrocytosis in the white matter of the cerebral cortex of the patient featured in **Figs 6.32** and **6.33**. *(Anti-GFAP × 200.)*

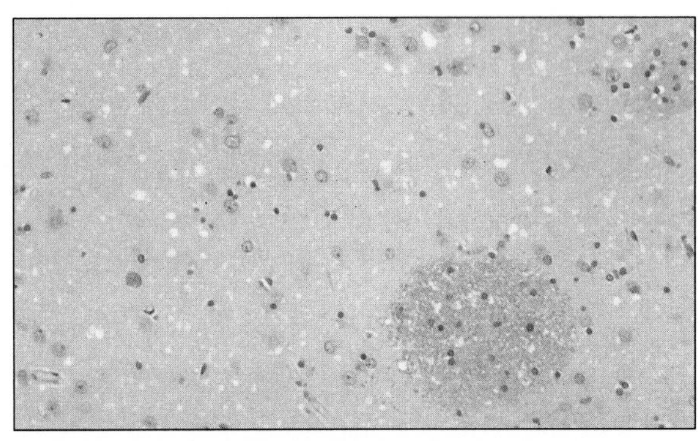

Fig. 6.35 Lack of vacuolation of the putamen of the patient featured in **Figs 6.32–6.34**. *(Haematoxylin–eosin × 200.)*

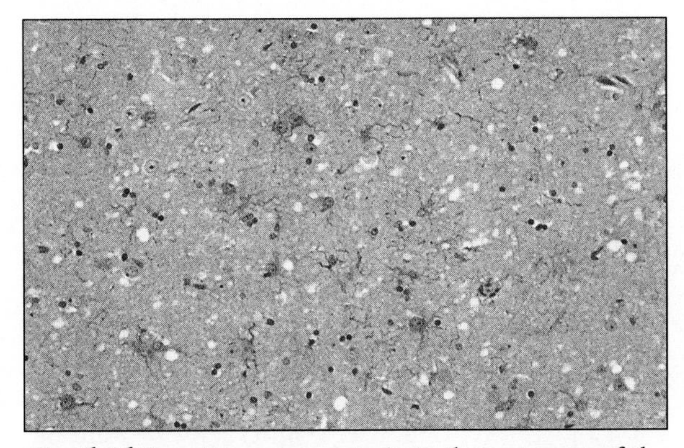

Fig. 6.36 Reactive astrocytosis in the putamen of the patient featured in **Figs 6.32–6.35**. *(Phosphotungstic acid–haematoxylin × 200.)*

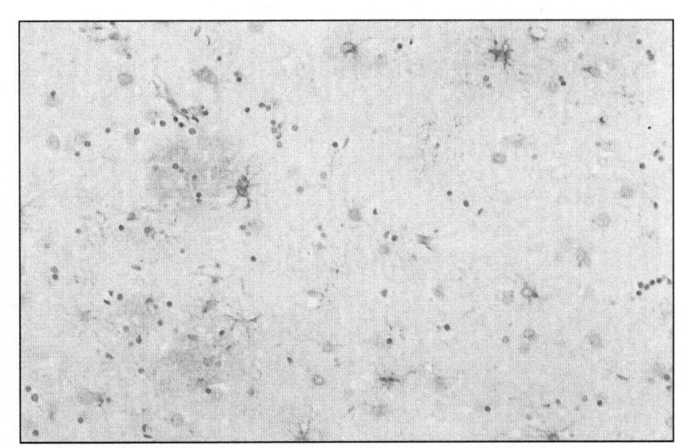

Fig. 6.37 Reactive astrocytosis in the putamen of the patient featured in **Figs 6.32–6.36**. As **Fig. 6.36**, but anti-GFAP. *(× 200.)*

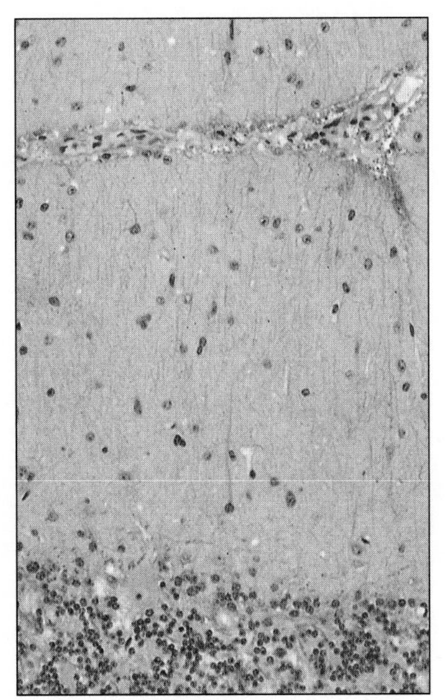

Fig. 6.38 (left) Lack of vacuolation in the molecular layer of the cerebellum of the patient featured in **Figs 6.32–6.37**.

Fig. 6.39 (right) Mild reactive astrocytosis in the molecular layer of the cerebellum of the patient featured in **Figs 6.32–6.38**.

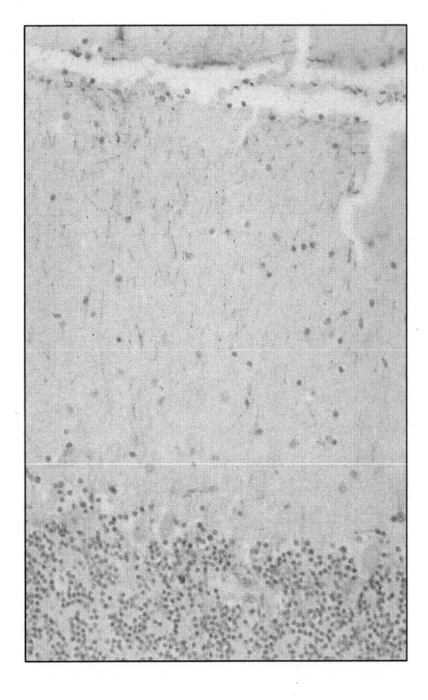

pare with **Figs 6.4–6.13** and **6.24**), possibly due to tissue 'collapse' when nerve cell loss is extreme and a heavy glial reaction prevails.

Amyloid deposition in prion diseases

In some patients (about 15% of those with CJD, but the majority with GSS), there are extracellular deposits of amyloid protein. These can be of two distinct types:

- Some deposits are recognised only by antibodies to β/A4 protein and appear as 'diffuse plaques' (**Fig. 6.40**). These are usually present in the more elderly patients and are probably age-related rather than indicative of a coincidental Alzheimer's disease; tangles are not usually present, except occasionally in the hippocampus. A congophilic angiopathy can also be found in some of these patients, but again the protein deposited is that of β/A4 protein (**Fig. 6.41**) and likely to be age-related.
- Other large, sometimes stellate or multicentric, deposits of the kind typically seen in kuru occur in some patients with CJD. These are particularly prevalent in the cerebellum, mostly within Purkinje (**Figs 6.42, 6.44, 6.48** and **6.49**) and granule cell (**Figs 6.43, 6.45, 6.48, 6.49** and **6.50**) layers, but are also common in the molecular layer (see **Figs 6.46** and **6.51**), and sometimes in the white matter (see **Fig. 6.47**). They are detectable with routine haematoxylin–eosin staining (see **Figs 6.42** and **6.43**), but stain particularly well with the periodic acid–Schiff method (**Figs 6.44–6.47**). These kinds

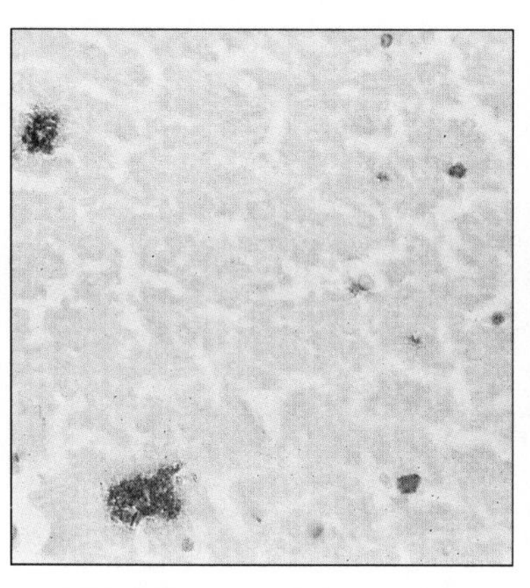

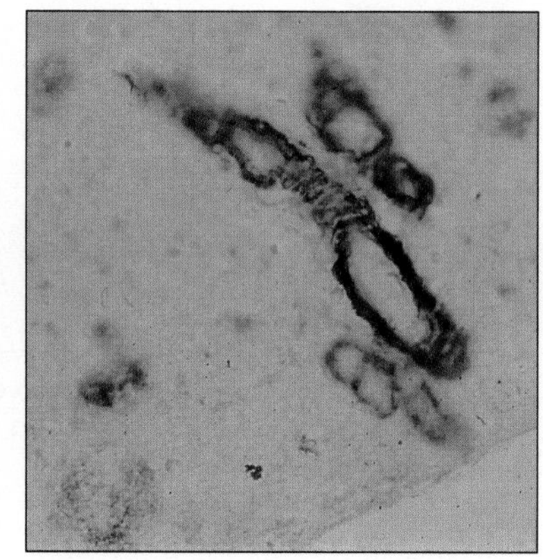

Fig. 6.40 (left) Deposition of amyloid proteins in the cortex of an elderly person with CJD. β/A4 protein is shown blue-green, prion protein deposits are brown. *(Double immunostaining anti-β/A4 and anti-prion protein × 100.)* (Courtesy of Dr G. W. Roberts.)

Fig. 6.41 (right) β/A4 protein deposition in the walls of blood vessels in an elderly person with CJD. *(Anti-β/A4 × 200.)* (Courtesy of Dr G. W. Roberts.)

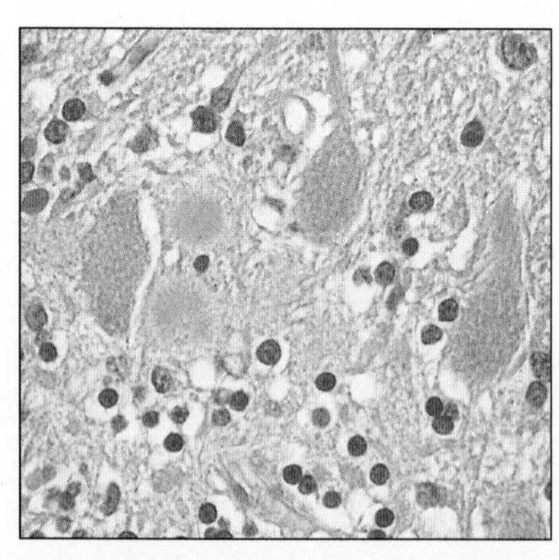

Fig. 6.42 Amyloid ('kuru') plaques in the Purkinje cell layer of the cerebellum. Note the 'stellate' appearance to the deposits. This 60-year-old woman had a methionine→valine polymorphism at codon 129 of the prion protein gene. *(Haematoxylin–eosin × 400.)*

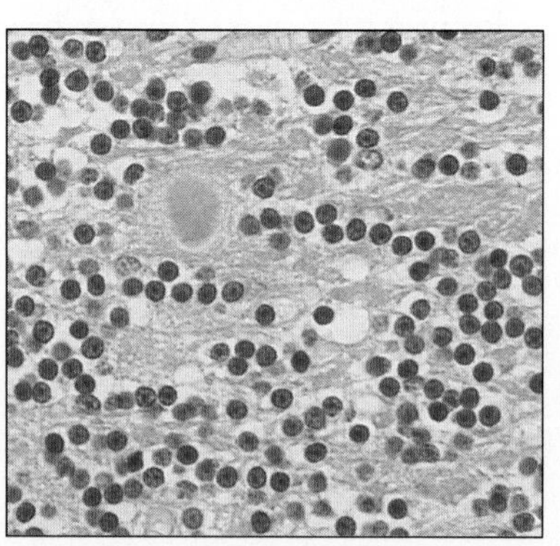

Fig. 6.43 Amyloid plaque in the granule cell layer of the cerebellum of the patient featured in **Fig.6.42.** *(Haematoxylin–eosin × 400.)*

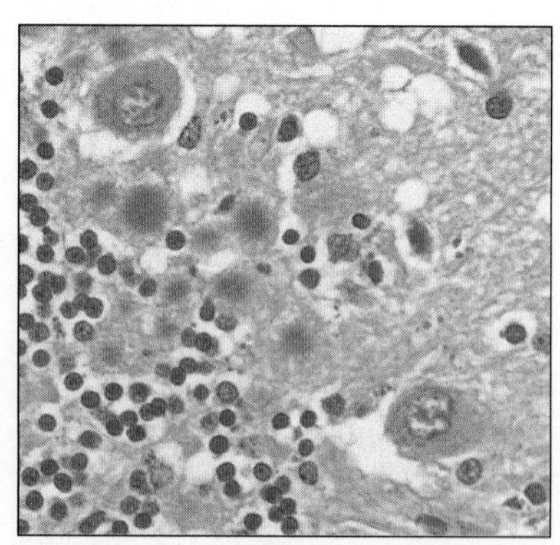

Fig. 6.44 Amyloid plaque in the Purkinje cell layer of the cerebellum. *(Periodic acid–Schiff × 400.)*

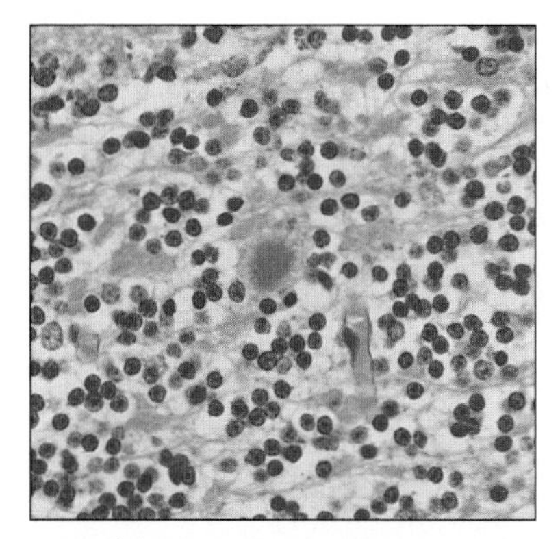

Fig. 6.45 Amyloid plaque in the granule cell layer of the cerebellum. *(Periodic acid–Schiff × 400.)*

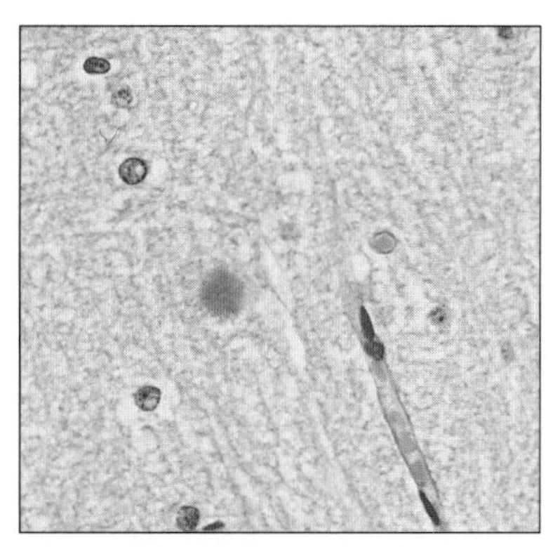

Fig. 6.46 Amyloid plaque in the molecular layer of the cerebellum. *(Periodic acid–Schiff × 400.)*

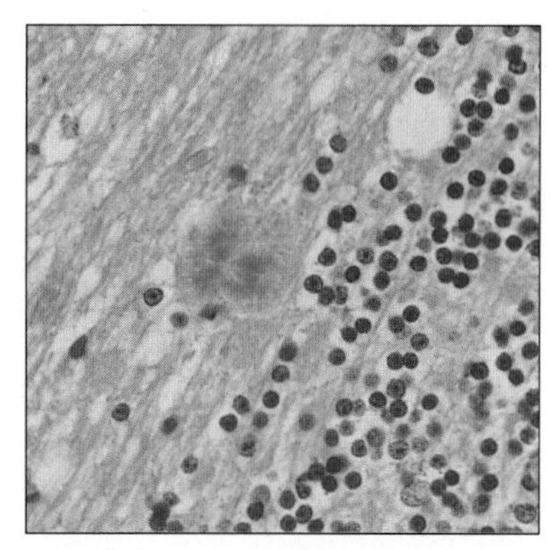

Fig. 6.47 Amyloid plaque in the white matter of the cerebellum. *(Periodic acid–Schiff × 400.)*

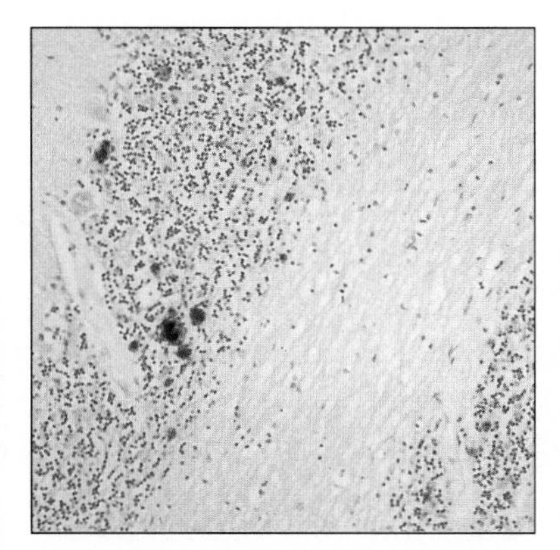

Fig. 6.48 Amyloid plaques in the cerebellum are immunoreactive with antibodies against prion-protein antigen. *(Anti-prion protein × 100.)*

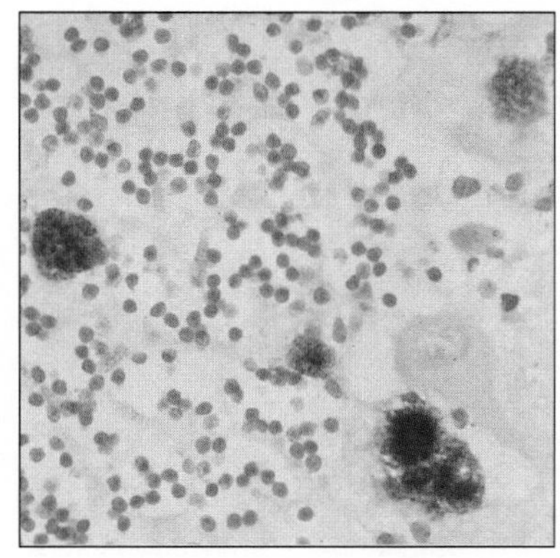

Fig. 6.49 Prion plaques in the Purkinje and granule cell layers of the cerebellum. *(Anti-prion protein × 400.)*

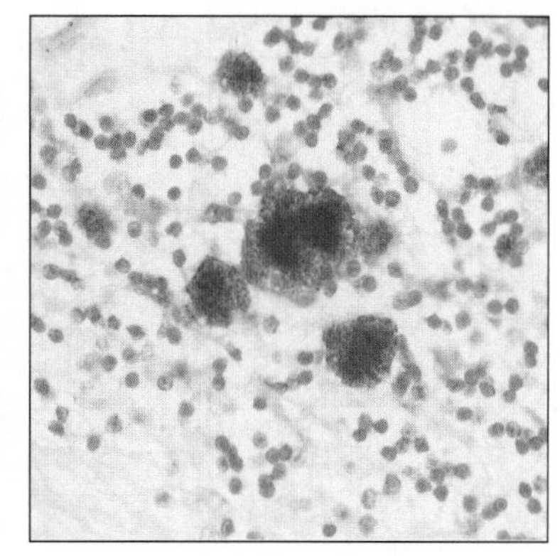

Fig. 6.50 Prion plaques in the granule cell layer of the cerebellum. *(Anti-prion protein × 400.)*

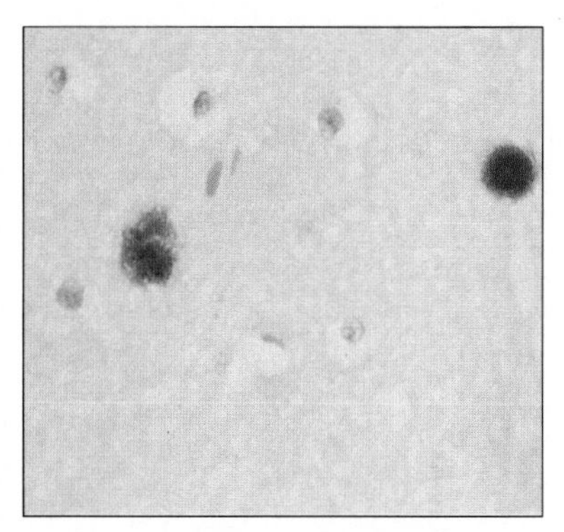

Fig. 6.51 Prion plaques in the molecular layer of the cerebellum. (Anti-prion protein x 400.)

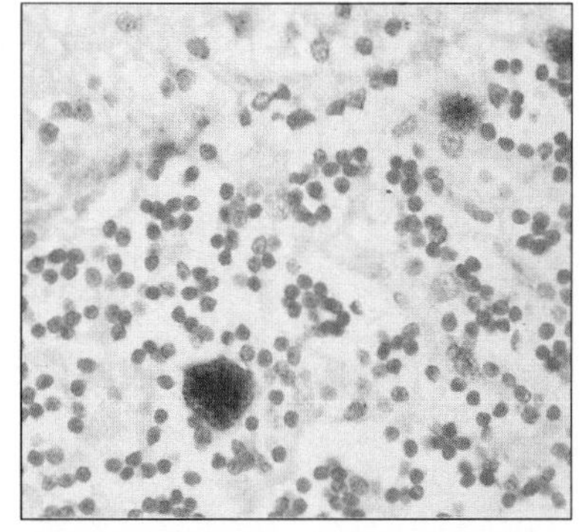

Fig. 6.52 Fine deposits of prion protein scattered along the Purkinje cell layer. *(Anti-prion protein × 400.)*

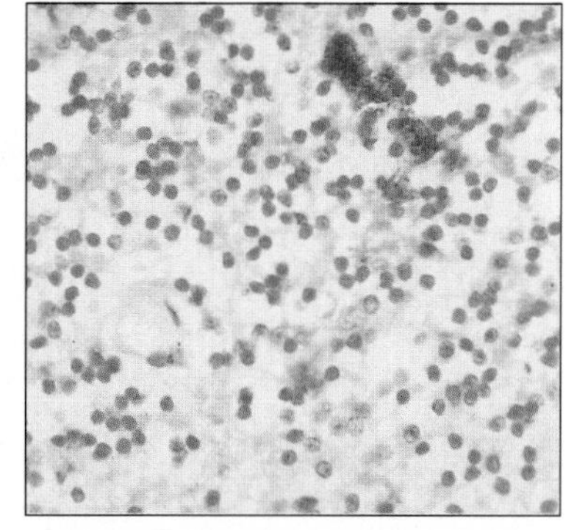

Fig. 6.53 Fine deposits of prion protein in the granule cell layer of the cerebellum. *(Anti-prion protein × 400.)*

of amyloid deposit are not age-related and are not reactive with antibodies against β/A4 protein. They do, however, react with antibodies against the so-called 'prion protein' (PrP) (**Figs 6.48–6.53**) (see page 159).

Finer deposits of PrP are scattered throughout the granule (see **Fig. 6.53**) and Purkinje cell (see **Fig. 6.52**) layers. Like the β/A4 amyloid plaques of Alzheimer's disease, the amyloid of these 'prion plaques' is associated with heparan sulphate proteoglycan (**Fig. 6.54**); they are also similarly reactive with Congo red due to the β–pleating of the PrP.

A mild microglial reaction surrounds, but does not infiltrate, the amyloid deposits (**Figs 6.55–6.57**). Ubiquitinated deposits, probably within enlarged nerve endings, are also present sometimes (**Fig. 6.58**) as is amyloid protein (APP). These swollen nerve terminals do *not* react with antibodies against tau protein (i.e. they do not contain neurites with PHF). There is also a mild astrocytic reaction around the deposits (**Figs 6.59–6.61**) and although the astrocytes appear to encircle the prion deposits completely, like microglia, their processes do not penetrate the amyloid to any great extent.

The presence of abnormal PrP within cortical sam-

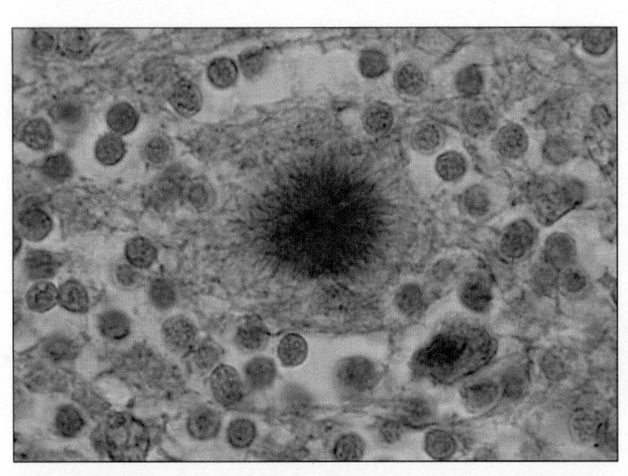

Fig. 6.54 Kuru-type prion plaques containing heparan sulphate proteoglycan. *(Sulphated Alcian blue stain × 400.)* (Courtesy of Dr A. Snow.)

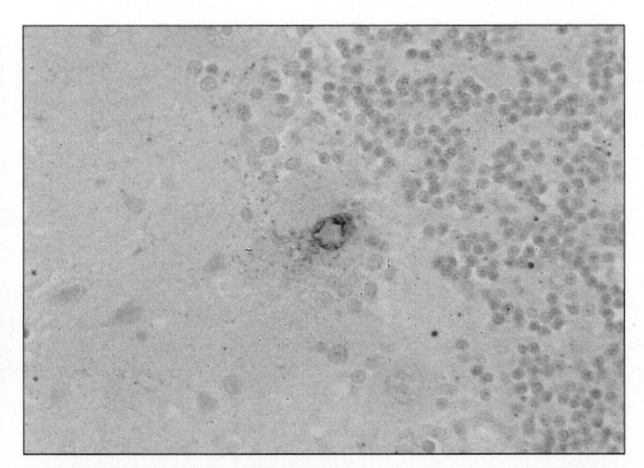

Fig. 6.55 Activated microglial cells surrounding prion plaques within the Purkinje cell layer of the cerebellum. *(Anti-ferritin × 400.)*

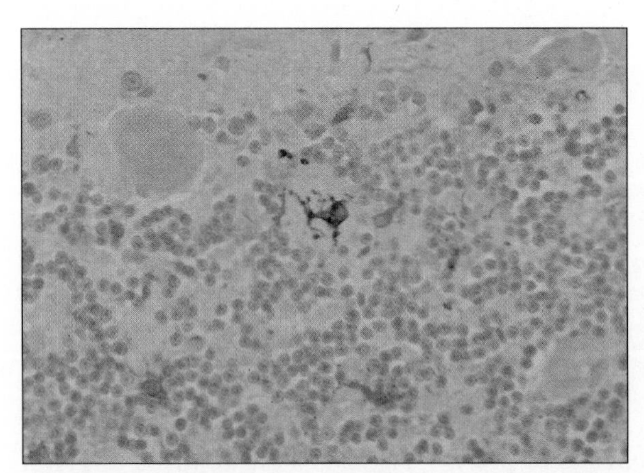

Fig. 6.56 Activated microglial cells surrounding prion plaques within the granule cell layer of the cerebellum. *(Anti-ferritin × 400.)*

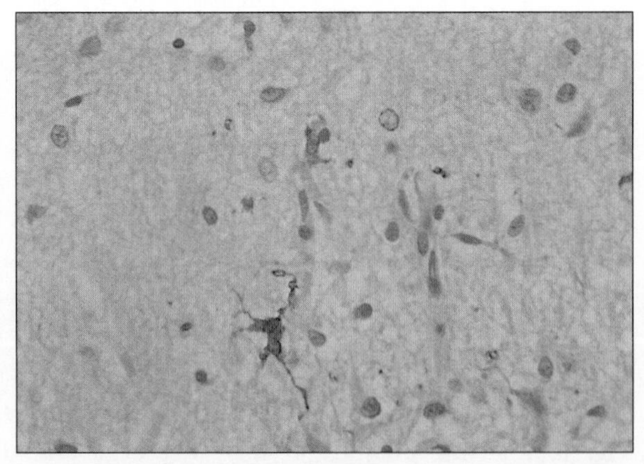

Fig. 6.57 Activated microglial cells surrounding prion plaques within the molecular layer of the cerebellum. *(Anti-ferritin × 400.)*

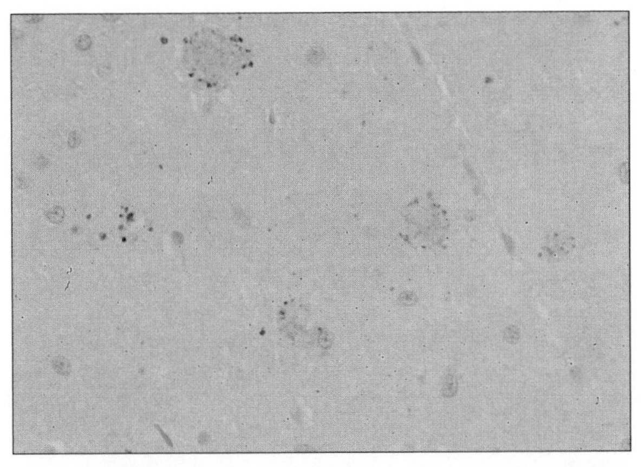

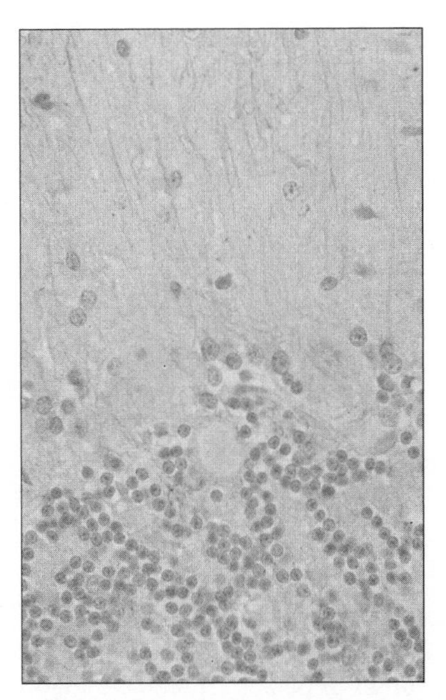

Fig. 6.58 Granular ubiquitin immunoreactivity within prion plaque regions in the molecular layer of the cerebellum. *(Anti-ubiquitin × 200.)*

Fig. 6.59 A mild astrocytic reaction surrounding prion deposits in the Purkinje cell layer. *(Anti-GFAP × 400.)*

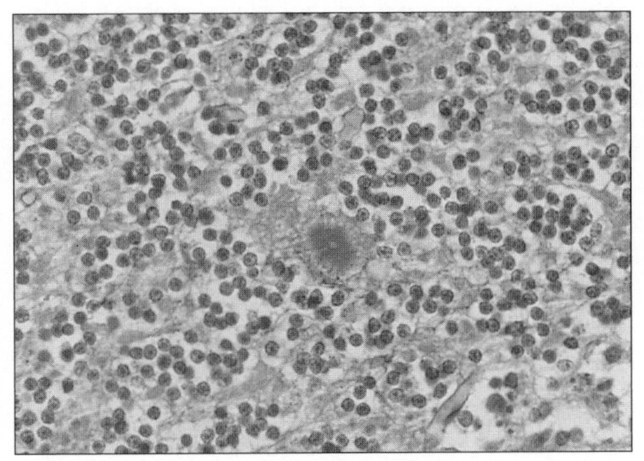

Fig. 6.60 A mild astrocytic reaction surrounding prion deposits in the granule cell layers of the cerebellum. *(Anti-GFAP counterstained with periodic acid–Schiff × 400.)*

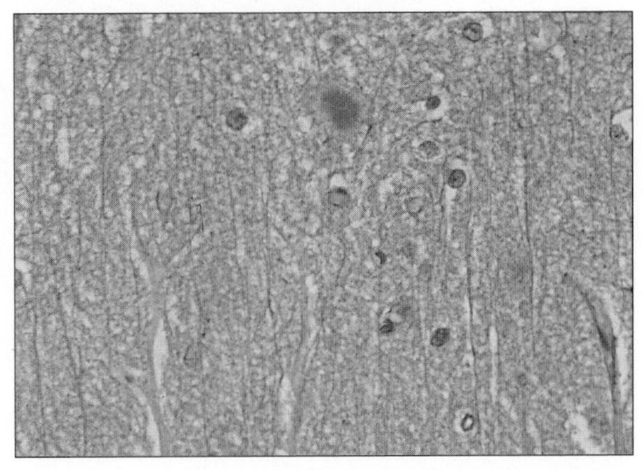

Fig. 6.61 A mild astrocytic reaction surrounding prion deposits in the molecular layers of the cerebellum. *(Anti-GFAP counterstained with periodic acid– Schiff × 400.)*

Fig. 6.62 Immunoblot showing the presence of abnormal prion protein in the cerebral cortex of four patients with Creutzfeldt–Jakob disease. Note lane '**P**' refers to the 51-year-old patient who showed only minimal histopathological changes featured in **Figs 6.32–6.39.**

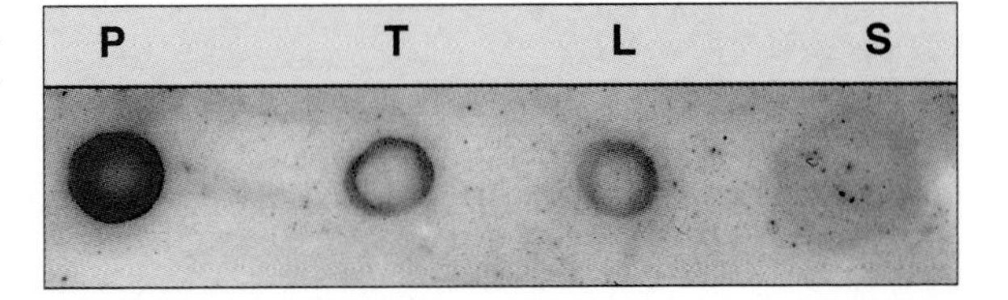

ples can be detected using a sensitive immunodot labelling method (**Fig. 6.62**), even when it cannot be detected microscopically in plaques by immunohistochemistry, and when there is minimal histopathological change (i.e. spongiosus, gliosis, nerve cell loss).

Similar deposits of prion protein occur in most patients with GSS, particularly in the cerebellum (**Figs 6.63** and **6.64**), but also in the cerebral cortex (**Fig. 6.65**) and basal ganglia (**Fig. 6.66**). These adopt various morphologies: stellate deposits

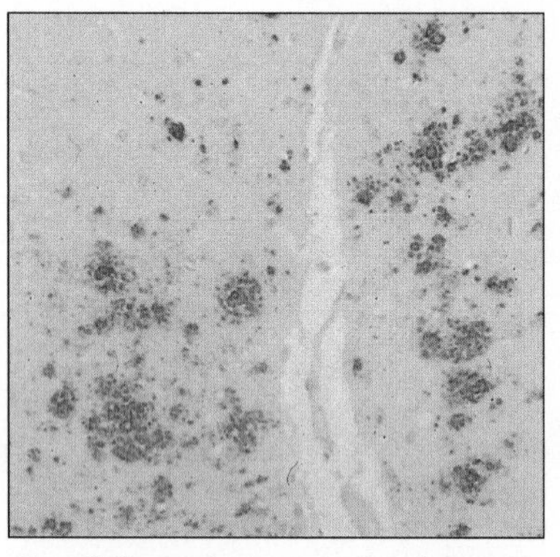

Fig. 6.63 Prion protein deposits in the cerebellum of a 70-year-old woman with GSS. The deposits appear as multicentric or conglomerate forms. *(Anti-prion protein × 100.)*

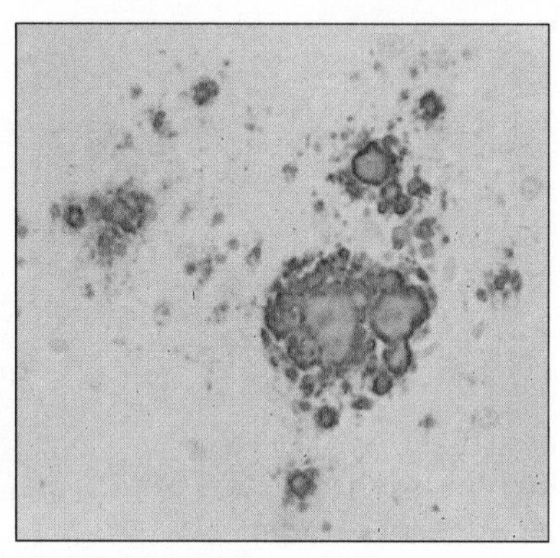

Fig. 6.64 Prion protein deposits in the cerebellum of the 70-year-old woman with GSS featured in **Fig. 6.63**, but × 200.

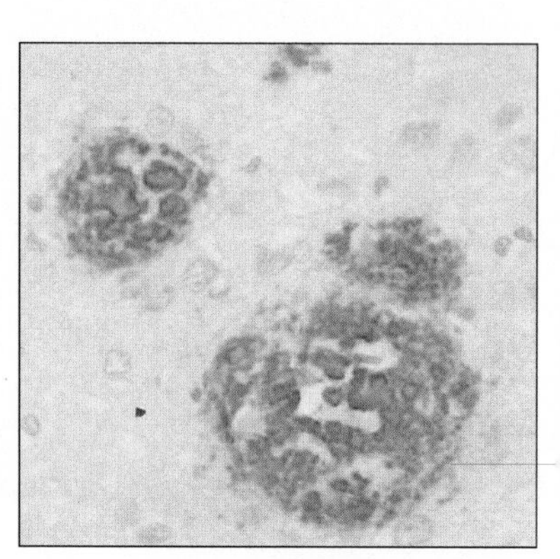

Fig. 6.65 Multicentric prion plaques in the cerebral cortex of the patient featured in **Figs 6.63** and **6.64**. *(Anti-prion protein × 200.)*

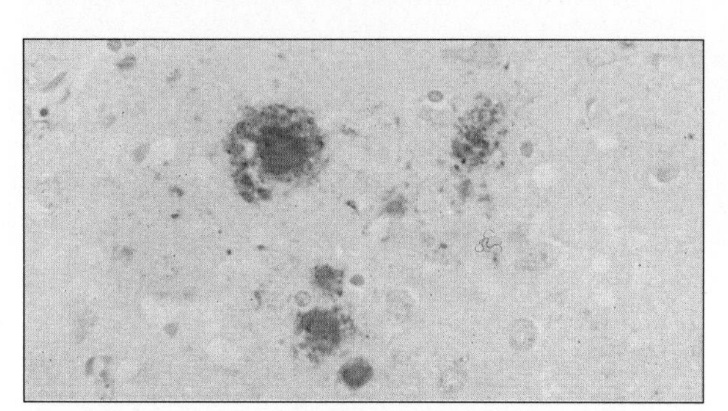

Fig. 6.66 Stellate and multicentric prion plaques in the putamen. *(Anti-prion protein × 200.)*

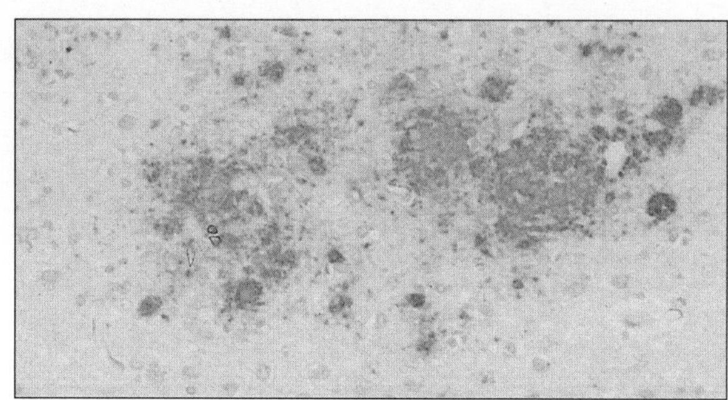

Fig. 6.67 Fine clouds of diffuse prion protein in the cerebral cortex of the patient featured in **Figs 6.63–6.65**. *(Anti-prion protein × 100.)*

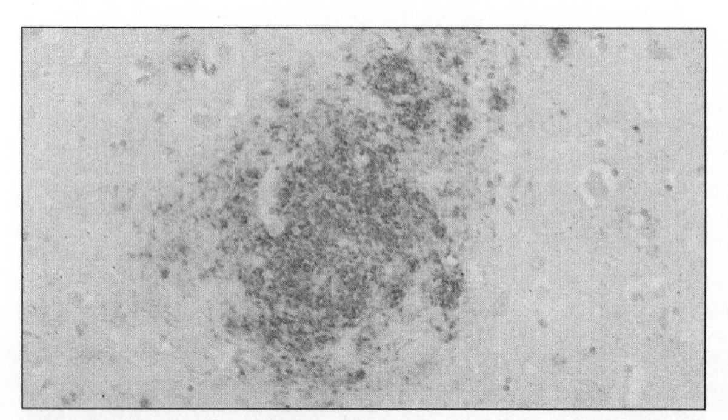

Fig. 6.68 Fine clouds of diffuse prion protein in the putamen of the patient featured in **Figs 6.63–6.65**. *(Anti-prion protein × 100.)*

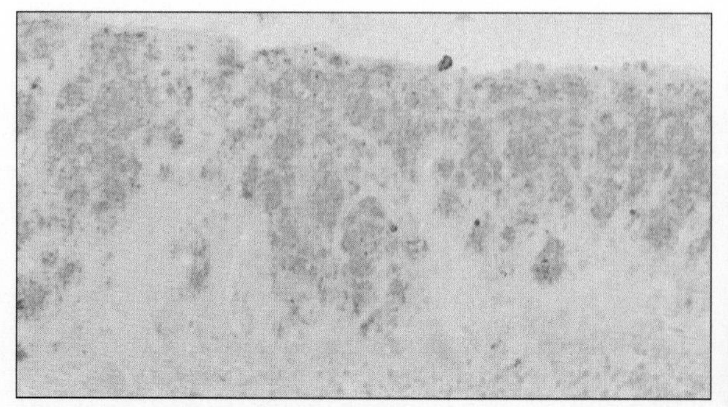

Fig. 6.69 Fine clouds of subpial deposit of prion protein in the cerebellum of the patient featured in **Figs 6.63–6.65**. *(Anti-prion protein × 100.)*

or multicentric conglomerates are the most common forms. Finer 'clouds' of diffuse deposit are also seen (**Figs 6.67 and 6.68**) and a large amount of protein can be deposited in subpial regions, especially in the cerebellum (**Fig. 6.69**). The deposits are again encircled by astrocytes (**Figs 6.70–6.74**), especially in the cerebral cortex, (see **Fig. 6.74**), but there is only limited penetration of the central core by their processes. Microglia are sparse (**Figs 6.75** and **6.76**). The amyloid

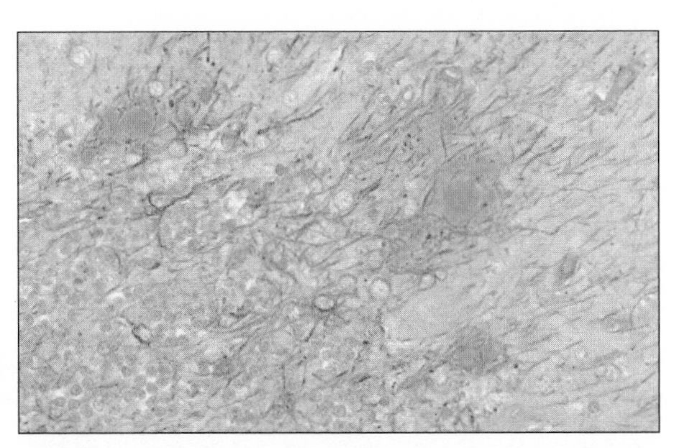

Fig. 6.70 Astrocytic reaction around prion plaques in the Purkinje cell layer. *(Anti-GFAP counterstained with periodic acid–Schiff × 200.)*

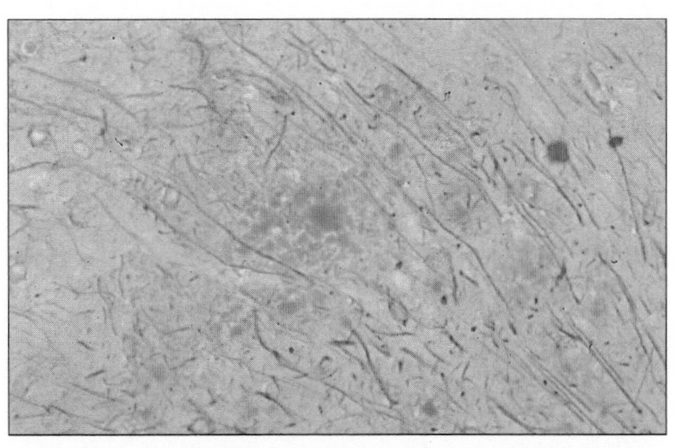

Fig. 6.71 Astrocytic reaction around prion plaques in the molecular layer. *(Anti-GFAP counterstained with periodic acid–Schiff × 200.)*

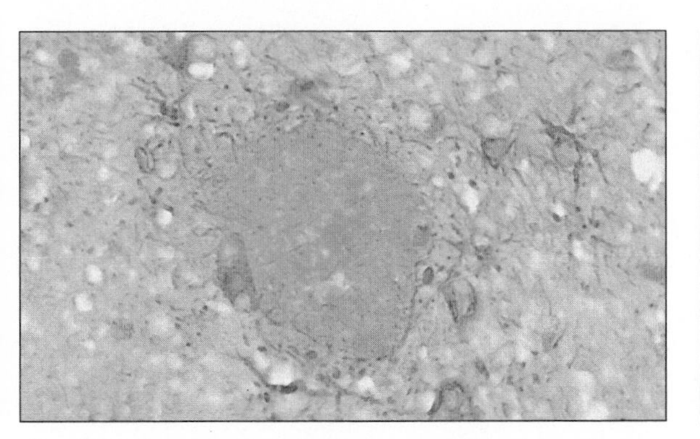

Fig. 6.72 Astrocytic reaction around prion plaques in the putamen. *(Anti-GFAP counterstained with periodic acid–Schiff × 200.)*

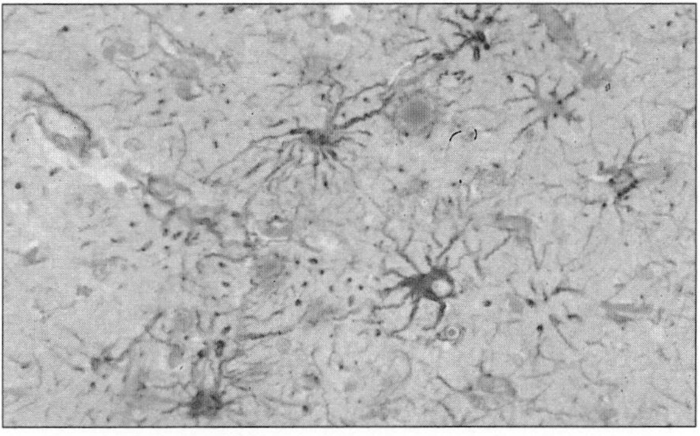

Fig. 6.73 Astrocytic reaction around prion plaques in the putamen. *(Anti-GFAP counterstained with periodic acid–Schiff × 200.)*

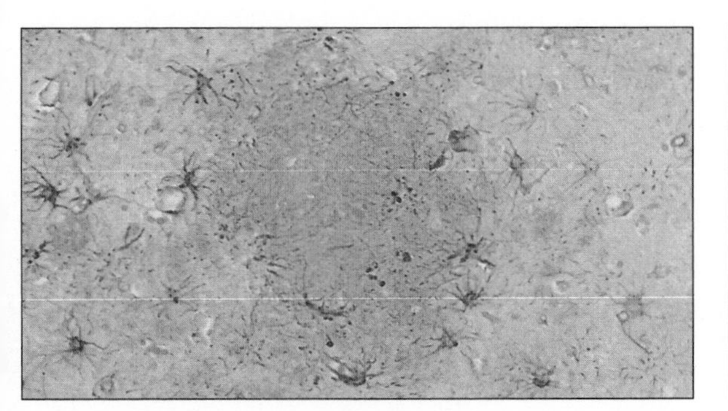

Fig. 6.74 Astrocytic reaction around a prion plaque in the cerebral cortex. *(Anti-GFAP counterstained with periodic acid–Schiff × 200.)*

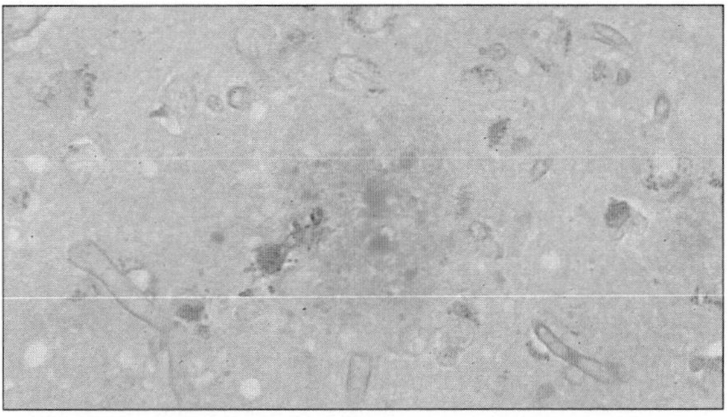

Fig. 6.75 A mild microglial reaction within prion plaques of the cerebral cortex. *(Anti-ferritin counterstained with periodic acid–Schiff × 200.)*

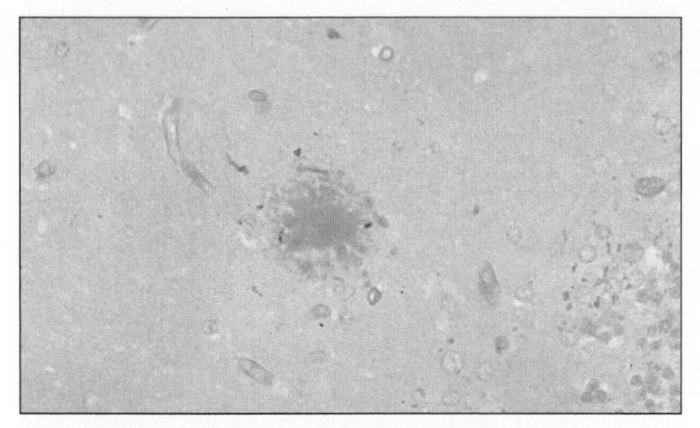

Fig. 6.76 A mild microglial reaction within prion plaques of the cerebellar cortex. *(Anti-ferritin counterstained with periodic acid–Schiff × 200.)*

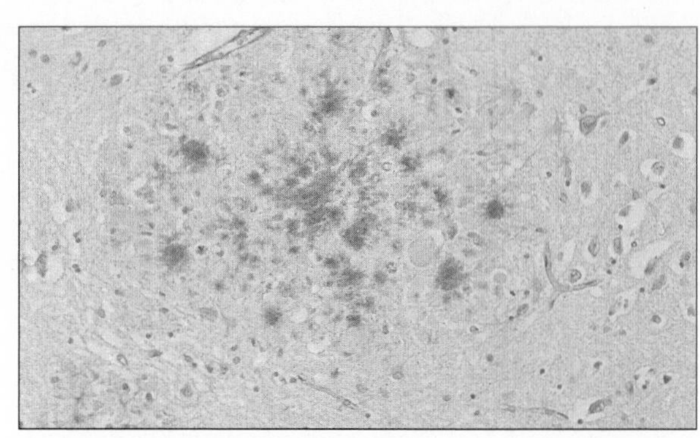

Fig. 6.77 Prion plaques contain heparan sulphate proteoglycan. *(Sulphated Alcian blue × 200.)* (Courtesy of Dr A. Snow.)

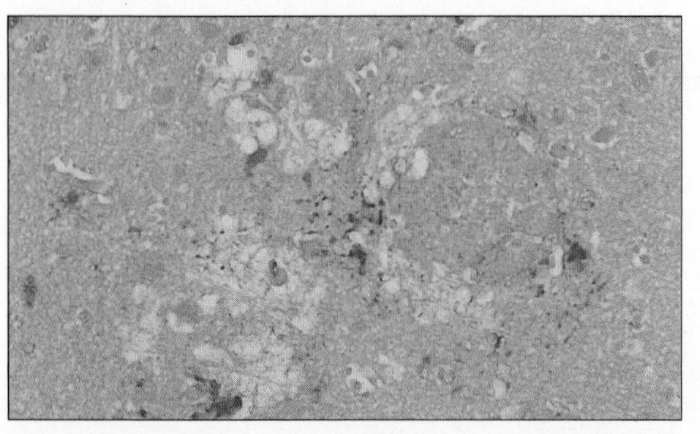

Fig. 6.78 Patchy vacuolation of the cerebral cortex with the astrocytic reaction relating to such areas of cavitation. *(Anti-GFAP counterstained with periodic acid–Schiff × 200.)*

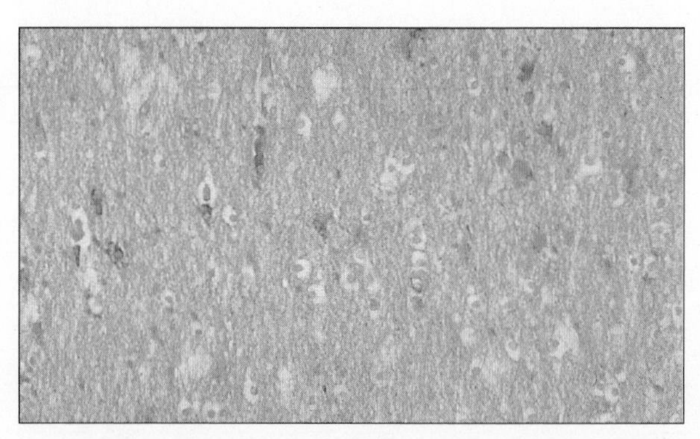

Fig. 6.79 Astrocytosis in the white matter of the temporal cortex. *(Anti-GFAP counterstained with periodic acid–Schiff × 200.)*

deposits in GSS also contain heparan sulphate proteoglycan (**Fig. 6.77**). Although spongiosus within the cortex is less pronounced and often patchy (see **Fig. 6.78**), astrocytosis occurs widely in white matter (**Fig. 6.79**).

Transmissibility of prion diseases

Like the spongiform encephalopathies of animals, human prion diseases can be transmitted from both humans to animals and from human to human. A wealth of experimental data shows that the passage of affected human nervous tissues into various animal species results, after a variable latency, in the development of a comparable disorder in the host species, with similar histopathological features to that of the human disease.

Human-to-human transmission has been recorded, particularly in the case of kuru, but also occasionally by the following iatrogenic routes:

- Contaminated instruments previously used in surgical procedures (biopsies) on patients with suspected CJD.
- Tissue donation of dural or corneal grafts from patients dying with CJD.

- Pituitary growth hormone or gonadotrophins from human cadavers, including presumably those with CJD. These were given to a large number of growth-retarded children and infertile women between 1963 and 1985.

Because of the long incubation times associated with such 'inefficient periphery to brain' transmissions, there will probably be future instances of disease associated with growth hormone or gonadotrophin treatment. Present autoclaving procedures preclude 'brain to brain' transmission in surgical procedures, tissue donations from suspect patients are no longer used, and synthetic hormones have replaced those extracted from human tissues.

Apart from these rare and inadvertent transmissions, there is no convincing evidence that the diseases can be transmitted from human to human, either in the community or in a non-surgical hospital setting. Most patients with the disease appear to develop it spontaneously or inherit it.

Molecular and genetic studies

The amyloid protein, which accumulates within the 'prion plaques' of kuru, CJD and GSS, is an unusual isoform of a normally produced membrane spanning glycoprotein and known as the previously described 'prion protein'. This is encoded by a gene on the short arm of chromosome 20 (in humans); the entire 253 codon open-reading frame exists within a single exon. In the brain, the highest levels of gene expression of PrP occur in neurones.

Like 'normal' prion protein the abnormal isoform has a molecular weight of 33–35kDa, these being designated PrP_{33-35}^{C} and PrP_{33-35}^{Sc} (c and Sc denoting its isolation from normal cells and scrapie-infected tissues, respectively). The function of PrP_{33-35}^{C} is not known; indeed, deletion of the prion gene in rodents is apparently without ill effect.

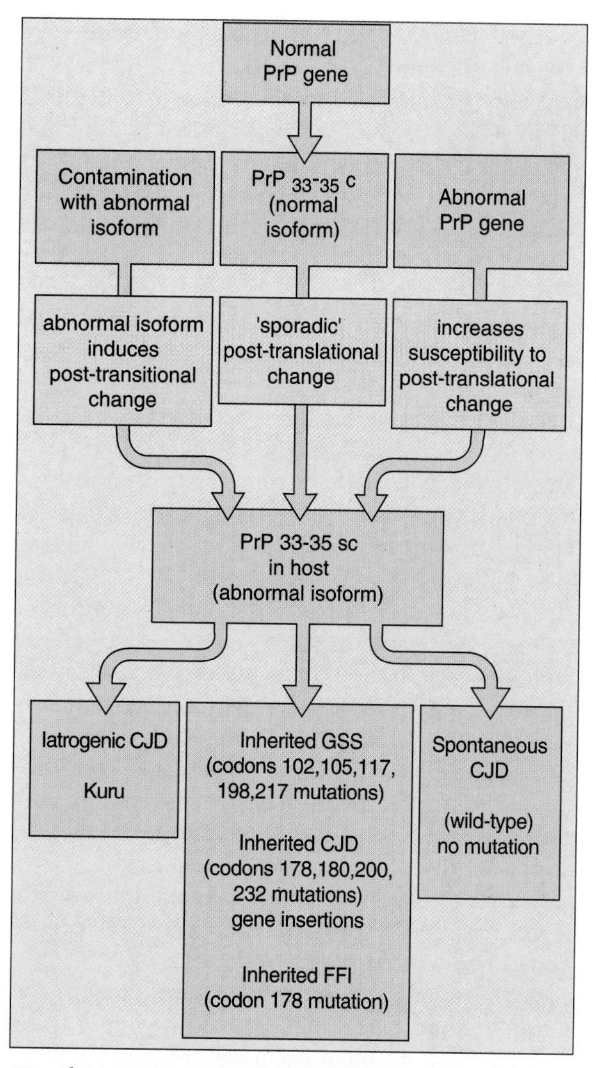

Fig. 6.80 Pathogenesis of iatrogenic, sporadic and inherited forms of prion disease.

In the human and animal spongiform encephalopathies the normal isoform PrP_{33-35}^{C} is post-translationally modified to give PrP_{33-35}^{Sc}; the level of PrP gene expression remains normal. This abnormal isoform is proteolytically resistant and unlike its normal counterpart, which *in vitro* can be digested completely by proteinase K, it can be only partially broken down to give a molecular species of 27–30kDa, known as PrP_{27-30}^{Sc}. It is this latter molecular species that accumulates in the prion plaques and is associated with disease transmissibility (**Fig. 6.80**).

How disease transmission is achieved is not clear, but it is postulated that when PrP_{27-30}^{Sc} is introduced into a host species it can act as a 'template' allowing the normally produced *host* PrP_{33-35}^{C} to undergo a conformational rather than chemical change becoming converted into PrP_{33-35}^{Sc}. This is subsequently partially catabolised and accumulates as PrP_{27-30}^{Sc}. The 'donated' PrP_{33-35}^{Sc} does not 'replicate' itself in the host as donor PrP. In this way transmission does not require the presence of an external agent or 'virus' as has been postulated.

The terms 'latent viral' or 'slow viral' transmission, which have been used in association with these disorders, are therefore inappropriate and should be discontinued. No nucleic acid has ever been extracted from the prion protein; transmisson of disease can still proceed even in tissues pretreated to hydrolyse or modify nucleic acid.

As the protein that accumulates on transmission is host- rather than donor-derived it is only to be expected that no immunological response will be triggered.

Alternatively, an increasing number of mutations within the prion gene have been detected in patients with familial CJD and GSS (**Figs 6.80** and **6.81**). These presumably act by increasing the probability that a post-translational modification of PrP_{33-35}^{C} occurs spontaneously in the person with the genetic defect.

- In GSS the most common mutation involves a proline→leucine change at codon 102 of the prion gene, although other mutations at codon 105 (also proline→leucine), at codon 117 (valine→alanine), and at codons 198 (phenylalanine→serine) and 217 (glutamine→arginine) in North American Indiana kindred and a Swedish kindred, have been identified. The codon 102 mutation has been found in 10 unrelated families and is probably due to a deamination event in a germline PrP gene, resulting in the substitution of a thymine for a cytosine with appropriate amino acid change.
- In familial CJD mutations are most common at codons 178 (aspartic acid→asparginine) and 200 (glutamine→lysine).
- A combination of the mutation at codon 178 with the codon 129 polymorphism (see below) is associated clinically with the disorder FFI.
- Other changes at codons 180 (valine→isoleucine) and 232 (methionine→arginine) have been reported in some Japanese GSS families.
- Transgenic mice expressing the equivalent 102 proline→leucine mutation spontaneously develop a neurological disease with spongiform degeneration and gliosis without any deposition of PrP.

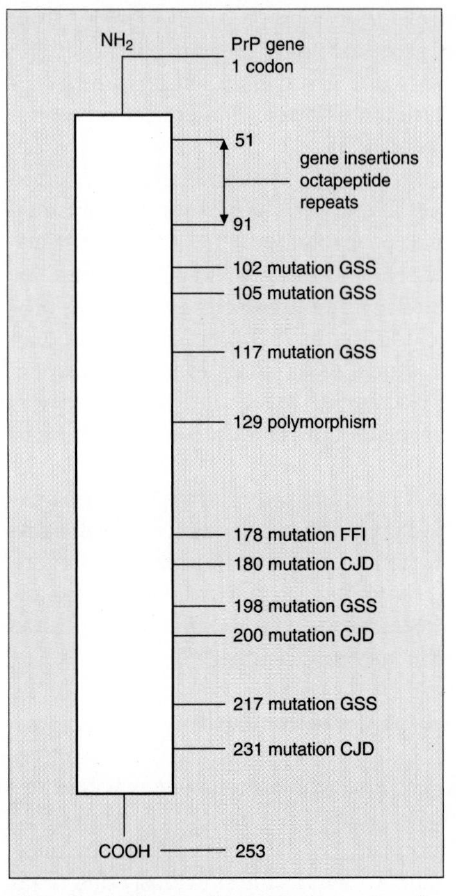

Fig. 6.81 Sites of mutations in the prion gene with clinical phenotype.

- In an extended British family with CJD, large insertions of 144 or 216 base pairs occur between codons 51 and 91 of the open reading frame of the prion gene. These insertions relate to a further 6 and 9 repeats of a particular 24 base pair (octapeptide) sequence, 5 repeats of which are *normally* present at this part of the prion gene. This particular mutation must have arisen through a complex series of events, since a *normal* sequence of 5 such repeats could not have led to an insertion of this size through a *single* recombination event. All British individuals affected by this mutation probably derive from a single founder born more than two centuries ago.
- Recently, an American family with an insert, again between codons 51 and 91 of the open reading frame, consisting of 168 base pairs (an additional 7 of the above octapeptide repeats), has been identified. Other unrelated American families with similar insertions in this same coding region have also been reported.
- Sequence of the PrP gene in Kuru fails to reveal any mutation.

Furthermore, it appears that a polymorphism (methionine→valine) exists within the prion gene at codon 129. Amongst Caucasians this polymorphism is common (methionine:valine = 0.62:0.38), though racial variations may occur. In Japan the polymorphism is uncommon, the equivalent ratio being 0.96:0.04. The presence of this particular polymorphism, or that of a homozygosity for either allele at codon 129 is an especially important change.

- It may increase susceptibility to non-familial forms of CJD (including kuru and *iatrogenic* CJD).
- It may be associated with the development of FFI in 'thalamic CJD'.
- It may influence the deposition of prion protein in 'wild-type' CJD (see below) and confer an earlier onset of disease in those individuals where a gene insertion occurs.

Conversely, the amino acid specified at codon 129 of the normal allele can modify the severity of disease in patients with 178 and 180 mutations, affecting either the duration or the age of onset of disease.

While it is plausible that these genetic disturbances producing mutant PrP isoforms may cause a spontaneous post-translational conversion of $PrP_{33-35}{}^{c}$, and that this same change may be induced by 'contamination' in iatrogenic cases, it is not clear how this change is brought about in spontaneous (wild-type) cases. About 85% of patients with CJD appear to develop it sporadically, and a genetic defect has yet to be detected in any 'sporadic' case. Furthermore, it is not known how the conversion of PrP_c into PrP_{Sc} relates to the wider provinces of neuronal dysfunction and loss, spongiosis and reactive astrocytosis.

Clinical, pathological and molecular considerations

Sometimes there are local differences of emphasis within the overall clinical symptomatology of CJD and GSS, presumably due to differences in the distribution and relative severity of the cerebral cortical and cerebellar pathology (e.g. cortical blindness when there is severe occipital involvement, fatal insomnia with thalamic disease, ataxia when there is GSS-type cerebellar emphasis). However, most patients do follow a broadly similar and well-defined clinical course (see page 18). Such a relative homogeneity of clinical presentation is seemingly at odds with the range of pathological changes that can occur, these varying from minimal through to extreme. Moreover, deposits of prion protein, as amyloid plaques, may or may not be present irrespective of the presence or extent of spongiosis or gliosis. Yet in all patients a devasting clinical picture prevails. This apparent paradox can be reconciled by an assumption that the widespread intellectual and behavioural derangement stems directly from a neuronal dysfunction brought about by a particular and presently unknown metabolic or physiological disturbance. How such a change might involve the prion protein is not clear. However, it can be assumed that the pathological changes relate to the abnormal accumulation of PrP^{SC}, rather than the absence of PrP^{C} (see mice experience, page 159). This putative 'functional' defect would, in turn, drive the pathological changes of the disorder. The differing aetiologies associated with CJD and GSS would therefore 'feed' a common physiological change involving the prion protein, with the eventual 'balance' of pathological alterations (i.e. phenotype) within the constellation of changes that seem to be possible dictated by the aetiological variant (**Fig. 6.63**).

In such a scheme, the clinical picture would depend not on the type, nor even necessarily the distribution, of pathological changes, but solely on the presence of this unifying physiological disturbance. Examples include the following:

- Most patients with the codons 102, 105, 117, 198, and 217 mutations (i.e. those with GSS) deposit a large amount of prion protein as plaques (see **Figs 6.63–6.69**). People with 'sporadic' CJD with the codon 129 met→val polymorphism also deposit prion protein as plaques (see **Figs 6.42–6.53**) and present a clinical picture similar to GSS.
- Patients without any point mutation, but with the normal codon 129 allele (i.e. wild-type CJD) do not deposit prion protein in plaques and run a clinically similar though more aggressive course.
- To what extent familial CJD and GSS with other missense protein variants (i.e. due to point mutations at codons 178 (FFI), 180, 200, and 232, and gene insertions) are linked to prion protein deposition is not clear. Usually, as with wild-type CJD, the abnormal PrP, although present in brain tissue, is not assimilated into clearly defined prion plaques, but may be more diffusely deposited as punctate deposits.
- The GSS associated mutations occur in putative α-helical portions of the prion gene and syntheti-c peptides containing such α-helical sequences spontaneous form amyloid fibrils. Mutations in these parts of the prion gene may promote this intrinsic amyloidogenicity causing plaques to form in vivo. Codon 200 is outside these α-helical regions and changes here, as with the normal wild-type gene, may preclude amyloidosis.
- Sporadic CJD, without a clear family history or genomic defect (wild-type), may be assocaited with the acquisition of the same physiological defect, possibly through rare environmental influences on prion metabolism leading to the abnormal modification of wild-type PrP, or perhaps more likely by the creation of a somatic mutation as a stochastic event within the prion gene, which then 'spreads' to direct the post-translational defect in the rest of the tissue. The presence and transmission of prions in the customary human food chain is an unlikely explanation

A similar situation to this exists in Alzheimer's disease (see page 65), where different aetiologies 'feed' a common pathogenetic process triggered by a 'mismetabolism' of APP (see **Fig. 3.175**). However, in contrast to prion diseases, no substantial pathological heterogeneity has as yet been found in Alzheimer's disease despite the diversity of initiating factors that have been linked to the disorder.

7. Diagnosis

The presence of 'disease-type' or 'disease-like' pathological changes in patients whose clinical features are inconsistent with those usually associated with such pathology presents a diagnostic problem that besets the dementias of adult life, especially for those in whom a primary neurodegenerative disease is the underlying cause. For example, those changes traditionally considered to be pathognomic for Alzheimer's disease (i.e. senile plaques and neurofibrillary tangles) can occur either separately, or in conjunction, in many other disorders. Similarly, the presence of inclusion bodies of different types or the appearance of a spongiform type of change seems to 'cross-react' between diseases. To what extent these concurrent pathologies represent co-existing disease within the same person is not known. It is possible that they reflect the range of pathological expressions (phenotypes) that can exist in any one disorder. Diagnostic uncertainties therefore can, and frequently do, arise when overlapping pathologies are present within a single patient.

Cerebral atrophy

Cerebral atrophy, seen either on brain scanning or at post mortem, is a feature that accompanies most neurodegenerative diseases causing dementia, although its extent and topographic distribution is extremely variable. Certain broad patterns of atrophy are, however, more commonly found in particular disorders, including the following:

- Fronto-temporal atrophy in fronto-temporal dementia.
- Medial temporal lobe atrophy of Alzheimer's disease.
- Striatal atrophy of Huntington's disease.

Not every patient with any one of these disorders always shows a common (average or typical) level of change and there is considerable variation. In addition, some patients with Alzheimer's disease show pronounced frontal lobe atrophy and some patients with fronto-temporal dementia display only a mild frontal lobe atrophy, while others have a severe striatal atrophy. Depigmentation of the substantia nigra is common to subcortical dementias with Parkinsonian-type features (Parkinson's disease, cortical Lewy body disease, progressive supranuclear palsy, cortico-basal degeneration), but can also be a feature in certain cortical dementias (e.g. fronto-temporal dementia), even when there are no apparent extrapyramidal signs.

Functional imaging of the brain during life, using either PET or SPET, can be informative in certain instances in detecting the abnormal posterior parietal lobe function of Alzheimer's disease or the frontal lobe defect in fronto-temporal dementia (see **Table 1.8**, page 20). However, a frontal lobe defect is common in some subcortical dementias, such as progressive supranuclear palsy, and not all patients with Alzheimer's disease display the posterior hemisphere defect. Furthermore, functional imaging detects regions of reduced neural activity, and this change is not always congruent with neuronal fallout and tissue loss.

The pattern of cerebral atrophy may, in many instances, lead to suspicion of a particular disease, but in itself is not a reliable guide; histopathological verification is required. This, in the main, is still provided by the presence of particular structural morphological changes in the brain that have traditionally been considered to 'segregate' with certain disorders. However, modern methods of detecting these changes show that classifications based upon such 'simplistic' markers of neurodegeneration are fraught with difficulties.

Plaques, tangles and amyloid β/A4 protein

The presence of 'excessive' quantities of plaques, tangles and amyloid β/A4 protein in the brain is usually considered to fulfil the diagnostic criteria for Alzheimer's disease (see page 56). However, any, or even all, of these very same changes can exist in the brain in other dementing and sometimes non-dementing (neurodegenerative) disorders. Indeed, they can also occur, though usually to a much lesser extent, in many elderly people who show no tangible evidence of psychiatric or neurological disorder, as illustrated by the following examples:

- β/A4 protein deposition in the form of diffuse plaques occurs with increasing frequency and severity in old age. It is rare before 50 years of age, but is seen in more than 75% of those over 75 years of age. Usually, the amyloid is confined to the cerebral cortex; the cerebellum, brain stem and basal ganglia are affected only rarely. The quantity is usually, but not always, much lower than that typically seen in Alzheimer's disease. In non-demented people only a few β/A4 protein plaques contain neurites. Neurofibrillary tangles are rare or absent in the neocortex but can be quite common in the hippocampus, especially within the CA1 region, and the entorhinal cortex. The presence of both tangles and diffuse β/A4 deposits, produces a pathological picture not unlike that seen in younger people (i.e. less than 50 years of age) with Down's syndrome. It has, therefore, been argued that such changes represent early or preclinical Alzheimer's disease and that if the patient had lived longer he or she would have developed full-blown pathological changes. Nonetheless, this still leaves some people with amyloid β/A4 protein *alone* within their brains; these people do not have tangles and it is not clear that they would ever have had tangles if they had lived longer. This particular situation is common in elderly people with other neurodegenerative disorders, such as the fronto-temporal dementias, progressive aphasia (page 90), progressive supranuclear palsy (page 102), Huntington's disease (page 107) and Parkinson's disease (page 112) and closed head trauma with prolonged survival (page 67) and in people on chronic renal dialysis (page 70). Are these changes best regarded as a reflection of the effects of 'pathological ageing' rather than incipient Alzheimer's disease or do they represent a prolonged prodromal phase of the disease that sometimes extends beyond life expectancy, so preventing full expression of the disease? It is not yet possible to answer this question.
- In cortical Lewy body disease (page 118) there is extensive β/A4 deposition in the cortex of most patients, and in many of these, but again not in all, there is some degree of neurofibrillary tangle formation. This can involve much of the cortex, but is usually severe only in the hippocampus and entorhinal cortex. Therefore, about one-third of patients have sufficient Alzheimer-type pathology in their brains to warrant an additional diagnosis of Alzheimer's disease (page 54). Do such changes represent a co-existing Alzheimer's disease, or is this particular disorder a variant of Alzheimer's disease in which Lewy bodies are widely present in the cortex and brain stem? Occasional Lewy bodies occur in the substantia nigra of about 40% of patients with Alzheimer's disease. Alzheimer's disease and certain Parkinson-type diseases (idiopathic Parkinson's disease and cortical Lewy body disease) may therefore lie on a continuum of pathological changes with prototypical Alzheimer's and Parkinson's disease occupying opposing poles. Disorders with a combined pathology (i.e. cortical Lewy body disease) would occupy a broad middle range.
- In the viral encephalitides of subacute sclerosing panenencephalitis and post-encephalitic Parkinsonism, neurofibrillary tangles occur without β/A4 protein. These tangles are ultrastructurally and immmunohistochemically identical to those of Alzheimer's disease. In some boxers, similar tangles can exist along with β/A4 deposition, although the anatomical distribution of both features does not always coincide (see page 67).

Pathological features such as neuritic plaques, neurofibrillary tangles and β/A4 amyloid therefore clearly do not provide precise markers for the unequivocal diagnosis of Alzheimer's disease. Typical disease can be easily identified by the usual criteria, but diagnosis may be less certain if the pathology is confounding (e.g. Lewy bodies) or in early, or incipient, disease when the quantity or distribution of Alzheimer-like changes may be restricted.

Intracellular inclusions

Intraneuronal inclusions other than the neurofibrillary tangles of Alzheimer's disease are common in neurodegenerative diseases as follows:

- Although pathognomic for idiopathic Parkinson's disease (page 110), Lewy bodies are widespread in the cerebral cortex in cortical Lewy body disease (page 116) and occasionally occur in the substantia nigra in Alzheimer's disease (page 54).
- Inclusions occur in the cortex and elsewhere in Pick's disease (page 74) and in fronto-temporal dementia with motor neurone disease (page 86).
- Structures similar to Alzheimer neurofibrillary tangles are present in progressive supranuclear palsy (page 98) and in cortico-basal degeneration (page 121).

As with plaques and tangles, occasional Lewy bodies also appear within the substantia nigra or cerebral cortex of a large number of asymptomatic elderly individuals.

Conventional neurohistological procedures, often based on silver impregnation methods, can usually detect the presence of these various inclusions, but frequently fail to discriminate between them and are poor diagnostic tools. Immunohistochemical procedures have begun to characterise these various inclusions and it is now clear that distinctions can be made according to their antigenic properties (**Table 7.1**). These can be helpful, not only in detecting their presence but also in providing a diagnosis.

Table 7.1 Immunohistochemical and other staining properties of pathological intraneuronal inclusions. (0, always unstained; 0/+, only occasionally stained; +, always, but weakly stained; ++, always, but moderately stained; +++, always strongly stained.)

Pathological change	Silver	Tau	Ubiquitin	αB crystallin	Phosphorylated neurofilament	Basophilia
Alzheimer's disease (neurofibrillary tangle)	+++	+++	++	0	+	0
Progressive supranuclear palsy (neurofibrillary tangle)	+++	+++	0/+	0	+	0
Cortico-basal degeneration ('tangle')	+	+++	0	0	+	+
Parkinson's disease (Lewy body)	0	0	+++	+	+	0
Cortical Lewy body disease (Lewy body)	0	+	+++	+	+	0
Pick's disease (Pick bodies)	+++	+++	+++	++	0	0
Motor neurone disease (+ dementia) (cortical inclusions)	0	0	+++	0	0	0
Creutzfeldt-Jakob disease, Pick's disease, Cortico-basal degeneration, Alzheimer's disease (ballooned cells)	++	++	+	+++	+++	0
Motor neurone disease (+ dementia) (spinal inclusions)	0	0	+++	0	0	0

The 'neurofibrillary' inclusions of Alzheimer's disease and cortico-basal degeneration are both tau-positive, but can be distinguished because those of cortico-basal degeneration are weakly argyrophilic and basophilic, and lack ubiquitin-immunoreactivity. In contrast, Alzheimer tangles are strongly argyrophilic and usually react well with anti-ubiquitin. The tangles of progressive supranuclear palsy, like those of Alzheimer's disease, are strongly argyrophilic and tau-immunoreactive, but those of progressive supranuclear palsy exhibit variable anti-ubiquitin reactivity; weak positivity is reported by some, but not others.

Although the cortical Lewy bodies in cortical Lewy body disease (page 116) react with anti-ubiquitin antisera, they do not react constantly with tau antisera, whereas the nigral inclusions in both Parkinson's disease (page 110) and cortical Lewy body disease react only with ubiquitin. Using anti-ubiquitin staining alone, it may therefore be difficult to differentiate between small tangles (if present) occurring in the cortex and the cortical Lewy bodies in cortical Lewy body disease. Double immunostaining for tau and ubiquitin helps, because only the tangles will usually be both tau- and ubiquitin-immunoreactive; alternatively, single-stained adjacent sections can be directly compared.

The inclusions of Pick's disease (page 74) and fronto-temporal dementia with motor neurone disease (page 86) are present in similar cell types (i.e. the granule cells of the dentate gyrus of the hippocampus and the layer II pyramidal cells of the frontal and temporal cortex) and are strongly ubiquitin-immunoreactive, but can be distinguished because those of fronto-temporal dementia with motor neurone disease lack tau-immunoreactivity and argyrophilia.

Pick bodies can usually be differentiated from Alzheimer tangles on the basis of their shape and location: Pick bodies are rounded and occur mainly in cortical layer II cells, while tangles in Alzheimer's disease are flame-shaped or globose and occur mainly in cortical layers III and V. Both are silver, tau- and ubiquitin-immunoreactive.

Pick bodies apparently identical to those of Pick's disease itself are occasionally found in patients with progressive aphasia and fronto-temporal dementia with motor neurone disease, and even in progressive supranuclear palsy.

As with plaques, tangles and β/A4 amyloid, a few Lewy bodies are found in the substantia nigra or cerebral cortex of many asymptomatic elderly individuals. It has been suggested that this presence of nigral Lewy bodies, in the absence of clinical Parkinsonism, reflects an incipient Parkinson's disease. By analogy, the presence of occasional cortical Lewy bodies may therefore be a pathological forerunner of cortical Lewy body disease. In view of the high prevalence of both disorders among the elderly, it is quite plausible that there is a large number of asymptomatic individuals with early disease who are identified only by chance at autopsy following death from unrelated causes (as for Alzheimer's disease). Again, as with Alzheimer's disease, this view remains to be proven and it is not clear whether this can be applied to all, or only a certain proportion, of such people.

'Inflated' or 'ballooned' neurones

Swollen (inflated or ballooned) cells represent, along with Pick bodies, a cardinal change in Pick's disease (page 78), but can be present in Creutzfeldt–Jakob disease (page 148) and cortico-basal degeneration (page 124), and sometimes in Alzheimer's disease. In all instances, such cells are strongly immunoreactive with antibodies to phosphorylated neurofilament protein, react less strongly with tau and silver stains, are only weakly immunoreactive with ubiquitin antisera, and react strongly with antisera against αB crystallin (a small 'heat-shock' protein of the hsp20–30 class).

Ballooned cells are characterised by an accumulation of neurofilament protein, possibly mediated by interactions with αB crystallin. This may reflect a reactive change by the neurone to damaging processes that involve or invoke a remodelling or regrowth of nerve cell processes. Their appearance may therefore represent a nerve cell response to a kind of injury that may be common to all these various disorders. Such cells should not be taken to indicate the presence of any particular disease (e.g. Pick's disease).

Cerebral (amyloid) angiopathy

Cerebral amyloid angiopathy (CAA) is usually regarded as one of the typical (if less consistent) pathological features of Alzheimer's disease (page 47), but it is again clear that, as with amyloid plaques and neurofibrillary tangles, it can occur, though to a much less extent, in the leptomeningeal and intraparenchymal arteries of about 50% of non-demented elderly people. In addition, the frequency and severity of CAA in patients with cortical Lewy body disease who show numerous parenchymal amyloid plaques and neurofibrillary tangles are similar to those patients with Alzheimer's disease alone experience, whereas the prevalence in patients with Lewy bodies but *without* plaques and tangles falls to match that of mentally able control subjects. This implies that the presence of CAA in Lewy body disease is not fundamental to the disorder, but, as with plaques and tangles, occurs in a certain proportion of individuals as part of the spectrum of Alzheimer-type changes. Whether these changes are indicative of a coincidental Alzheimer's disease or reflect 'pathological ageing' remains unclear.

Spongiform changes

The terms 'spongiform change' or 'status spongiosus' are used to describe the vacuolation of the neuropil that is often present in certain neurodegenerative disorders. However, the two terms are *not* interchangeable.

- *Spongiform change* refers to vacuolation of the cortex that is a result of neuronal *shrinkage* (atrophy) and loss. To avoid potential confusion the term 'microvacuolation' might be preferable (see page 79).
- *Status spongiosus* on the other hand describes a *swelling* of cells and processes to produce the widespread sieve-like appearance of tissue in the prion disorders of Creutzfeldt–Jakob disease and Gerstmann– Sträussler–Sheinker syndrome (page 145).

Sometimes, a vacuolation of the neuropil, similar to that typically seen in the outer laminae of the cortex in frontal dementia (with or without motor neurone disease) occurs diffusely throughout all cortical laminae in Alzheimer's disease or in the striatum in Huntington's disease, when nerve cell loss and atrophy are severe. Sometimes tissue vacuolation can be seen in autopsied brains regardless of the presence of these diseases. Such a change is probably artefactually produced through differential fixational and tissue processing changes, because when present it is randomly dispersed, showing no preferential anatomical (i.e. laminar) or regional distribution. Pathological vacuolation is always topographically located, with regions of non-vacuolated tissue in those parts of the brain unaffected by disease.

Specificity

It is therefore quite clear that the pathological changes discussed above in either neurones or neuropil in these neurodegenerative disorders are unsatisfactory markers of disease. Neuronal inclusions or extracellular deposits once thought to be specific for certain disorders may reflect adaptive or reactive cellular and cytoskeletal changes that have the capacity to co-exist, to a greater or lesser extent, across conventional disease boundaries according to prevailing aetiological factors. Such changes probably represent the pathological 'end-stages' of particular disease processes, any one of which can be driven by diverse aetiologies that 'feed' a defined and restricted pathological cascade. The overlapping presence of certain changes in different disorders may reflect the fact that neural tissue possesses only a limited repertoire of responses to the diverse range of damaging factors to which it may be exposed.

The presence of intracellular inclusions may relate to a secondary 'collapse' of the cytoskeleton, with a broadly similar mix of structural and molecular components becoming enmeshed within them (thereby providing similar or overlapping antigenic properties). Emphasis on one or other component may perhaps be related to the particular cause of the damage. None may in fact represent a specific disease product relationship.

Similarly, deposition of β/A4 amyloid protein may reflect a reactive change by the neurone to 'stresses' of all kinds, be they 'metabolic' or 'physical'. The common feature may be that they trigger the overproduction or catabolism of amyloid precursor protein (APP), this being broken down and accumulating as amyloid β/A4 protein plaques.

New and unequivocal markers of disease are needed. Some may come from refining immunohistochemical approaches, others from molecular biological studies. Ultimately, many of these disorders will prove to have a genomic origin for which DNA analysis will reveal the presence of a particular mutation, expansion or an insertion within relevant genes, providing an irrefutable diagnostic marker. A start has been made with some inherited forms of Alzheimer's disease (page 54), Huntington's disease (page 103) and for the prion disorders (page 160) where such genetic factors are clear. It will in time become possible to evaluate the relevance to the diagnosis of the pathological end-products that by necessity are currently used to define each disorder.

PRACTICAL METHODS FOR DIAGNOSIS

This section is intended as a working guide to examining the brain in dementia and provides an outline of the methods we have found helpful in demonstrating, and discriminating between, the principal pathological changes associated with the different types of dementia.

Brain preparation

The fresh brain is fixed by suspension in 10% neutral formalin for a minimum of 3–4 weeks. The cerebellum and brain stem are then removed at the level of the oculomotor nucleus and the cerebral hemisphere is sliced coronally at intervals of 1–2 cm. Blocks of fixed tissue are cut from prescribed regions of the brain, compatible with the clinical history, and processed 'by hand' or by tissue processor through graded alcohols into paraffin wax. Sections are cut on a rotary microtome at a thickness of 6 μm and mounted onto cleaned glass slides. These may be coated with poly-l-lysine, or APES if immunohistochemical procedures are to be used or if the section may 'float off' during staining.

If Creutzfeldt–Jakob or another prion disease is suspected clinically the blocks should be 'decontaminated' in 90% formic acid for 4 hours before processing through alcohols. This, as well as initial fixation and subsequent processing, should be carried out within appropriate microbiological containment facilities.

To provide a full diagnostic survey of major brain structures in dementia, blocks should be cut routinely from the following regions:

1 Frontal pole including orbitofrontal and superior frontal gyri.
2 Anterior parietal cortex including cingulate gyrus.
3 Temporal pole.
4 Temporal cortex (all three gyri) including amygdaloid nucleus.
5 Temporal cortex (all three gyri) including anterior hippocampus and entorhinal cortex.
6 Temporal cortex (all three gyri) including posterior hippocampus (Ammon's horn).
7 Posterior parietal cortex.
8 Occipital cortex including calcarine gyrus.
9 Caudate/putamen at the level of the nucleus accumbens.
10 Globus pallidus including insular cortex and nucleus basalis of Meynert.
11 Thalamus.
12 Substantia nigra at the level of the oculomotor nucleus.
13 The cerebellar hemisphere including dentate nucleus.
14 Pons at the levels of the locus caeruleus and trigeminal nucleus.
15 Medulla at the level of the hypoglossus nucleus.
16 Spinal cord, if available.

From these sections a basic *minimum* of blocks can be chosen according to the clinical history. When subjected to an appropriate range of staining techniques these will usually provide sufficient data for a 'safe' diagnosis while at the same time economising preparation time, technical labour, and reagent cost.

For the various diseases considered here, it is recommended that the schedule in **Table 7.2** is adopted as a basic minimum.

Table 7.2 Recommended brain sampling according to clinically suspected disease

Disease	Recommended tissue blocks (minimum)
Alzheimer's disease	1, 4, 5, 6, 13
Fronto-temporal dementia (FTD)	1, 2, 3, 6, 8, 9, 12
FTD + motor neurone disease	1, 2, 3, 6, 9, 12, 14, 15, 16
Progressive aphasia	1, 2, 3, 6, 8, 9 (left + right), 12
Creutzfeldt–Jakob disease, GSS	1, 6, 8, 9, 11, 13
Huntington's disease	1, 6, 9, 10, 12
Parkinson's disease	2, 6, 12, 14
Cortical Lewy body disease	1, 2, 5, 6, 12
Cortico-basal degeneration	2, 7, 10, 12, 13, 14
Progressive supranuclear palsy	5, 6, 10, 12, 13, 14
Cerebrovascular disease	According to regions of cerebral softening
Alcoholism	1, 5, 11 + mammillary bodies
Dementia where clinical history is unknown	1, 2, 5, 6, 8, 9, 12, 13

Staining techniques

There is a bewildering array of neurohistological and immunohistochemical procedures of potential value in revealing the diagnostic pathological features associated with each type of dementia. It is, however, quite impractical and unnecessary to apply all possible methods to a single brain. Experience shows that the first seven basic histopathological procedures listed below are usually sufficient to reveal most if not all neuropathological changes that are generally present in dementia. However, depending on the clinical history and suspected diagnosis, not all of the methods are equally informative and therefore necessary.

1 **Weigert's haematoxylin–eosin** for general cytology.
2 **Cresyl violet** for neurones and glia.
3 **Luxol fast blue/neutral red** for myelin.
4 **Palmgren silver** stain for axons, neurofibrillary changes, some inclusions (Pick bodies).
5 **Methenamine silver** stain for amyloid β/A4 protein.
6 **Phosphotungstic acid–haematoxylin** for reactive astrocytes and processes.
7 **Congo Red** stain for amyloid

These basic methods can be augmented if desired by immunohistochemical procedures which localise molecular features that the basic methods do not specifically detect:

8 **Anti-prion protein** immunostaining for prion plaques.
9 **Anti-tau** staining for inclusions and filamentous changes.
10 **Anti-ubiquitin** staining for inclusions and filamentous changes.
11 **Anti-αB crystallin** for ballooned neurones.
12 **Anti-β/A4** staining for amyloid β/A4 protein in plaques and cerebral vessels.
13 **Anti-GFAP** staining for astrocytic processes.
14 **Anti-ferritin** for reactive microglial cells.

According to the clinical history (suspected diagnosis) a combination of sample blocks (**Table 7.2**) and staining procedures (**Table 7.3**) can be chosen to maximise the diagnostic information from a minimum of stained sections. Clinical diagnoses are not infallible, however, and often the brain tissue is received with little or no helpful clinical information. The guide for 'dementia without history' should then be followed to allow diagnosis.

Table 7.3 Recommended staining schedules for each disease

Disease	Essential basic stains	Other (recommended) supplementary stains	Optional stains
Alzheimer's disease	1,4,5	7,9,10,12	3,6,13,14
Fronto-temporal dementia (FTD)	1,4,6	3,9,10,11,13	5,12
FTD + motor neurone disease	1,4,6,10	3,9,11,13	5,12
Progressive aphasia	1,4,6	3,13	5
Creutzfeldt–Jakob disease, GSS	1,4,6,8	5,12,13,14	3
Huntington's disease	1,6	4,5,13	3
Parkinson's disease	1,10	4,5	3,6,12
Cortical Lewy body disease	1,4,5,10	7,9,12	3
Cortico-basal degeneration	1,2,4,6	5,9,11,12,13	3
Progressive supranuclear palsy	1,4,5	9,10,12	3
Cerebrovascular disorders	1,3,6,7	4,5	9,12
Alcoholism	1,3,6	4,5	9,12
Dementia where clinical history is unknown	1,3,4,5,6	9,10,12,13	7,11,14

Routine staining procedures

1 Weigert's haematoxylin–eosin

Reagents
Solution A (stain)
Haematoxylin 1 g; absolute alcohol 100 ml

Solution B (mordant)
30% aqueous ferric chloride (anhydrous) 4 ml; concentrated hydrochloric acid 1 ml; distilled water 95 ml

Mixing the reagents
The two solutions (A and B) are stored separately and mixed immediately before use because the prepared stain keeps for only a few hours. Equal volumes of the two solutions are mixed to make the iron–haematoxylin solution. If they are not fresh a less than equal volume should be used. The colour of the mixture is a deep purplish-black.

Method
1 Dewax sections and rehydrate.
2 Stain sections with iron–haematoxylin mixture for 5–15 minutes.
3 Wash sections in tap water.
4 Examine sections microscopically and if required 'differentiate' in acid alcohol (0.5–1% hydrochloric acid in 70% alcohol) for a few seconds and then re-examine.
5 Wash sections thoroughly in running tap water.
6 Counterstain sections in 1% aqueous eosin.
7 Dehydrate, clear, and mount sections in DPX.

Results
- Nuclei: brownish-black to black.
- Cytoplasm: shades of pink.
- Myelin: blue.

2 Cresyl fast violet stain for Nissl substance

Method
1 Dewax and rehydrate sections
2 Immerse sections in 1% aqueous cresyl fast violet containing glacial acetic acid, 0.25 ml/100 ml stain. Stain sections at room temperature (approximately 20°C) for 20–30 minutes.
3 Rinse sections in distilled water and pass through 95% alcohol to 'differentiate', checking microscopically, until Nissl substance is obvious and background neuropil is clear.
4 Wash sections in 95% alcohol.
5 Dehydrate, clear and mount sections in DPX.

Results
- Nissl: violet.
- Nuclei/nucleoli: blue.
- Background: clear.

Note
Sections may be stained in an oven at 55°C for 5_6 minutes and allowed to cool before washing and differentiating.

3 Luxol fast blue (LFB)

Reagents
- Luxol fast blue 0.1 g
- 10% acetic acid 0.5 ml
- 95% alcohol 100 ml

The resulting solution is filtered.

Method
1 Dewax sections and take to absolute alcohol.
2 Stained sections in LFB overnight (8–16 hours) at 60°C.
3 Rinse sections in 95% alcohol, followed by distilled water.
4 Commence differentiation by rinsing for a few seconds in 0.05% lithium carbonate.
5 Continue differentiation in 70% alcohol for 20–30 seconds.
6 Rinse sections in distilled water. Control differentiation microscopically and repeat steps 4, 5, and 6 as necessary. Decolorisation in 70% alcohol is slow and controllable. This can be continued until there is a clear distinction between the blue staining of the white matter and the colourless grey matter.
7 Wash sections well in distilled water.
8 Counterstain sections in 1% neutral red for 5 minutes.
9 Rinse sections in distilled water.
10 Differentiate the counterstain in 95% alcohol.
11 Dehydrate, clear and mount sections in DPX.

Results
- Myelin and erythroctyes: deepish purplish-blue.
- Nuclei and Nissl substance: red.

4 Mallory's phosphotungstic acid–haematoxylin (PTAH)

Mallory's bleach (steps 2–6).

Reagents
- Haematein 1 g
- Phosphotungstic acid 20 g
- Distilled water 1000 ml
- Potassium permanganate 0.18 g

Dissolve separately in distilled water with gentle heat. Combine and make up to 1 litre of PTAM stain.
- Lugol's iodine
- 3% sodium thiosulphate
- 0.25% potassium permanganate
- 5% oxalic acid

Method
1 Dewax sections and rehydrate.
2 Treat with iodine for 2 minutes, rinse in water, treat with sodium thiosulphate for three minutes, rinse in water for 3 minutes.
3 Treat with 0.25% potassium permanganate for 3 minutes.
4 Wash in water for 2 minutes.
5 Rinse in distilled water.
6 Treat with 5% oxalic acid for 10 minutes.
7 Wash in water for 5 minutes, then rinse in distilled water.
8 Stain in PTAH for 12–24 hours.

Routine staining procedures (continued)

9 Dehydrate rapidly through 95% and absolute alcohol to conserve red stain.
10 Clear in xylene, and mount in DPX.

Results
- Nuclei, astrocytes and astrocytic fibres: blue.
- Collagen and reticulin: yellow to brick red.

5 Methenamine silver stain

Reagents: staining solution
- 5% methenamine 100 ml
- 5% silver nitrate 5 ml
- 5% sodium tetraborate 5 ml

Mix well and place in a glass dish in 60°C oven to warm up.
- 10% neutral formalin
- 2.5% sodium thiosulphate

Method
1 Dewax and rehydrate sections.
2 Use a glass rack and place sections in staining solution in the 60°C oven for up to 2 hours.
3 Wash sections briefly in tap water and immerse in 10% neutral buffered formalin for 10 minutes at room temperature (approximaely 20°C).
4 Rinse sections briefly in tap water and immerse in 2.5% sodium thiosulphate for 2 minutes at room temperature.
5 Wash sections in tap water.
6 Dehydrate, clear, and mount in DPX.

Results
- Amyloid β/A4 protein: black.

Note
All glassware is washed in 5% nitric acid and rinsed in distilled water before use.

6 Palmgren's silver impregnation method

Reagents: Palmgren's silver solution
- Silver nitrate 45 g
- Potassium nitrate 30 g (oxidiser)
- Distilled water 300 ml
- 5% glycine 3 ml

The solution is filtered before use.

Reagents: Palmgren's reducer
- Pyrogallol 25 g
- Distilled water 1125 ml
- Absolute alcohol 1375 ml
- 1% nitric acid 5 ml

Method
1 Place two pots of the reducer in a 37°C oven ready for use later in the procedure.
2 Dewax and rehydrate sections.
3 Immerse sections in 1% solution of aqueous ammonia at room temperature for 5 minutes.
4 Wash sections thoroughly in at least three changes of distilled water.
5 Place sections in Palmgren's silver solution in the dark for 90 minutes at room temperature (approximately 20°C).
6 Place sections in the reducer and agitate for a few seconds. The solution goes black and the sections brown. Then place the sections in the second reducer and agitate for 30 seconds.
7 Wash sections in tap water and rinse in distilled water.
8 Fix sections with 5% sodium thiosulphate solution.
9 Wash sections in tap water, dehydrate clear and mount in DPX.

Note
All glassware is washed in 5% nitric acid and rinsed in distilled water before use.

Results
- Neurofibrillary tangles: black.
- Axons: black.
- Neuritic plaques: black.
- Background: pale brown.

7 Alkaline Congo Red

Reagents
- Sodium chloride saturated 80% alcohol
- 0.5 Congo Red in sodium chloride saturated 80% alcohol
- 1% Sodium hydroxide

When making reagents add 80 ml alcohol to 20 ml of 15% sodium chloride to ensure the alcohol is saturated. To make Congo Red stain add 0.5 g Congo Red to 20 ml of 15% sodium chloride to dissolve before adding 80 ml of alcohol. These stock solutions deteriorate. It is necessary to add 1 ml of 1% sodium hydroxide before use.

Method
1 Dewax sections and rehydrate
2 Stain nuclei in Mayer's haemtoxylin for 5 minutes. Rinse in water and 'blue'.
3 Incubate sections in sodium chloride saturated in 80% alcohol fo 20 minutes.
4 Without rinsing, transfer section to freshly filtered Congo Red stain for 20 minutes.
5 Rinse in 80%, 90% and 100% alcohol, clean amd mount in DPX

Results
- Amyloid – pink
- Nuclein – blue-black
- Amyloid in polarised light - yellow green birefringence

8 Periodic acid–Schiff (PAS)

Reagents
- Pararosaniline (CI 42500)
- 0.25M hydrochloric acid
- Sodium metabisulphite
- Decolorising charcoal

Routine staining procedures (continued)

Preparation of Schiff's reagent
Dissolve 2 g pararosaniline in 100 ml 0.25M hydrochloric acid. Add 3.9 g sodium metabisulphite and stir for2 hours. Next add 2 g of decolorising charcoal and stir for 5 minutes. Filter and use. This solution can be diluted 1:1 with distilled water.

Method
1 Dewax sections and rehydrate.
2 Treat with 1% periodic acid for 4–5 minutes.
3 Wash in distilled water.
4 Treat with 'cold' Schiff reagent: 10 minutes 50% Schiff's; 7.5 minutes 100% Schiff's. (Note that 10 minutes with the 100% reagent gives very sharp staining of basement membranes, but there may also be some background staining.)
5 Develop the colour over 10 minutes in *warm* running water.
6 Stain nuclei using Mayer's haematoxylin for 30 seconds.
7 Wash in running water.
8 Differentiate in acid alcohol for 8 seconds.
9 'Blue' in saturated lithium carbonate.
10 Wash, dehydrate, clear, and mount in DPX.

Results
- Amyloid - pink
- Basement membrane, lipofuscin-pink
- Nuclei-blue
- Background pale-pink

9 Immunohistochemistry

Reagents
Stock x 10, 0.05M tris buffered saline (TBS)
Tris-(hydroxymethyl)-aminomethane (mol wt 121.1) 121.1g
Sodium chloride 170.0 g

Mixing the reagents
Dissolve in 1500 ml distilled water.
Add 75 ml of concentrated hydrochloric acid (specific gravity 1.18).
Make up the total volume to 2000 ml.
Check the pH and adjust to 7.4–7.6 with concentrated hydrochloric acid.

Working solution
Dilute 1 in 10 with distilled water.

3,3'-diaminobenzidine tetrahydrochloride dihydrate (DAB) substrate
3,3'-diaminobenzidine tetrahydrochloride dihydrate 1.5 g
0.05M TBS (dilute stock 1 in 10) 200 ml
Adjust to pH 7.2 with concentrated hydrochloric acid. Filter if necessary.

Working solution
Add 20 ml of DAB to 280 ml 0.05M TBS. Just before use add 1 ml hydrogen peroxide (30 vol). Use within 30 minutes.

Avidin–Biotin indirect method for immunohistochemistry

Method
1 Dewax and rehydrate sections and pass to 70% methanol with 0.3% v/v hydrogen peroxide added for 30 minutes.
2 Rinse sections in running tap water and blott off excess tap water.
3 Incubate sections in 20% normal swine serum (NSS) (about 250 microlitres/slide) for 30 minutes.
4 Wipe off excess NSS and apply the primary antibody, at the appropriate dilution (about 250 microlitres/slide), overnight at 4°C.
5 Wash sections in three changes of 0.05M TBS for 5 minutes each wash.
6 Apply secondary antibody (biotinylated IgG), at the appropriate dilution, for 30 minutes at room temperature.
7 Wash sections in three changes of 0.05M TBS for 5 minutes each wash.
8 Apply avidin-peroxidase (in 0.125M TBS) for 60 minutes at room temperature (approximately 20°C).
9 Wash sections in three changes of 0.05M TBS for 5 minutes each wash.
10 Incubate sections in DAB solution.
11 Wash sections in running tap water, counterstain briefly in Mayer's haematoxylin, differentiate in acid alcohol for 30 seconds, dehydrate, clear, and mount. Alternatively, sections can be couner-sained with Periodic-acid-Schiff stain (see Method 8).

Notes
- For amyloid β/A4 protein, immunohistochemistry sections are treated with 80% formic acid for 10 minutes after step 1 and then rinsed well in distilled water. Such treatment will enhance the β/A4 protein immunoreactivity.
- For prion protein immunohistochemistry, sections are treated with formic acid as above before step 2 *or* autoclaved for 10 minutes in a vessel containing 0.9 mm Hydrochloric acid. Either of these procedures can be used to enhance prion protein (PrP) immunoreactivity.
- The source and working dilution of the antibodies used by us are given in **Table 7.4**.

Table 7.4 Source and working dilution of antibodies used for immunohistochemistry

Antibody	Source	Dilution
Biotinylated IgG	Sigma	1/300
Avidin peroxidase	Sigma	1/400
Anti-β/A4	K Beyreuther[1]	1/500
Anti-tau	Sigma	1/750
Anti-PHF	Y Ihara[2]	1/500
Anti-GFAP	Sigma	1/750
Anti-PrP	J Hope[3]	1/500
Anti-ubiquitin	Dako	1/750

Addresses

[1] Z.M.B.H. Im Neuenheimerfeld 282, University of Heidelberg, Heidelberg, Germany

[2] Department of Neuropathology, University of Tokyo, Tokyo, Japan

[3] AFRC & MRC Neuropathogenesis Unit, University of Edinburgh, West Mains Road, Edinburgh, Scotland

8. Dementia clinic

A dementia clinic has the following functions:

- To combine the management of patients with the accurate diagnosis of individual disorders.
- To define homogeneous groups of patients for therapeutic strategies.
- To advance basic knowledge in the aetiology and pathogenesis of brain disorders leading to dementia.

A dementia clinic is ideally set in a neuroscientific centre for referral of patients and liaison with referring groups, the social services and charitable organisations.

Structure of the clinic

The patients are managed as far as possible in an outpatient setting conveniently divided into a new patient and follow-up patient clinic.

The clinics are staffed by a consultant neurologist, a psychiatrist and a geneticist, with trainees in neurology, psychiatry, psychogeriatrics and geriatrics. Neuropsychologists and dedicated social workers are essential to team management.

The clinic has access to imaging, both structural (CT and MRI) and functional (SPET and PET), and electroencephalography.

Follow-up to autopsy is essential. After full discus-

Investigation of dementia using single-photon emission computed tomography (SPET)

SPET is a new diagnostic imaging methodology that allows the investigation of brain morphology and function by producing three-dimensional images of the distribution of a radiopharmaceutical. Like radiographic computed axial tomography (CT) it is a method of displaying images in sections on slices (transaxial, sagittal and coronal) so that the organ under investigation can be more critically assessed.

There are several different radiopharmaceuticals for imaging the brain. These include the following:

- Those that do not pass the blood–brain barrier and are taken up by brain areas only when the blood–brain barriers have been damaged.
- Those that cross the blood–brain barrier and accumulate in the neurones of the cortical and subcortical areas of the brain (perfusion tracers).
- Those that are taken up by specific receptors.

At present the most common procedures in clinical practice are those that employ perfusion tracers. The most readily available of these compounds is technetium labelled hexamethyl propylene amine oxime (^{99m}Tc-HMPAO), a lipophilic compound. After intravenous injection, HMPAO passes through the intact blood–brain barrier and is distributed according to blood flow. It has a high extraction efficiency, and once trapped by the neurones remains unchanged for a sufficient period of time to allow imaging of its distribution in the brain.

The images presented in this book were obtained using a Toshiba GCA-901A/SA rotating gamma camera. This is an integrated digital gamma camera and computer system that has a single rotating detector fitted with a low energy high resolution collimator. The gamma camera rotates 360° in an elliptical orbit around the patient's head. Sixty 20-second views are acquired on a 64 × 64 matrix with a ×2 magnification given a pixel size of 4 mm.

Transaxial slices of 1 or 2 pixels (4 mm or 8 mm thick) are produced using the filtered back projection technique and the data is reformatted to provide 2 pixel thick sagittal and coronal slices. These slices are displayed interpolated onto a 128 × 128 matrix. The pixel with most activity is considered to be 100% (upper display level) and the lower display level is 45% of the most active pixel.

From the point of view of clinical diagnosis this technique is highly sensitive, demonstrating small changes in perfusion at a very early stage. It is, however, nonspecific and has to be used in conjunction with other diagnostic modalities – in the case of dementia, including neuropsychological tests.

sion carers are encouraged to sign a pre-mortem consent form, which is then attached to all the patient's present and future medical records. This is accompanied by a document containing the names, addresses and telephone numbers of individual members of the team who can be contacted for brain harvesting from the patient's hospital or residential home. Brain retrieval is directed by a consultant neuropathologist who can dedicate tissue for both neuropathological and neurochemical analysis. Usually, a half brain is dedicated for each form of study, although dissection of specific regions for neurochemical purposes before fixing the rest for pathological investigation is necessary when lesions are asymmetrically distributed.

During life, blood samples are stored for genetic and molecular biological investigation.

Weekly clinical meetings allow comparison of neurological and psychological findings with the results of imaging and electroencephalography. Three-monthly clinico-pathological meetings reinforce the diagnostic precision of the multi-disciplinary team.

Diagnosis

Clinical examination and investigations categorise the patient as having an *extrinsic, metabolic* or *intrinsic* encephalopathy. Further management of patients with *extrinsic encephalopathy* requires the collaboration of neurosurgery, whereas *metabolic encephalopathies* are the province of the appropriate specialist within general medicine.

It is important in the diagnosis of *intrinsic encephalopathy* to consider the complicating features of the following:

- A co-existent metabolic encephalopathy.
- The co-existence of anxiety, depression and functional psychosis.
- The co-existence of a sensory deficit such as deafness or impaired vision.

The precise diagnosis of intrinsic encephalopathy is carried out as indicated on pages 12–20. The presence of new and previously undiagnosed disorders must be constantly considered.

Patient management

General management

The dementia clinic acts as a diagnostic centre and also follows up longitudinally potentially informative patients. Most patients' on-going care will continue in geriatrics, psychogeriatrics, psychiatry or general medicine. Links with the social services and charitable institutions enable greater support for carer and patient.

Individual management

The patient and carers must be given precise diagnostic information and an expected prognosis. Advice is given about the importance of habitual routine both in the home and in institutional care and on aspects of retirement, the ability to drive, and personal and family finance. Full support within the home must be established in the form of home-helps, meals-on-wheels, district nurses, laundry service and appropriate social benefits. The carers require relief from caring in the form of day-centre, holiday, and respite accommodation; and finally require advice on the painful decision to obtain long-term care in a nursing home or hospital unit.

Drug therapy

Symptomatic remedies are required for the effective treatment of depression, confusion, agitation and insomnia. Specific remedies to slow decline or arrest dementia are lacking and the endeavour of research into this area is to determine the precise aetiology and pathogenesis in order to apply rational remedies. Accurate diagnosis is essential to the therapeutic enterprise.

Index

nb - page numbers in *italics* refer to figures and tables